IVF Technologies and Infertility - Current Practices and New Perspectives

Edited by Iavor K. Vladimirov

Published in London, United Kingdom

IVF Technologies and Infertility - Current Practices and New Perspectives
http://dx.doi.org/10.5772/intechopen.102193
Edited by Iavor K. Vladimirov

Contributors
Sirin Aydın, Mehmet Eflatun Deniz, Suchada Mongkolchaipak, Delia Hutanu, Ioana Rugescu, Jean-Claude Emperaire, J. Charles Eldridge, Timothy J. Gelety, Bassim Alsadi, Mehdi Yousefi, Javad Ahmadian-Heris, Shahla Danaii, Samaneh Abdolmohammadi-Vahid, Leili Aghebati-Maleki, Iavor K. Vladimirov, Antonio Díez-Juan, Martin Vladimirov

First published in London, United Kingdom, 2023 by IntechOpen
IntechOpen is the global imprint of INTECHOPEN LIMITED, registered in England and Wales, registration number: 11086078, 5 Princes Gate Court, London, SW7 2QJ, United Kingdom

British Library Cataloguing-in-Publication Data
A catalogue record for this book is available from the British Library

Additional hard and PDF copies can be obtained from orders@intechopen.com

IVF Technologies and Infertility - Current Practices and New Perspectives
Edited by Iavor K. Vladimirov
p. cm.
Print ISBN 978-1-80356-719-8
Online ISBN 978-1-80356-720-4
eBook (PDF) ISBN 978-1-80356-721-1

For EU product safety concerns:
IN TECH d.o.o., Prolaz Marije Krucifikse Kozulić 3, 51000 Rijeka, Croatia,
info@intechopen.com or visit our website at intechopen.com.

Meet the editor

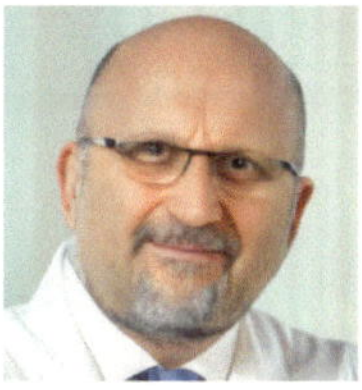

Dr. Iavor K. Vladimirov is the founder and medical director of the Sofia IVF clinic (SBALAGRM-SOFIA). He is an honorary lecturer at "St. Kliment Ohridski" University, Bulgaria. Dr. Vladimirov is one of the authors of "Theory about the Embryo Cryo-Treatment," which is the first theory giving a scientific explanation for the high success rate in some infertility cases using the embryo freezing and thawing procedure. He has introduced the following methods in Bulgaria: assessment of the ovarian reserve, in vitro maturation, and determination of the so-called implantation window using endometrial receptivity analysis (ERA). He is a member of numerous professional and scientific organizations relating to the problem of infertility and has received various prestigious awards and accolades.

Contents

Preface

More than 45 years have passed since the successful application of in vitro fertilization (IVF) technologies and the birth of the world's first baby. Over the past few decades, assisted reproductive technologies (ARTs) have become one of the fastest-growing branches of medicine, with IVF becoming the main approach to treating infertility.

Numerous significant discoveries and improvements have helped increase the effectiveness of IVF technology such as the intracytoplasmic sperm injection (ICSI) procedure and the freezing of gametes, embryos, and reproductive tissue via vitrification. These innovations aim to increase the success rate of fertilization and reduce patient risk and service costs. They have led to the optimization of some phases of the treatment process, such as the development and implementation of stimulation protocols to reduce patient risk and innovations in the IVF laboratory to establish the embryo with the greatest potential for implantation and the birth of a healthy baby. At the heart of this approach is the thesis, which I follow, that each and every embryo is a living organism, not a group of cells, for which we must take care, creating optimal conditions for its development and treating it as needed, as we do for our patients.

This book focuses on the application of various methods and techniques for the diagnosis and treatment of infertility through IVF technologies. The authors consider topics such as sperm analysis and new modern diagnostic approaches, clinical and laboratory aspects of the in vitro maturation method, oocyte freezing, as well as the quality management system in assisted reproduction, in accordance with modern European standards. The book also discusses topics such as immunology and infertility and artificial intelligence in ovarian stimulation. Finally, it examines ovarian reproductive aging and rejuvenation strategies, the new challenge in the treatment of infertility through IVF technologies.

This book is a useful resource for embryologists and physicians concerned with the diagnosis and treatment of infertility through in vitro technologies.

Iavor K. Vladimirov
IVF Clinic (SBALAGRM-SOFIA),
Sofia, Bulgaria

Section 1

Introduction

Chapter 1

Introductory Chapter: IVF Technology and Perspectives

Iavor K. Vladimirov and Martin Vladimirov

1. Introduction

Assisted reproductive technologies (ART) is the main method of treating infertility, which occurs in 10–15% of people of reproductive age. In recent decades, ART has become one of the most rapidly developing interdisciplinary technologies in medicine. Doctor Patrick Steptoe and biologist Robert Edwards are the pioneers of the *in vitro* method. After 60 unsuccessful attempts, Louise Brown was born on July 25, 1978, the world's first "baby in a test tube."

Currently, almost 10 million children have been born in the world thanks to *in vitro* methods, and during this period of 45 years, the success rate in treatment has increased many times: ranging in the first years from less than 10%, reaching today more than 50% in certain groups of patients. The reason for this rapid increase is the introduction of new medications and stimulation protocols, improvement of embryo culture media, and use of laboratory equipment that all provide better conditions for embryo development. Last but not least, the introduction of modern methods for genetic analysis and new techniques for freezing gametes, embryos, and tissue has improved the diagnostic and therapeutic possibilities of ART.

Regardless of the relatively high success rate of ART, the method has certain limitations. The final result, the birth of a healthy child, depends on many factors, such as the age of the partners, cause of infertility, lifestyle and diet, harmful habits, accompanying diseases, and, last but not least, heredity.

Currently, one out of every three embryos created through *in vitro* fertilization has chromosomal abnormalities that interfere with the development of the pregnancy and the birth of a healthy baby. Advances in genetics and genome sequencing enable the introduction of genetic analysis for each created embryo. This makes it possible to detect genes that correlate with the implantation and normal development of the embryo, as well as genes that correlate with early or late implantation failure. The effects of screening and selection of embryos, as well as improved outcomes, are under debate [1]. However, there has been steady progress on this front. On the other hand, genetic screening methods can better define the underlying genetic diseases and expand screening to cover a larger group of congenital conditions and diseases. Solving this task is complex from both a medical and ethical point of view, but the future convergence of well-defined genomes and very effective embryo testing make the application of genetic screening and selection inevitable [2].

A major criterion for good ART practice is reducing the risk to the patient and the pregnancy and increasing the success rate, which is determined based on live births. Ovarian hyperstimulation syndrome (OHSS) is a major risk for the woman during treatment and is a consequence of gonadotropin stimulation. It is also the most common

IntechOpen

complication that can end in a fatal outcome. Currently, OHSS occurs relatively rarely and most often in mild or moderate form. This is a consequence of the more frequent application of stimulation protocols: light stimulation and the so-called *in vitro* spontaneous cycle procedure. On the other hand, the use of GnRH-agonists as an ovulation trigger in GnRH-antagonist and progestin priming ovarian stimulation protocols with subsequent embryo freezing makes an OHSS-free clinic a real concept [3].

Reducing the number of transferred embryos leads to a reduction in the percentage of multiple pregnancies, respectively reducing the risk for the fetus and the mother [4]. For this reason, it has become increasingly beneficial in practice to apply a strategy for single embryo transfer (SET), resulting in the birth of one baby. This approach also defends the hypothesis that the embryo is not a group of developing cells, but is a patient like any other who should receive the best possible conditions for development and help, if necessary. Many patients express concern that single embryo transfer (SET) may reduce their already low chances of conceiving. However, recent studies have refuted such a statistically significant relationship, showing that SET has no real impact on pregnancy rates, compared to embryo transfer of two or more embryos [5].

Safety remains a major topic of debate, with some believing that children born after IVF are at greater risk of complications than those born after natural conception. However, a recent study published in *Lancet* [6] showed that the increased risk of pregnancy and birth complications seen in children conceived as a consequence of IVF may be the result of the parent's underlying infertility problems, rather than the technology itself.

Another important question to be answered is how to reduce the cost of ART treatment. It is in the interest of the patient and of society to reduce the direct and indirect costs incurred by infertility treatment. With in vitro treatment, the costs of drugs and procedures are well-known and can be budgeted. Side costs are not few and can be difficult to predict. Direct nonmedical costs, as well as indirect costs, connected to the IVF treatment itself, have been found to vary between 45% and 52% of total costs [7]. This figure includes the costs of travel, food, hotel, and the time a person spends visiting the clinic, which is why they are inclined to take vacations or sick leave. Studies have shown that the time cost alone of performing the entire in vitro procedure averages around 162 hours [8]. Another research article, authored by colleagues from Ireland points out that, depending on the distance to the clinic, patients can lose between 15 and 75 hours in travel, and expenses for local food and accommodation which amount to 104–703 euros [9].

To reduce these costs, new methods are being developed to manage ovarian stimulation during *in vitro* treatment. They are based on the determination of urinary estrone-3-glucuronide levels [10, 11] and salivary hormone oestradiol and progesterone measurements [12]. Currently, two main stimulation approaches have been developed: Self-Operated Endovaginal Telemonitoring (SOET) [13] and Controlled Ovarian Stimulation Monitoring by Self-Determination of Estrone-3-Glucuronide and Single Ultrasound (COSSESU). The implementation of these approaches is carried out with the active participation of patients [14].

Advantages of these two approaches to ovarian stimulation include the reduction of:

1. Costs of regular ultrasound and hormone tests.

2. Stress is incurred by frequent blood sampling to determine serum hormone levels.

3. Time wasted in frequent clinic visits and traveling.

4. Direct nonmedical expenses related to the use of a car, bus, train, hotel accommodation, and food.

5. Risk of infection in situations similar to COVID-19.

The two approaches described above use elements of telemedicine. Although much has been published in terms of telemedicine in the fields of cardiology, diabetes, dermatology, and general practice, little has been reported regarding reproductive medicine. Interest has also increased tremendously due to the recent COVID-19 pandemic. Telemedicine has a place in the treatment of infertility with the use of *in vitro* technologies [15].

Another step in reducing costs and the human factor in IVF treatment is the automation of the laboratory. Technologies and methods from the 80s are currently being used, that is, the embryologist opens the incubator door, removes the petri dish, closes the incubator door, then works on the embryo or medium, opens the incubator door again, puts it back the dish, and closes the incubator door. This series of steps is repeated for each IVF case. The inclusion of Artificial Intelligence for Ovarian Stimulation is also of interest, which is part of the modern trend of introducing artificial intelligence into medicine and, in particular, in vitro technologies. Automation of the IVF lab and other future technological developments will make IVF treatment more efficient and optimized [16].

The trends in assisted reproductive technologies outlined above have found a place in some of the chapters of this book. Readers will be introduced to the modern techniques of seminal analysis and the different methods of sperm processing in various ART techniques. The authors of this book examine some modern technologies, such as egg freezing and the *in vitro* maturation method, as well as the application of artificial intelligence in ovarian stimulation. A current topic will be discussed here, namely ovarian aging and the modern strategy of treating women with this problem. Also, an important place is given to the quality management system in assisted reproductive technologies, which is decisive in modern quality control in ART. This book also addresses the problem of infertility from an immunological perspective, with the authors covering a large number of diagnostic tests and clinical behaviors, including those whose effectiveness continues to be debated in the scientific community.

Author details

Iavor K. Vladimirov[1,2]* and Martin Vladimirov[1]

1 IVF Unit, SBALAGRM-Sofia, Bulgaria

2 Faculty of Biology, Sofia University "St. Kliment Ohridski", Bulgaria

*Address all correspondence to: vladimirov@ivf.bg

References

[1] Pagliardini L, Viganò P, Alteri A, Corti L, Somigliana E, Papaleo E. Shooting STAR: Reinterpreting the data from the 'single embryo TrAnsfeR of Euploid embryo' randomized clinical trial. Reproductive Biomedicine Online. 2020;**40**:475-478

[2] Church G. Compelling reasons for repairing human germlines. The New England Journal of Medicine. 2017;**377**:1909-1911

[3] Mourad S, Brown J, Farquhar C. Interventions for the prevention of OHSS in ART cycles: An overview of Cochrane reviews. Cochrane Database of Systematic Reviews. 2017;**1**(1):CD012103

[4] Multiple gestation pregnancy. The ESHRE Capri workshop group. Human Reproduction. 2000;**15**(8):1856-1864

[5] McLernon DJ, Harrild K, Bergh C, Davies MJ, de Neubourg D, Dumoulin JC, et al. Clinical effectiveness of elective single versus double embryo transfer: Meta-analysis of individual patient data from randomised trials. Version 2. BMJ. 2010;**341**:c6945

[6] Liv Bente Romundstad, Pål R Romundstad, Arne Sunde, Vidar von Düring, Rolv Skjærven, David Gunnell et all. Effects of technology or maternal factors on perinatal outcome after assisted fertilisation: A population-based cohort study. Lancet Vol 372, Issue 9640, 2008, p 737-743.

[7] Le KD, Vuong LN, Ho TM, Dang VQ, Pham TD, Pham CT, et al. A cost-effectiveness analysis of freeze only or fresh embryo transfer in IVF of non-PCOS women. Human Reproduction. 2018;**33**(10):1907-1914

[8] Wu AK, Elliott P, Katz PP, Smith JF. Time costs of fertility care: The hidden hardship of building a family. Fertility and Sterility. 2013;**99**:2025-2030. DOI: 10.1016/j.fertnstert.2013.01.145

[9] Kelly J, Hughes CM, Harrison RF. The hidden costs of IVF. Irish Medical Journal. 2006;**99**:142-143

[10] Vladimirov, V Martin, T Desislava. Urine estrone–3-glucuronide (E3G) assay: Is there any place during ovarian stimulation for IVF cycles? Human Reproduction, Volume 36, Issue Supplement_1, deab130.669, 2021

[11] Hart RJ, D'Hooghe T, Dancet EAF, Aurell R, Lunenfeld B, Orvieto R, et al. Self-monitoring of urinary hormones in combination with telemedicine - a timely review and opinion piece in medically assisted reproduction. Reproductive Sciences. 2021;**29**:1-14. DOI: 10.1007/s43032-021-00754-5

[12] Sakkas D, Howles CML, Atkinson L, Borini A, Bosch EA, Bryce C, et al. A multi-Centre international study of salivary hormone Oestradiol and progesterone measurements in ART monitoring. Reproductive Biomedicine Online. 2020;**42**:421-428

[13] Gerris J, Annick DA, Dhont N, Frank VF, Madoc B, Magaly BM, et al. Self-operatedEndovaginalTelemonitoring versus traditional monitoring of ovarian stimulation in assisted reproduction: An RCT. Human Reproduction. 2014;**29**:1941-1948. DOI: 10.1093/humrep/deu168

[14] Vladimirov IK, Vladimirov M, Tacheva D. A new protocol for controlled ovarian stimulation monitoring by self-determination of Estrone-3-glucuronide

and single ultrasound (COSSESU) open journal of. Obstetrics and Gynecology. 2021;**11**:1217-1228

[15] Berg WT, Goldstein M, Melnick AP, Rosenwaks Z. Clinical implications of telemedicine for providers and patients. Fertility and Sterility. 2020;**114**(6):1129-1134. DOI: 10.1016/j.fertnstert.2020.10.048

[16] Costa-Borges N, Giralt G, Albó E, Alvarez A, Ramos J, Hernandez I, et al. ICSI in a box: Development of a successful automated sperm injection robot with external supervision and minimal manual intervention. Human Reproduction. 2021;**36**(Supplement_1):deab126.047

Section 2

Semen Analysis, Techniques and Evaluation

Chapter 2

Semen Analysis and Infertility

Suchada Mongkolchaipak

Abstract

Male factor infertility contribute approximately at 50% for the cause of infertility. The steady declination of semen quality in men for all over the world might be from various factors such as life style changes, environmental toxicity, dietary contribution and social problems. Assisted reproduction is the main treatment of choice for male infertility; However, in severe male factor infertility, the treatment outcomes could end up with recurrent implantation failure or recurrent pregnancy loss. Basic semen analysis still has limitation to explain the cause of failure for the part of male factors. The purposes of developing new sperm evaluation methods are to improve the diagnostic tools for identifying the sperm defects, appraise of fertility potential and provide suitable treatment for an infertile couple, explain the cause of treatment failure from male factor part and measure the efficacy of male contraception.

Keywords: male factor infertility, sperm DNA fragmentation, sperm oxidative stress, semen analysis, total antioxidant capacity, sperm motility, sperm morphology, sperm concentration

1. Introduction

According to the World Health Organization (WHO), infertility is a reproductive system disease that is defined as "a failure to conceive naturally after regular sexual intercourse without the use of contraception for at least a year" [1]. It is estimated that 8–12% of people who are of reproductive age encounter infertility problems [2]. The male factor is responsible for 50% of infertility cases [3].

Furthermore, the incidence of male factor infertility in men in the active reproductive age bracket has been reported to be as high as 15% [4]. The causes of male factor are multifactorial. The pathophysiology of the causes is not fully understood, and most of them are idiopathic [5]. Initial investigation of the male partner consists of a history, physical examination, and semen analysis; however, some may require specific hormonal investigations to determine the causes of male infertility [4].

Semen analysis is a basic method to investigate the cause of infertility in the male. Six versions of a semen assessment methods guideline have been created by WHO. The first manual was published in 1980 based on clinical experience and research. The following versions were published in 1987, 1992, 1999, 2010, and 2021. The reasons for revising the manual included improving the semen analysis methods and updating the semen parameters to be more compatible with normal male fertility [6–9].

Nevertheless, at least 15% of infertile men are found to have a normal semen analysis according to WHO criteria [10]. However, further abnormalities were detected by a sperm DNA integrity test [11–13]. In the latest edition of WHO's laboratory manual for human semen evaluation, revisions have been made to improve the accuracy of the test and eliminate the unnecessary steps of the evaluation [14].

2. Semen sample assessment

Semen analysis is the method of evaluating the ejaculate composed of sperm, which originates from the testes and seminal fluid secreted from the accessory glands. Components in seminal fluid facilitate the sperm's access to the female genital tract and its ability to fertilize the mature oocyte *in vivo* [15]. In the sixth edition of WHO's laboratory manual for human semen examination, the procedure is divided into three parts. The first part is a basic semen examination. The second is an extended analysis, which is specialized for specific clinical applications. The last part is an advanced procedure, which is not used in routine practice. It must be done in a special laboratory, and it is mainly used in research studies [16]. The basic assessment includes the measurement of ejaculate volume, macroscopic evaluation, and microscopic examination.

In the sixth WHO manual, revisions to the basic assessment are based on evidence-based practices that improve the process of assessment, reduce the workload in the laboratory, and promote inter-laboratory quality assurance. The WHO manual emphasizes the importance of precisely measuring the ejaculate volume, which reflects the true total sperm count and examining the extent of sperm motility, which is clinically related to the male fertility potential.

3. Basic examination of semen sample parameters

General semen quality has shown a steady decline across the world [17] due to various factors, such as lifestyle changes, environmental toxicity, dietary contribution, and social problems [18–20]. Today, there are multiple tools to evaluate the semen quality and find suitable treatments for each infertile couple. Each semen parameter reflects the individual cause that needs to be clarified.

3.1 Gross appearance

Normal ejaculate has a homogeneous grayish color. In the case of pale color or colorlessness, the patient should be asked if there is orgasm during seminal collection because the semen component might only be from the Cowper's glands, not the prostate gland, seminal vesicle, or seminiferous tubule. The former occurs from sexual arousal, while the latter occurs from an orgasm. The color could be a deep yellow in patients with jaundice or those taking vitamin supplements. Normally, the ejaculate is odorless and can be liquefied within 30 min at room temperature. A strong smell is not normal and should be noted in the report.

3.2 Volume

The ejaculate volume is clinically significant for the diagnosis of male infertility, as it reflects the total sperm count in the ejaculate. The sixth WHO manual focuses on the accuracy of the volume measurement by instructing to weigh the ejaculate (pre-weighing the container and subtracting it from the total weight of the final specimen) and calculate back into the volume. The formula for calculating semen density is 1 g per 1 ml. Total sperm count is related to the sperm produced directly from the seminiferous tubules. This count is used as an indicator of spontaneous conception and treatment success in intrauterine insemination [21].

3.3 Microscopic examination

3.3.1 Sperm concentration

The clinical value of sperm concentration is less than the total sperm count per ejaculate because the sperm concentration depends on the amount of accessory gland secretion activity. Sperm concentration does not indicate the chance of success in intracytoplasmic sperm injection (ICSI) cycles [22].

3.3.2 Sperm motility

In the sixth WHO manual, the assessment of sperm motility has reverted to the four categorizations presented in the fourth WHO manual: rapidly progressive ($\geq$25 μ m/s), slowly progressive (5 to <25 μ m/s), nonprogressive (<5 μ m/s) and immotile (no active tail movement) (they are classified as grade a, b, c, and d, respectively) movement. However, in the fifth edition, sperm motility was classified into just three categories: progressive motility, nonprogressive motility, and immotile.

The total number of progressively motile spermatozoa indicates the chance of success in intrauterine insemination [23], and the presence of rapidly progressive motile sperm is clinically significant [24]. Asthenozoospermia is a medical term defined as "lower sperm motility than the reference values." It could result from several factors.

3.3.2.1 Varicocele

Varicocele is a chronic disease involving the pampiniform plexus of veins. It creates the tortious vessels in the spermatic cord [25]. The mechanisms involved in sperm function in the case of varicocele have not been clearly explained. However, some mechanisms might be related to sperm motility. The most likely pathophysiologic cause of sperm impairment is increased scrotal temperature caused by tortious veins, which increase oxidative stress, and reflux of toxic substances from the kidneys and adrenal glands into the testes [26]. There is evidence that varicoceles impair sperm motility [27–29]. While a varicocelectomy can improve sperm motility, other sperm parameters are still controversial [30–33]. Adjuvant therapy using antioxidant supplements to improve sperm quality [34, 35] has had conflicting outcomes [36].

3.3.2.2 Sexual abstinence

The duration of abstinence impacts sperm quality, including sperm motility [37]. Consequently, the male partner should be advised to be abstinent for 2–7 days to maintain sperm analysis accuracy among patients and between laboratories [16]. The sperm kinematics was improved when the duration of abstinence was 2 hr. compared to 4–7 days, both in normal semen [38] and oligozoospermic semen [39].

However, contradictory outcomes were still reported, as some studies revealed that the duration of abstinence at 4–5 days had higher sperm motility than 2–3 days and 6–7 days of abstinence [40].

3.3.2.3 Lifestyle factors

A recent systematic review of the literature shows that smoking is a strong factor impacting sperm concentration and motility [41]. Even a moderate amount of smoking can impair progressive motility. The pathophysiology of tobacco that results in diminished sperm motility could be oxidative stress that leads to the axonemal and mitochondrial damage on the midpiece of the spermatozoa [42, 43]. Both smoking and alcohol consumption had a detrimental effect on sperm motility and other sperm parameters [44]. When considering alcohol consumption alone, it is shown to have some association with decreased sperm quality when the amount of consumption is significant and chronic [45]. In men with obesity, sperm quality is diminished in concentration and morphology but not sperm motility [46].

3.3.2.4 Genetic causes of male infertility

Some genetic defects, such as Kartagener's syndrome and primary ciliary dyskinesia, directly cause abnormal sperm motility due to their effects on the flagellar structure and function [46–48].

3.3.2.5 Mitochondrial DNA mutation

Mitochondria are the bioenergetic source for sperm activity. They are required for natural conception and *in vitro* fertilization. The mitochondrial DNA mutation could be one cause of male infertility [49–51]. Mitochondrial DNA is vulnerable to damage from reactive oxygen species due to the lack of histone protein. It is physically associated with the inner mitochondrial membrane, where free oxygen radicals are generated [50]. Recently, an association was discovered between the single nucleotide variants of the mitochondria cytochrome B gene (MT-CYB) and male infertility [52].

3.3.2.6 Anti-sperm antibody

The presence of an anti-sperm antibody in the ejaculate is correlated with semen quality—sperm count, motility, and morphology in terms of oligoasthenoteratozoospermia [53, 54]. However, the screening of an anti-sperm antibody test before ICSI is not meaningful because the process of ICSI already bypasses the natural ability of sperm to fertilize the oocyte [55].

3.3.2.7 Medication's effects on sperm motility

Several kinds of medications have deleterious effects on spermatogenesis. For example, chemotherapeutic drugs have a strong negative effect on sperm production [56–58]. However, the effect of chemotherapeutic drugs on sperm motility is still controversial. While psychotherapeutic drugs, such as imipramine hydrochloride, chlorpromazine, trifluoperazine are commonly used medications, there is strong evidence that they negatively affect sperm motility [59]. Additionally, acetaminophen, which is used as an antipyretic drug, and non-steroid anti-inflammatory drugs

(NSAIDs) affect sperm motility [60, 61]. Moreover, regular consumption of marijuana also results in decreased sperm motility [62].

3.3.2.8 Heat exposure

Normal spermatogenesis requires environmental temperatures to be 32 to 35°C, which is lower than human core temperature, around 2–5°C. Research in animal models has shown that that heat stress could impact sperm motility by downregulating mitochondria activity and decreasing ATP activity [63]. Furthermore, increasing whole body temperature could induce damage to the epididymal spermatozoa's membrane, resulting in apoptosis [64]. These findings support the conclusion that heat exposure can damage spermatozoa productivity and function.

3.3.2.9 Environmental factors

Due to the rapidly growing industrial and agricultural countries around the world, the environment is polluted with pesticides, herbicides, petrochemical agents, and volatile organic compounds. These are all endocrine-disrupting agents that can interfere with normal spermatogenesis and male endocrine function. Several published data support that pesticides [65], dioxins [66], phthalates [65], perfluorinated compounds [67], polychlorinated biphenyls [65], heavy metals [68], dichloro-diphenyl trichloroethane [69], and plasticizers [70] impact sperm motility.

3.3.3 Sperm morphology

Sperm morphology is an important indicator of male fertility. Teratozoospermia is the nomenclature in the fifth WHO edition that means "lower sperm morphology than the reference value."

In the sixth edition, there is no nomenclature such as teratozoospermia to clarify the semen quality (the sperm morphology is less than the reference value). However, the editors used the lower fifth percentile value of the sperm from men with a female counterpart who has had a spontaneous pregnancy within a year without contraception with a 95% confidence interval. In clinical practice, the clinician might need to use the reference value to discriminate between fertile and infertile men, as demonstrated in the fifth WHO edition that the normal morphology is less than 4% according to the strict Kruger's criteria [9]. The sperm morphology alone cannot be used to predict the success of intrauterine insemination [71]. Therefore, in teratozoospermia without other sperm abnormalities, the couple should not be excluded from the process of intrauterine insemination. In contrast, in a retrospective study in 22,000 assisted reproductive technologies cycles, there was a predictive value of sperm morphology with fertilization rate, clinical pregnancy rate, and live birth rate [72].

3.3.4 Sperm vitality

The sperm vitality test is not a routine step in the sperm assessment process. Vitality tests should be done in semen samples that have very low motile sperm. The purpose of sperm vitality is to distinguish the immotile living sperm from the immotile dead sperm (necrozoospermia). A high percentage of dead sperm in the ejaculate indicates pathology in the epididymis (testicular cause) [73, 74] or sperm damage from infection (extra-testicular cause) [75]. The vitality can be assessed by an eosin-nigrosin (E-O) stain by evaluating sperm membrane integrity and permeability. The hypoosmotic swelling test is used to directly test the viability of the sperm without staining and evaluate the sperm membrane permeability [76].

4. Potential extended and advanced examination of semen sample parameters

4.1 Sperm DNA fragmentation

Conventional or basic semen analysis is used to identify male factor infertility. However, at least 15% of the infertile male partners have normal semen analysis based on conventional semen analysis [77, 78] However, basic semen analysis cannot detect some additional issues related to the fertilization rate, embryo development rate, and success rate in *in vitro* fertilization. Further investigation should be done on semen. Sperm DNA integrity is necessary for reproducing healthy offspring from one generation to the next generation. A DNA integrity test is a biomarker of intact chromatin and one of the independent tests available in male infertility besides basic semen analysis [79].

Reactive oxygen species (ROS) are free radicals of oxygen-producing hydroxyl radicals, superoxide anion, and hydrogen peroxide. During natural conception, low levels of reactive oxygen species are needed to maintain sperm capacitation, hyperactivation, acrosome reaction, and fertilization. DNA fragmentation occurs when there are more reactive oxygen species in the spermatozoa environment than the natural seminal antioxidant [80]. Some other external factors that impact the DNA fragmentation rate are as follows: obesity, psychogenic stress, smoking, alcoholic consumption, medication, and advanced paternal age [81].

DNA fragmentation is an important factor in detecting further male factor beyond basic semen analysis, which plays a role in IVF or ICSI failure. One publication demonstrated that the DNA fragmentation test is a useful tool for male factor evaluation [82]. High DNA fragmentation in the semen can interfere with the fertilization rate, embryo development rate, and implantation rate. Furthermore, it can increase the chance of spontaneous miscarriage [83–85]. The generation of sperm DNA fragmentation is initiated during maturation in the seminiferous tubule [86] and during sperm chromatin packaging in spermiogenesis [86–88].

In spermatozoa with low-level chromatin damage, fertilization capability remains intact due to the self-repairing action of the oocyte [89]. However, with higher chromatin damage, reproductive success depends on the extent of DNA damage and the repairing ability of the oocyte [90]. Young oocytes have a better repairing capacity than older oocytes [91]. In cases of severe sperm chromatin damage beyond repair, the embryo's development might fail to implant or be developmentally delayed [91, 92]. The sperm's DNA damage might not impact the fertilization rate, but the damage of the paternal part can have an effect later (late paternal effect), resulting in delayed embryo development during genomic activation—at the stage of development when there are 4–8 cells [93]—or later, at the time of implantation, leading to implantation failure or miscarriage.

Today's sperm DNA fragmentation tests have a variety of methods. The most commonly used tests in andrology laboratories are the sperm chromatin structural assay (SCSA), terminal deoxynucleotidyl transferase (TdT) dUTP nick-end labeling (TUNEL) assay, sperm chromatin dispersion (SCD) test, and the alkaline Comet test.

There are variations in clinical thresholds with cut-off level among these tests as well as the sites of the damaged DNA detected [94]. The best assay for DNA fragmentation has not been determined yet. In a systematic review and meta-analysis study, a threshold of 20% of fragmented DNA in the semen sample regarding the SCSA, TUNEL, and SCD tests can be used to differentiate between infertile and fertile men, with a sensitivity of 79% and specificity of 86% [95]. A threshold level of 20–30% of SCSA and SCD tests correlate with the duration of infertility, decreasing the chance of success in intrauterine insemination (IUI), in vitro fertilization (IVF), and intracytoplasmic sperm injecton (ICSI) and increasing the risk of miscarriage [96, 97]. The fragmented DNA is similar to the tip of the iceberg. The hidden part of the fragmented DNA cannot be detected; however, they are prone to be damaged during the process of *in vitro* manipulation of the sperm during assisted reproductive technology.

A DNA fragmentation test behaves the same as semen analysis in that it cannot discriminate between infertile from fertile men, nor can it be used to detect the success in assisted reproductive technology (ART) cycles. The test is not independent in that it still relies on the partner's factors—for example, oocyte quality and age. Basic semen analysis and sperm DNA fragmentation tests complement each other in the diagnosis of male infertility; however, they play a different part in the aspect of male fertility care.

In the clinical setting, sperm DNA fragmentation plays a role in fulfilling the diagnosis of male infertility, especially in the male partner who has specific conditions that require further analysis beyond the basic semen analysis.

4.1.1 Varicocele

Spermatozoa from a male partner with varicocele have a high potential to be affected by osmotic stress due to high temperature in the testicular environment. These factors result in sperm DNA fragmentation in at least 50% of cases [98]. A systematic review and meta-analysis demonstrated an improved DNA fragmentation rate after varicocelectomy and achievement of pregnancy in comparison to no surgery [99]. After varicocelectomy, a DNA fragmentation test can be a valuable prognostic tool to guide a suitable infertility treatment for a couple. A lower DNA fragmentation than the threshold can indicate a better outcome for natural conception, IVF, and ICSI. The type of treatment depends on the female factor. In the case of persistently high DNA fragmentation, the appropriate treatment can be assisted reproductive technology (ART), either with or without specific sperm selection for better sperm quality [100].

Sperm DNA fragmentation and male infertility are identified in subclinical varicocele. However, the controversial issue related to varicocele is that apparent vein dilation is not found upon examination; it is detected by doppler ultrasound. There was no significant difference in sperm DNA fragmentation rates between fertile and infertile men with subclinical varicocele [101]. A systematic review and meta-analysis study provided evidence that sperm DNA fragmentation rate is comparable between clinical and subclinical varicocele. However, varicocelectomy can only improve the fragmentation rate significantly in clinical varicocele [102].

4.1.2 Idiopathic infertility and unexplained infertility

Unexplained infertility is responsible for 15–30% of infertile patients. It means they have been investigated using a conventional diagnostic approach for the cause of infertility, but no clear cause of infertility was found [103]. However, about 40–50% of unexplained or idiopathic infertile couples have elevated sperm DNA fragmentation [104]. Likewise, men who have been diagnosed with idiopathic infertility are more likely to have abnormal semen parameters based on basic semen analysis without any obvious abnormality [105]. This information implies that an extended or advanced investigation might be necessary to uncover the causes of infertility in this group [105].

Sperm DNA damage might be one of the main causes of male infertility, especially in cases where infertility is idiopathic or unexplained. The added benefit of the sperm DNA fragmentation evaluation, apart from basic semen analysis, is that it might improve the chance of pregnancy, both natural conception and assisted reproduction that uses adjunctive treatment to improve sperm DNA integrity.

4.1.3 Recurrent pregnancy loss

The European Society of Human Reproduction and Embryology (ESHRE) has defined the terms of recurrent pregnancy loss as "at least two spontaneous miscarriages starting from natural conception until 24 weeks of gestation" [106]. The sperm DNA fragmentation rate is significantly higher in men with female partners who have had recurrent pregnancy loss than in a fertile female control group having at least one ongoing pregnancy or live birth [107, 108]. The mechanism of sperm fragmented DNA that initiates recurrent pregnancy loss has not been determined yet. However, one hypothesis is that the oocyte repair mechanism might be the main culprit, leading to poor blastocyst development, recurrent implantation failure, and pregnancy loss [108].

4.1.4 Intrauterine insemination

There is evidence that men with a sperm DNA fragmentation rate diagnosed above 27% by SCSA have higher early pregnancy loss and a lower pregnancy rate than the general infertile population with a lower sperm DNA fragmentation [109, 110]. According to this information, the sperm DNA fragmentation test has an additional benefit of guiding the clinician to choose the treatment of choice for each infertile couple. In case of the sperm DNA fragmentation being higher than the threshold, the couples should have complementary treatment before IUI to ameliorate the sperm DNA fragmentation rate. However, in couples with advanced female age, assisted reproduction should be considered early on due to the oocyte's diminished repair ability and the risk of chromosome abnormality, which are the main causes of treatment failure [94].

4.1.5 Assisted reproduction (in vitro fertilization (IVF), intracytoplasmic sperm injection (ICSI)

High sperm DNA fragmentation impacts the likelihood of successful pregnancy in a natural cycle, intrauterine insemination, and advanced treatments such as IVF and ICSI. There are several studies demonstrating that elevated sperm DNA fragmentation adversely impacts IVF and ICSI. Mainly, it increases spontaneous abortion and recurrent implantation failure. Additionally, it decreases the live birth rate [111–113]. Evidence suggests that the impact of sperm DNA fragmentation might be higher in IVF than in ICSI [114]. It was postulated that the sperm needs to be incubated with the oocyte *in vitro* longer in IVF than in ICSI. The duration of exposure of sperm to the external environment during IVF might generate more DNA damage than ICSI, which requires only a short time after ejaculation until successful fertilization [115]. Additionally, the sperm is a significant source of reactive oxygen species. IVF requires the direct contact of at least one hundred thousand sperms and an oocyte for natural fertilization. The exposure of the oocyte to oxidative stress from sperm could adversely impact the embryo's development [116, 117].

Likewise, high sperm DNA fragmentation has an adverse effect that results in these couples having more spontaneous pregnancy losses than couples with low sperm DNA fragmentation [118]. The authors concluded that using a sperm selection method during assisted reproduction to choose sperm with low fragmented DNA could improve the pregnancy rate and decrease the miscarriage rate [118].

The pathophysiologic cause of an increasing rate of spontaneous abortion in high sperm DNA fragmentation in couples undergoing IVF or ICSI is still inconclusive. One proposed mechanism is that the genetic and epigenetic effects of sperm DNA damage could cause mutation or dysregulation of DNA methylation processes that are crucial for embryo development [119–121]. The other proposed mechanism is the oocyte's ability to repair the sperm DNA defect. In oocyte donation cycles, it was found that a good quality oocyte can counteract the defected sperm DNA. However, oocytes from women of advanced maternal age have diminished repair functions compared to young women [122]. Single-stranded DNA breakage is more likely to be repaired than double-stranded DNA breakage [123, 124]. Therefore, the final impact of sperm DNA fragmentation on the pregnancy outcome still relies on the balance of the oocyte repairing system and the extent of sperm DNA damage [90].

Persistent high sperm DNA fragmentation is one of the leading causes of IVF and ICSI failure. Detection of sperm DNA damage is crucial for treatment success. In cases where no causative factor of elevated sperm fragmented DNA is identified, testicular spermatozoa are the suggested method to improve treatment success in ICSI [125–132]. ICSI uses testicular spermatozoa instead of ejaculated spermatozoa, which could be related to the lower sperm DNA damage in the testicular sperm compared to ejaculated sperm that must transit from the epididymis to the male reproductive tract [132–136].

4.1.6 Other risk factors

Some lifestyle factors can increase sperm DNA fragmentation. Some examples are smoking, drinking, cannabis consumption, exposure to air pollutants, pesticides, polyaromatic hydrocarbons, and fertilizers. Among these factors, smoking has the most impact on sperm DNA fragmentation [137, 138]. Cannabis consumption also impairs sperm DNA integrity [139]. Advanced paternal age above 40 years also reduces the sperm DNA quality [140–142].

Obesity is another common problem that leads to poor sperm quality due to peripheral aromatization from testosterone to estradiol in the subcutaneous fat. The increasing testicular temperature from subpubic fat and the high estradiol levels in obese men might cause hypogonadism and sperm DNA damage [143].

4.1.7 Sperm cryopreservation

Sperm cryopreservation is a method to preserve male fertility for future use. This method allows men to preserve their semen. Candidates for sperm cryopreservation include men who have cancer and require chemotherapy or radiation treatments or healthy men who need to preserve semen for future purposes before a vasectomy or after assisted reproduction. This technique is required for sperm donation. However, the process of sperm freezing and thawing can be harmful to sperm quality. It impacts the sperm's motility, viability, and normal morphology. Additionally, it increases osmotic stress on the spermatozoa and leads to sperm DNA damage [144, 145].

The vitrification technique has recently been developed for sperm cryopreservation. It has the potential to reduce sperm DNA damage compared to conventional slow freezing [146, 147]. However, more research is needed.

Sperm DNA fragmentation tests should be done before and after sperm cryopreservation to help improve the method to reduce the impact of cryopreservation on sperm parameters. Moreover, the tests provide the optimal treatment based on sperm quality. The addition of an antioxidant to the sperm freezing media is one technique to protect the sperm from the harsh conditions of the freezing and thawing process by reducing the osmotic stress-induced DNA damage [148].

4.2 Reactive oxygen species measurement

One of the causes of male infertility and sperm DNA damage is osmotic stress to the spermatozoa. Reactive oxygen species are derived from the metabolism of oxygen. They play a vital role in cellular signaling pathways, sperm maturation processes, and capacitation [149]. Excessive ROS can have a significant detrimental effect on sperm fertility potential [150]. All along the journey initiated from the seminiferous tubule and through the epididymis, *vas deferens,* and finally to the outlet of the male reproductive tract, spermatozoa are potentially assaulted from oxidative stress, which diminishes fertilizing capability and leads to recurrent implantation failure and pregnancy loss. External osmotic stress interferes with the sperm membrane, while internal osmotic stress acts on lipid peroxidation mechanisms, resulting in sperm DNA damage.

Possible mechanisms of oxidative damage to the spermatozoa are sperm membrane and DNA damage, which decrease sperm motility and fertilization ability. These types of damage can also cause poor embryo development, recurrent implantation failure, and early pregnancy loss [84, 151]. Sperm damage by ROS reduces sperm motility, as demonstrated in both conventional and computer-assisted semen analyses [152, 153].

Human semen consists of various kinds of cells, including mature and immature spermatozoa, epithelial cells, and leukocytes. The main sources of ROS in semen are leukocytes (i.e., extrinsic source) and spermatozoa (i.e., intrinsic source). In addition, environmental factors, such as heavy metals, smoking, varicocele, obesity, chronic illness, and genitourinary tract infection are potential sources of ROS, affecting sperm DNA and resulting in DNA fragmentation and damage [154].

Oxidative stress has been demonstrated to be a main factor responsible for male infertility via sperm dysfunction. Oxidative stress on spermatozoa mainly derives from the excessive ROS and inadequate antioxidants to counteract them. Excess ROS can damage sperm by several mechanisms via the oxidative pathway. Approximately 30–40% of infertile men have oxidative stress that causes male infertility [155].

Spermatozoa are unique biological cells in the human body that have limited self-repair capability due to the lack of a cytoplasmic repairing mechanism. This is the most important reason that spermatozoa are vulnerable to internal and external ROS damage [156]. In addition, the membrane of spermatozoa is composed of polyunsaturated fatty acid that is susceptible to oxygen-induced damage and, hence, lipid peroxidation. One consequence of lipid peroxidation is damage to the axoneme and midpiece of spermatozoa, resulting in diminished sperm motility [157, 158]. High levels of ROS are detected in at least 25–40% of infertile men [159, 160] Levels of ROS above the semen's antioxidants result in oxidative stress to the sperm [160]. Currently, ROS measurement by chemiluminescence is the most well-described, advanced method of ROS detection in the seminal fluid [161–163].

4.3 Total antioxidant capacity measurement

Total antioxidant capacity (TAC) is a diagnostic test to measure enzymatic and non-enzymatic kinds of antioxidants in the seminal fluid during a male infertility work up. The value reflects the redox potential an antioxidant has to osmotic stress. There is substantial evidence that the utility of the TAC measurement lies in its ability to detect a lower TAC in infertile men than in a fertile control [164]. The imbalance between osmotic stress and TAC lead to male infertility. TAC is also used to detect who should have antioxidant supplementation before ICSI, especially in case of previously failed ICSI [165]. The role of an antioxidant supplement in male infertility has been reviewed with the potential to lead to a successful pregnancy [166].

4.4 Assessment of the presence of leukocytospermia and hematospermia

Normal leukocyte production occurs mainly in the epididymis, where they take responsibility for the immunosurveillance of abnormal sperm via phagocytosis. Leukocytes are composed of granulocytes at 50–60%, macrophages at 20–30%, and T-lymphocytes at 2–5% [167]. Leukocytospermia is an excessive amount of leukocytes—more than the threshold, according to the fifth WHO manual—which can impact the sperm quality, as leukocytes are the main source of ROS [154].

The best laboratory guideline for leukocyte assessment in semen is immunohistochemical staining against the various kinds of leukocytes; however, the method is complicated, time-consuming, and not well standardized [168]. The European Association of Urology recommends antibiotic treatment; however, evidence for improving pregnancy outcomes was not demonstrated [169]. Likewise, there is no clear evidence that either antioxidant or antibiotic treatment improves treatment success in infertile men with leukocytospermia [170].

Hematospermia is a term referring to the presence of gross and microscopic examination in the ejaculate. The pathophysiologic causes can be disorders in the ejaculatory ducts, accessory glands, and urethra. Alternatively, it can have iatrogenic causes. The extensive investigations in the case of hematospermia have been well-documented [171, 172]. There is some evidence of the relationship between hematospermia and male infertility [173, 174]. Red blood cells might be the main source of toxic substances leading to a decline in sperm quality. Hemolysis especially occurs during sperm cryopreservation and thawing [175].

5. Other extended and advanced examination of semen sample parameters

5.1 Sperm aneuploidy test

The sperm aneuploidy test is a direct evaluation of sperm chromosome complements that has been used in a couple with recurrent pregnancy loss. The test evaluates both structural and numerical chromosome abnormality in spermatozoa. A systematic review and meta-analysis demonstrated the increasing incidence of aneuploidy in spermatozoa in cases of recurrent pregnancy loss [176]. The real benefit and implementation of sperm aneuploidy in a routine laboratory for male infertility has yet to be determined, as molecular analysis in miscarriage has revealed that most chromosome aneuploidy occurs during female meiosis, resulting in meiotic non-disjunction [177]. In addition, the final evaluation of chromosome abnormality on the blastocyst can provide both the meiotic and mitotic origin—from either oocyte or spermatozoa—with no need to investigate the oocyte or sperm before fertilization.

5.2 Cytokine assessment in the semen

Infection and inflammation of the male genitourinary tract play an important role in male infertility due to inflammatory mediators and ROS causing damage to the spermatozoa. Any suspicious male genitourinary tract infection should be thoroughly investigated; otherwise, irreversible sperm damage might occur. The biological markers of infection and inflammation in the ejaculate are leukocyte numbers>1 million/ml, granulocyte elastase >280 ng/ml, and proinflammatory cytokines (e.g., interleukin (IL)-6 > 30 pg./ml, IL-8 > 7000 pg./ml) [178]. Cytokine detection might play a potential role and be a sensitive marker of male genitourinary tract infection and inflammation, especially in asymptomatic and silent cases.

5.3 Immature germ cell assessment

Immature germ cells can be differentiated from leukocytes by Papanicolaou staining. There is no longer a cut-off value of immature germ cells provided in the fifth and sixth WHO manuals, as there is not a sufficient number of studies to confirm the clinical importance of the value. However, elevation of immature germ cell to more than 15% of total sperm in the ejaculate might be significant and indicative of sperm chromatin immaturity [179]. Investigation into the pathophysiologic cause of high shedding of immature germ cells in the ejaculate and the consequences that ensue are not warranted [179].

6. Conclusion

Currently, semen analysis has become a standard tool for evaluating male infertility and guiding clinicians to provide appropriate treatments for couples. The sperm parameters in the ejaculate are the biological markers of male fertility. A basic semen analysis provides the initial information related to identifying whether a man is fertile or infertile; however, there is no absolute cut-off value for the inability to achieve conception.

In the modern era of assisted reproduction and molecular genetics, new diagnostic techniques reveal the deeply detailed causes of male infertility to improve the treatment outcome. In the modern world, there is more likely to be an association between men's general health and the environment regarding sperm parameters than previously. Having knowledge of the consequences of these factors on sperm parameters can possibly lead to the development of pharmaceutical components or supplements that improve male fertility.

DOI: http://dx.doi.org/10.5772/intechopen.107625

Author details

Suchada Mongkolchaipak
Chada IVF Fertility Clinic, Chonburi, Thailand

*Address all correspondence to: doctorsuchada@gmail.com

References

[1] Zegers-Hochschild F, Adamson GD, de Mouzon J, et al. International Committee for Monitoring Assisted Reproductive Technology (ICMART) and the World Health Organization (WHO) revised glossary of ART terminology, 2009. Fertility and Sterility. 2009;**92**(5):1520-1524. DOI: 10.1016/j.fertnstert.2009.09.009

[2] Sciarra J. Infertility: An international health problem. International Journal of Gynaecology and Obstetrics. 1994;**46**(2):155-163. DOI: 10.1016/0020-7292(94)90230-5

[3] Agarwal A, Mulgund A, Hamada A, Chyatte MR. A unique view on male infertility around the globe. Reproductive Biology and Endocrinology. 2015;**13**(1):37. DOI: 10.1186/s12958-015-0032-1

[4] Esteves SC, Miyaoka R, Agarwal A. An update on the clinical assessment of the infertile male. [corrected]. Clinics (Sao Paulo). 2011;**66**(4):691-700. DOI: 10.1590/s1807-59322011000400026

[5] Brandes M, Hamilton CJCM, de Bruin JP, Nelen WLDM, Kremer JAM. The relative contribution of IVF to the total ongoing pregnancy rate in a subfertile cohort. Human Reproduction. 2010;**25**(1):118-126. DOI: 10.1093/humrep/dep341

[6] World Health Organization. WHO Laboratory Manual for the Examination and Processing of Human Semen. 2th ed. Cambridge: World Health Organization; 1987

[7] World Health Organization. WHO Laboratory Manual for the Examination and Processing of Human Semen. 3th ed. Cambridge: World Health Organization; 1992

[8] World Health Organization. WHO Laboratory Manual for the Examination and Processing of Human Semen. 4th ed. Cambridge: World Health Organization; 1999

[9] World Health Organization. WHO Laboratory Manual for the Examination and Processing of Human Semen. 5th ed. Geneva: World Health Organization; 2010

[10] Hamada A, Esteves SC, Nizza M, Agarwal A. Unexplained male infertility: Diagnosis and management. International Brazilian Journal of Urology. 2012;**38**(5):576-594. DOI: 10.1590/s1677-55382012000500002

[11] Zini A, Bielecki R, Phang D, Zenzes MT. Correlations between two markers of sperm DNA integrity, DNA denaturation and DNA fragmentation, in fertile and infertile men. Fertility and Sterility. 2001;**75**(4):674-677. DOI: 10.1016/s0015-0282(00)01796-9

[12] Ahmad G, Moinard N, Esquerré-Lamare C, Mieusset R, Bujan L. Mild induced testicular and epididymal hyperthermia alters sperm chromatin integrity in men. Fertility and Sterility. 2012;**97**(3):546-553. DOI: 10.1016/j.fertnstert.2011.12.025

[13] Brahem S, Mehdi M, Elghezal H, Saad A. The effects of male aging on semen quality, sperm DNA fragmentation and chromosomal abnormalities in an infertile population. Journal of Assisted Reproduction and Genetics. 2011;**28**(5):425-432. DOI: 10.1007/s10815-011-9537-5

[14] Björndahl L, Kirkman Brown J. Other editorial board members of the WHO Laboratory manual for the examination

and processing of human semen. The sixth edition of the WHO Laboratory manual for the examination and processing of human semen: Ensuring quality and standardization in basic examination of human ejaculates. Fertility and Sterility. 2022;**117**(2):246-251. DOI: 10.1016/j.fertnstert.2021.12.012

[15] Schjenken JE, Robertson SA. Seminal fluid Signalling in the female reproductive tract: Implications for reproductive success and offspring health. Advances in Experimental Medicine and Biology. 2015;**868**:127-158. DOI: 10.1007/978-3-319-18881-2_6

[16] World Health Organization, editor. WHO Laboratory Manual for the Examination and Processing of Human Semen. 6th ed. Geneva: World Health Organization; 2021

[17] Levine H, Jørgensen N, Martino-Andrade A, et al. Temporal trends in sperm count: A systematic review and meta-regression analysis. Human Reproduction Update. 2017;**23**(6):646-659. DOI: 10.1093/humupd/dmx022

[18] Jafarabadi M. Episodic air pollution is associated with increased DNA fragmentation in human sperm without other changes in semen quality. Human Reproduction. 2007;**22**(12):3263 ; author reply 3264. DOI: 10.1093/humrep/dem329

[19] Agarwal A, Desai NR, Makker K, et al. Effects of radiofrequency electromagnetic waves (RF-EMW) from cellular phones on human ejaculated semen: An in vitro pilot study. Fertility and Sterility. 2009;**92**(4):1318-1325. DOI: 10.1016/j.fertnstert.2008.08.022

[20] Sikka SC, Wang R. Endocrine disruptors and estrogenic effects on male reproductive axis. Asian Journal of Andrology. 2008;**10**(1):134-145. DOI: 10.1111/j.1745-7262.2008.00370.x

[21] Hajder M, Hajder E, Husic A. The effects of total motile sperm count on spontaneous pregnancy rate and pregnancy after IUI treatment in couples with male factor and unexplained infertility. Medical Archives. 2016;**70**(1):39. DOI: 10.5455/medarh.2016.70.39-43

[22] Yang C, Zhou ZH, Zheng DN, et al. Sperm origins and concentration do not impact the clinical outcomes in intracytoplasmic sperm injection cycles. Asian Journal of Andrology. 2018;**20**(5):454-458. DOI: 10.4103/aja.aja_27_18

[23] Ok EK, Doğan OE, Okyay RE, Gülekli B. The effect of post-wash total progressive motile sperm count and semen volume on pregnancy outcomes in intrauterine insemination cycles: A retrospective study. Journal of the Turkish German Gynecological Association. 2013;**14**(3):142-145. DOI: 10.5152/jtgga.2013.52280

[24] Barratt CLR, Björndahl L, Menkveld R, Mortimer D. ESHRE special interest group for andrology basic semen analysis course: A continued focus on accuracy, quality, efficiency and clinical relevance. Human Reproduction. 2011;**26**(12):3207-3212. DOI: 10.1093/humrep/der312

[25] Miyaoka R, Esteves SC. A critical appraisal on the role of varicocele in male infertility. Advances in Urology. 2012;**2012**:597495. DOI: 10.1155/2012/597495

[26] Blumer CG, Restelli AE, Giudice PT, et al. Effect of varicocele on sperm function and semen oxidative stress. BJU International. 2012;**109**(2):259-265.

DOI: 10.1111/j.1464-410X.2011.
10240.x

[27] Agarwal A, Sharma R, Harlev A, Esteves SC. Effect of varicocele on semen characteristics according to the new 2010 World Health Organization criteria: A systematic review and meta-analysis. Asian Journal of Andrology. 2016;**18**(2):163-170. DOI: 10.4103/1008-682X.172638

[28] Abd-Elmoaty MA, Saleh R, Sharma R, Agarwal A. Increased levels of oxidants and reduced antioxidants in semen of infertile men with varicocele. Fertility and Sterility. 2010;**94**(4):1531-1534. DOI: 10.1016/j.fertnstert.2009.12.039

[29] Zargooshi J. Sperm count and sperm motility in incidental high-grade varicocele. Fertility and Sterility. 2007;**88**(5):1470-1473. DOI: 10.1016/j.fertnstert.2007.01.016

[30] Malasevskaia I, Ali Al-Awadhi A, Ali RF. Fertility outcomes after varicocele repair: Are there any benefits? A traditional review. Fortune Journal of Health Sciences. 2021;**04**(02):284-298. DOI: 10.26502/fjhs022

[31] Kantartzi PD, Goulis CD, Goulis GD, Papadimas I. Male infertility and varicocele: Myths and reality. Hippokratia. 2007;**11**(3):99-104

[32] Chu DI, Zderic SA, Shukla AR, et al. Does varicocelectomy improve semen analysis outcomes in adolescents without testicular asymmetry? Journal of Pediatric Urology. 2017;**13**(1):76.e1-76.e5. DOI: 10.1016/j.jpurol.2016.09.010

[33] Shabana W, Teleb M, Dawod T, et al. Predictors of improvement in semen parameters after varicocelectomy for male subfertility: A prospective study. Canadian Urological Association Journal. 2015;**9**(9-10):E579-E582. DOI: 10.5489/cuaj.2808

[34] Wang J, Wang T, Ding W, et al. Efficacy of antioxidant therapy on sperm quality measurements after varicocelectomy: A systematic review and meta-analysis. Andrologia. 2019;**51**(10):e13396. DOI: 10.1111/and.13396

[35] Chen YW, Niu YH, Wang DQ, et al. Effect of adjuvant drug therapy after varicocelectomy on fertility outcome in males with varicocele-associated infertility: Systematic review and meta-analysis. Andrologia. 2018;**50**(8):e13070. DOI: 10.1111/and.13070

[36] Pyrgidis N, Sokolakis I, Palapelas V, et al. The effect of antioxidant supplementation on operated or non-operated varicocele-associated infertility: A systematic review and meta-analysis. Antioxidants (Basel). 2021;**10**(7):1067. DOI: 10.3390/antiox10071067

[37] Comar VA, Petersen CG, Mauri AL, et al. Influence of the abstinence period on human sperm quality: analysis of 2,458 semen samples. JBRA Assist Reprod. 2017;**21**(4):306-312. Published 2017 Dec 1. DOI: 10.5935/1518-0557.20170052

[38] Alipour H, Van Der Horst G, Christiansen OB, et al. Improved sperm kinematics in semen samples collected after 2 h versus 4-7 days of ejaculation abstinence. Human Reproduction. 2017;**32**(7):1364-1372. DOI: 10.1093/humrep/dex101

[39] Dupesh S, Pandiyan N, Pandiyan R, Kartheeswaran J, Prakash B. Ejaculatory abstinence in semen analysis: Does it make any sense? Therapeutic Advances in Reproductive Health.

2020;**14**:2633494120906882. DOI: 10.1177/2633494120906882

[40] Elzanaty S, Malm J, Giwercman A. Duration of sexual abstinence: Epididymal and accessory sex gland secretions and their relationship to sperm motility. Human Reproduction. 2005;**20**(1):221-225. DOI: 10.1093/humrep/deh586

[41] Ventimiglia E, Montorsi F, Salonia A. Re: Reecha Sharma, Avi harlev, Ashok Agarwal, Sandro C. esteves. Cigarette smoking and semen quality: A new meta-analysis examining the effect of the 2010 world health organization laboratory methods for the examination of human semen. Eur urol 2016;70:635-45. European Urology. 2017;**71**(1):e19-e20. DOI: 10.1016/j.eururo.2016.05.051

[42] Linck RW, Chemes H, Albertini DF. The axoneme: The propulsive engine of spermatozoa and cilia and associated ciliopathies leading to infertility. Journal of Assisted Reproduction and Genetics. 2016;**33**(2):141-156. DOI: 10.1007/s10815-016-0652-1

[43] Kurkowska W, Bogacz A, Janiszewska M, et al. Oxidative stress is associated with reduced sperm motility in normal semen. American Journal of Men's Health. 2020;**14**(5):1557988320939731. DOI: 10.1177/1557988320939731

[44] Silva JV, Cruz D, Gomes M, et al. Study on the short-term effects of increased alcohol and cigarette consumption in healthy young men's seminal quality. Scientific Reports. 2017;7:45457. DOI: 10.1038/srep45457

[45] Ricci E, Al Beitawi S, Cipriani S, et al. Semen quality and alcohol intake: A systematic review and meta-analysis. Reproductive Biomedicine Online. 2017;**34**(1):38-47. DOI: 10.1016/j.rbmo.2016.09.012

[46] Leigh MW, Pittman JE, Carson JL, et al. Clinical and genetic aspects of primary ciliary dyskinesia/Kartagener syndrome. Genetics in Medicine. 2009;**11**(7):473-487. DOI: 10.1097/GIM.0b013e3181a53562

[47] Chemes HE, Rawe VY. The making of abnormal spermatozoa: Cellular and molecular mechanisms underlying pathological spermiogenesis. Cell and Tissue Research. 2010;**341**(3):349-357. DOI: 10.1007/s00441-010-1007-3

[48] Gupta S, Handa KK, Kasliwal RR, Bajpai P. A case of Kartagener's syndrome: Importance of early diagnosis and treatment. Indian Journal of Human Genetics. 2013;**19**(2):266-269. DOI: 10.4103/0971-6866.116107

[49] Kumar DP, Sangeetha N. Mitochondrial DNA mutations and male infertility. Indian Journal of Human Genetics. 2009;**15**(3):93-97. DOI: 10.4103/0971-6866.60183

[50] Venkatesh S, Deecaraman M, Kumar R, Shamsi MB, Dada R. Role of reactive oxygen species in the pathogenesis of mitochondrial DNA (mtDNA) mutations in male infertility. The Indian Journal of Medical Research. 2009;**129**(2):127-137

[51] Amor H, Hammadeh ME. A systematic review of the impact of mitochondrial variations on male infertility. Genes (Basel). 2022;**13**(7):1182. DOI: 10.3390/genes13071182

[52] Saleh Jaweesh M, Hammadeh ME, Dahadhah FW, Al Zoubi MS, Amor H. Association between the single nucleotide variants of the mitochondrial cytochrome B gene (MT-CYB) and the male infertility. Molecular Biology Reports. 2022;**49**(5):3609-3616. DOI: 10.1007/s11033-022-07200-y

[53] Kamphorst K, Faber J, van der Linden PJQ. The presence of antisperm antibodies in semen of subfertile men—Positive ASA in subfertile men. Open Journal of Obstetrics and Gynecology. 2021;**11**(02):88-101. DOI: 10.4236/ojog.2021.112011

[54] Garcia PC, Rubio EM, Pereira OCM. Antisperm antibodies in infertile men and their correlation with seminal parameters: Antisperm antibodies versus seminal parameters. Reproductive Medicine and Biology. 2007;**6**(1):33-38. DOI: 10.1111/j.1447-0578.2007.00162.x

[55] El-Sherbiny AF, Ali TA, Hassan EA, Mehaney AB, Elshemy HA. The prognostic value of seminal anti-sperm antibodies screening in men prepared for ICSI: A call to change the current antibody-directed viewpoint of sperm autoimmunity testing. Therapeutic Advances in Urology. 2021;**13**:1756287220981488. DOI: 10.1177/1756287220981488

[56] Williams DH 4th, Karpman E, Sander JC, Spiess PE, Pisters LL, Lipshultz LI. Pretreatment semen parameters in men with cancer. The Journal of Urology. 2009;**181**(2):736-740. DOI: 10.1016/j.juro.2008.10.023

[57] Agarwal A, Dias T, Pushparaj P, Ahmad G, Sharma R. Reduced semen quality in patients with testicular cancer seminoma is associated with alterations in the expression of sperm proteins. Asian Journal of Andrology. 2020;**22**(1):88. DOI: 10.4103/aja.aja_17_19

[58] Hendry WF, Stedronska J, Jones CR, Blackmore CA, Barrett A, Peckham MJ. Semen analysis in testicular cancer and Hodgkin's disease: Pre- and post-treatment findings and implications for cryopreservation. British Journal of Urology. 1983;**55**(6):769-773. DOI: 10.1111/j.1464-410x.1983.tb03423.x

[59] Levin RM, Amsterdam JD, Winokur A, Wein AJ. Effects of psychotropic drugs on human sperm motility. Obstetrical & Gynecological Survey. 1982;**37**(7):484-486. DOI: 10.1097/00006254-198207000-00017

[60] Banihani SA. Effect of paracetamol on semen quality. Andrologia. 2018;**50**(1):10.1111/and.12874. DOI: 10.1111/and.12874

[61] Stutz G, Zamudio J, Santillán ME, Vincenti L, de Cuneo MF, Ruiz RD. The effect of alcohol, tobacco, and aspirin consumption on seminal quality among healthy young men. Archives of Environmental Health. 2004;**59**(11):548-552. DOI: 10.1080/00039890409603432

[62] du Plessis SS, Agarwal A, Syriac A. Marijuana, phytocannabinoids, the endocannabinoid system, and male fertility. Journal of Assisted Reproduction and Genetics. 2015;**32**(11):1575-1588. DOI: 10.1007/s10815-015-0553-8

[63] Gong Y, Guo H, Zhang Z, Zhou H, Zhao R, He B. Heat stress reduces sperm motility via activation of glycogen synthase kinase-3α and inhibition of mitochondrial protein import. Frontiers in Physiology. 2017;**8**:718. Published 2017 Sep 22. DOI: 10.3389/fphys.2017.00718

[64] Wechalekar H, Setchell BP, Peirce EJ, Ricci M, Leigh C, Breed WG. Whole-body heat exposure induces membrane changes in spermatozoa from the cauda epididymidis of laboratory mice. Asian Journal of Andrology. 2010;**12**(4):591-598. DOI: 10.1038/aja.2010.41

[65] Hauser R, Williams P, Altshul L, Calafat AM. Evidence of interaction between polychlorinated biphenyls

and phthalates in relation to human sperm motility. Environmental Health Perspectives. 2005;**113**(4):425-430. DOI: 10.1289/ehp.7305

[66] Mocarelli P, Gerthoux PM, Patterson DG Jr, et al. Dioxin exposure, from infancy through puberty, produces endocrine disruption and affects human semen quality. Environmental Health Perspectives. 2008;**116**(1):70-77. DOI: 10.1289/ehp.10399

[67] Governini L, Guerranti C, De Leo V, et al. Chromosomal aneuploidies and DNA fragmentation of human spermatozoa from patients exposed to perfluorinated compounds. Andrologia. 2015;**47**(9):1012-1019. DOI: 10.1111/and.12371

[68] Mendiola J, Moreno JM, Roca M, et al. Relationships between heavy metal concentrations in three different body fluids and male reproductive parameters: A pilot study. Environmental Health. 2011;**10**(1):6. DOI: 10.1186/1476-069X-10-6

[69] Pant N, Kumar R, Mathur N, Srivastava SP, Saxena DK, Gujrati VR. Chlorinated pesticide concentration in semen of fertile and infertile men and correlation with sperm quality. Environmental Toxicology and Pharmacology. 2007;**23**(2):135-139. DOI: 10.1016/j.etap.2006.07.012

[70] Fredricsson B, Möller L, Pousette A, Westerholm R. Human sperm motility is affected by plasticizers and diesel particle extracts. Pharmacology & Toxicology. 1993;**72**(2):128-133. DOI: 10.1111/j.1600-0773.1993.tb00303.x

[71] Stanhiser J, Mersereau JE, Dock D, et al. Sperm morphology from the actual inseminated sample does not predict clinical pregnancy following intrauterine insemination. F & S Reports. 2021;**2**(1):16-21. DOI: 10.1016/j.xfre.2020.11.007

[72] Villani MT, Morini D, Spaggiari G, et al. Are sperm parameters able to predict the success of assisted reproductive technology? A retrospective analysis of over 22,000 assisted reproductive technology cycles. Andrology. 2022;**10**(2):310-321. DOI: 10.1111/andr.13123

[73] Wilton LJ, Temple-Smith PD, Baker HW, de Kretser DM. Human male infertility caused by degeneration and death of sperm in the epididymis. Fertility and Sterility. 1988;**49**(6):1052-1058. DOI: 10.1016/s0015-0282(16)59960-9

[74] Mahfouz RZ, du Plessis SS, Aziz N, Sharma R, Sabanegh E, Agarwal A. Sperm viability, apoptosis, and intracellular reactive oxygen species levels in human spermatozoa before and after induction of oxidative stress. Fertility and Sterility. 2010;**93**(3):814-821. DOI: 10.1016/j.fertnstert.2008.10.068

[75] Nduwayo L, Barthélémy C, Lansac J, Tharanne MJ, Lecomte P. Conduite à tenir devant une nécrozoospermie [Management of necrospermia]. Contraception, Fertilité, Sexualité (1992). 1995;**23**(11):682-685

[76] Agarwal A, Gupta S, Sharma R. Hypoosmotic swelling test (HOS). In: Agarwal A, Gupta S, Sharma R, editors. Andrological Evaluation of Male Infertility. Cham: Springer; 2016. DOI: 10.1007/978-3-319-26797-5_12

[77] Sharma RK, Said T, Agarwal A. Sperm DNA damage and its clinical relevance in assessing reproductive outcome. Asian Journal of Andrology. 2004;**6**(2):139-148

[78] Agarwal A, Said TM. Oxidative stress, DNA damage and apoptosis in male infertility: A clinical approach. BJU

International. 2005;**95**(4):503-507. DOI: 10.1111/j.1464-410X.2005.05328.x

[79] Raheem OA, Ana M, Urol M, Walsh TJ. Clinical utility of sperm DNA fragmentation testing: Practice recommendations based on clinical scenarios. Translational Andrology and Urology. 2017;**6**(Suppl. 4):S322-S323. DOI: 10.21037/tau.2017.08.14

[80] Alahmar A. Role of oxidative stress in male infertility: An updated review. Journal of Human Reproductive Sciences. 2019;**12**(1):4. DOI: 10.4103/jhrs.jhrs_150_18

[81] Durairajanayagam D. Lifestyle causes of male infertility. Arab Journal of Urology. 2018;**16**(1):10-20. DOI: 10.1016/j.aju.2017.12.004

[82] Bungum M, Humaidan P, Axmon A, et al. Sperm DNA integrity assessment in prediction of assisted reproduction technology outcome. Human Reproduction. 2007;**22**(1):174-179. DOI: 10.1093/humrep/del326

[83] Lewis SEM, John Aitken R, Conner SJ, et al. The impact of sperm DNA damage in assisted conception and beyond: Recent advances in diagnosis and treatment. Reproductive Biomedicine Online. 2013;**27**(4):325-337. DOI: 10.1016/j.rbmo.2013.06.014

[84] Simon L, Murphy K, Shamsi MB, et al. Paternal influence of sperm DNA integrity on early embryonic development. Human Reproduction. 2014;**29**(11):2402-2412. DOI: 10.1093/humrep/deu228

[85] Gosálvez J, López-Fernández C, Fernández JL, Esteves SC, Johnston SD. Unpacking the mysteries of sperm DNA fragmentation: Ten frequently asked questions. Journal of Reproductive Biotechnology and Fertility. 2015;**4**:205891581559445. DOI: 10.1177/2058915815594454

[86] Sakkas D, Moffatt O, Manicardi GC, Mariethoz E, Tarozzi N, Bizzaro D. Nature of DNA damage in ejaculated human spermatozoa and the possible involvement of apoptosis. Biology of Reproduction. 2002;**66**(4):1061-1067. DOI: 10.1095/biolreprod66.4.1061

[87] Shamsi MB, Kumar R, Dada R. Evaluation of nuclear DNA damage in human spermatozoa in men opting for assisted reproduction. The Indian Journal of Medical Research. 2008;**127**(2):115-123

[88] Aitken RJ, De Iuliis GN. On the possible origins of DNA damage in human spermatozoa. Molecular Human Reproduction. 2010;**16**(1):3-13. DOI: 10.1093/molehr/gap059

[89] Zenzes MT, Puy LA, Bielecki R, Reed TE. Detection of benzo[a]pyrene diol epoxide-DNA adducts in embryos from smoking couples: Evidence for transmission by spermatozoa. Molecular Human Reproduction. 1999;**5**(2):125-131. DOI: 10.1093/molehr/5.2.125

[90] Champroux A, Torres-Carreira J, Gharagozloo P, Drevet JR, Kocer A. Mammalian sperm nuclear organization: Resiliencies and vulnerabilities. Basic and Clinical Andrology. 2016;**26**(1):17. DOI: 10.1186/s12610-016-0044-5

[91] Horta F, Catt S, Ramachandran P, Vollenhoven B, Temple-Smith P. Female ageing affects the DNA repair capacity of oocytes in IVF using a controlled model of sperm DNA damage in mice. Human Reproduction. 2020;**35**(3):529-544. DOI: 10.1093/humrep/dez308

[92] Martin JH, Aitken RJ, Bromfield EG, Nixon B. DNA damage and repair in

the female germline: Contributions to ART. Human Reproduction Update. 2019;**25**(2):180-201. DOI: 10.1093/humupd/dmy040

[93] Tesarik J, Greco E, Mendoza C. Late, but not early, paternal effect on human embryo development is related to sperm DNA fragmentation. Human Reproduction. 2004;**19**(3):611-615. DOI: 10.1093/humrep/deh127

[94] Esteves SC, Zini A, Coward RM, et al. Sperm DNA fragmentation testing: Summary evidence and clinical practice recommendations. Andrologia. 2021;**53**(2):e13874. DOI: 10.1111/and.13874

[95] Santi D, Spaggiari G, Simoni M. Sperm DNA fragmentation index as a promising predictive tool for male infertility diagnosis and treatment management—Meta-analyses. Reproductive Biomedicine Online. 2018;**37**(3):315-326. DOI: 10.1016/j.rbmo.2018.06.023

[96] Nicopoullos J, Vicens-Morton A, Lewis SEM, et al. Novel use of COMET parameters of sperm DNA damage may increase its utility to diagnose male infertility and predict live births following both IVF and ICSI. Human Reproduction. 2019;**34**(10):1915-1923. DOI: 10.1093/humrep/dez151

[97] Majzoub A, Agarwal A, Cho CL, Esteves SC. Sperm DNA fragmentation testing: A cross sectional survey on current practices of fertility specialists. Translational Andrology Urology. 2017;**6**(S4):S710-S719. DOI: 10.21037/tau.2017.06.21

[98] Telli O, Sarici H, Kabar M, Ozgur BC, Resorlu B, Bozkurt S. Does varicocelectomy affect DNA fragmentation in infertile patients? Indian Journal of Urology. 2015;**31**(2):116-119. DOI: 10.4103/0970-1591.152811

[99] Smit M, Romijn JC, Wildhagen MF, Veldhoven JLM, Weber RFA, Dohle GR. Decreased sperm DNA fragmentation after surgical varicocelectomy is associated with increased pregnancy rate. The Journal of Urology. 2013;**189**(Suppl. 1):S146-S150. DOI: 10.1016/j.juro.2012.11.024

[100] Roque M, Bedoschi G, Esteves SC. Effect of varicocele repair on sperm DNA fragmentation: A systematic review and meta-analysis. Fertility and Sterility. 2018;**110**(4):e162. DOI: 10.1016/j.fertnstert.2018.07.481

[101] Ni K, Steger K, Yang H, et al. A comprehensive investigation of sperm DNA damage and oxidative stress injury in infertile patients with subclinical, normozoospermic, and astheno/oligozoospermic clinical varicocoele. Andrology. 2016;**4**(5):816-824. DOI: 10.1111/andr.12210

[102] García-Peiró A, Ribas-Maynou J, Oliver-Bonet M, et al. Multiple determinations of sperm DNA fragmentation show that varicocelectomy is not indicated for infertile patients with subclinical varicocele. BioMed Research International. 2014;**2014**:181396. DOI: 10.1155/2014/181396

[103] Gelbaya TA, Potdar N, Jeve YB, Nardo LG. Definition and epidemiology of unexplained infertility. Obstetrical & Gynecological Survey. 2014;**69**(2):109-115. DOI: 10.1097/OGX.0000000000000043

[104] Gill K, Jakubik J, Rosiak-Gill A, et al. Utility and predictive value of human standard semen parameters and sperm DNA dispersion for fertility potential. International Journal of Environmental Research and Public

Health. 2019;**16**(11):2004. DOI: 10.3390/ijerph16112004

[105] Gunes S, Esteves SC. Role of genetics and epigenetics in male infertility. Andrologia. 2021;**53**(1):e13586. DOI: 10.1111/and.13586

[106] ESHRE Guideline Group on RPL, Bender Atik R, Christiansen OB, et al. ESHRE guideline: recurrent pregnancy loss. Human Reproduction Open. 2018;**2018**(2):hoy004. DOI: 10.1093/hropen/hoy004

[107] McQueen DB, Zhang J, Robins JC. Sperm DNA fragmentation and recurrent pregnancy loss: A systematic review and meta-analysis. Fertility and Sterility. 2019;**112**(1):54-60.e3. DOI: 10.1016/j.fertnstert.2019.03.003

[108] Tan J, Taskin O, Albert A, Bedaiwy MA. Association between sperm DNA fragmentation and idiopathic recurrent pregnancy loss: A systematic review and meta-analysis. Reproductive Biomedicine Online. 2019;**38**(6):951-960. DOI: 10.1016/j.rbmo.2018.12.029

[109] Rilcheva VS, Ayvazova NP, Ilieva LO, Ivanova SP, Konova EI. Sperm DNA integrity test and assisted reproductive technology (art) outcome. Journal of Clinical & Biomedical Research. 2016;**9**(1):21-29. DOI: 10.1515/jbcr-2016-0003

[110] Chen Q, Zhao JY, Xue X, Zhu GX. The association between sperm DNA fragmentation and reproductive outcomes following intrauterine insemination, a meta analysis. Reproductive Toxicology. 2019;**86**:50-55. DOI: 10.1016/j.reprotox.2019.03.004

[111] Osman A, Alsomait H, Seshadri S, El-Toukhy T, Khalaf Y. The effect of sperm DNA fragmentation on live birth rate after IVF or ICSI: A systematic review and meta-analysis. Reproductive Biomedicine Online. 2015;**30**(2):120-127. DOI: 10.1016/j.rbmo.2014.10.018

[112] Simon L, Emery BR, Carrell DT. Review: Diagnosis and impact of sperm DNA alterations in assisted reproduction. Best Practice & Research. Clinical Obstetrics & Gynaecology. 2017;**44**:38-56. DOI: 10.1016/j.bpobgyn.2017.07.003

[113] Deng C, Li T, Xie Y, et al. Sperm DNA fragmentation index influences assisted reproductive technology outcome: A systematic review and meta-analysis combined with a retrospective cohort study. Andrologia. 2019;**51**(6):e13263. DOI: 10.1111/and.13263

[114] Lewis SEM. The place of sperm DNA fragmentation testing in current day fertility management. Middle East Fertility Society Journal. 2013;**18**(2):78-82. DOI: 10.1016/j.mefs.2013.01.010

[115] Gosálvez J, López-Fernández C, Fernández JL, Gouraud A, Holt WV. Relationships between the dynamics of iatrogenic DNA damage and genomic design in mammalian spermatozoa from eleven species. Molecular Reproduction and Development. 2011;**78**(12):951-961. DOI: 10.1002/mrd.21394

[116] Gosálvez J, López-Fernández C, Hermoso A, Fernández JL, Kjelland ME. Sperm DNA fragmentation in zebrafish (Danio rerio) and its impact on fertility and embryo viability — Implications for fisheries and aquaculture. Aquaculture. 2014;**433**:173-182. DOI: 10.1016/j.aquaculture.2014.05.036

[117] Johnston SD, López-Fernández C, Arroyo F, et al. Reduced sperm DNA longevity is associated with an increased incidence of still born; evidence from a multi-ovulating sequential artificial insemination animal model. Journal of Assisted Reproduction and Genetics.

2016;**33**(9):1231-1238. DOI: 10.1007/s10815-016-0754-9

[118] Zhao J, Zhang Q, Wang Y, Li Y. Whether sperm deoxyribonucleic acid fragmentation has an effect on pregnancy and miscarriage after in vitro fertilization/intracytoplasmic sperm injection: A systematic review and meta-analysis. Fertility and Sterility. 2014;**102**(4):998-1005.e8. DOI: 10.1016/j.fertnstert.2014.06.033

[119] Dada R. Sperm DNA damage diagnostics: When and why. Translational Andrology and Urology. 2017;**6**(Suppl. 4):S691-S694. DOI: 10.21037/tau.2017.05.26

[120] Aitken RJ. DNA damage in human spermatozoa; important contributor to mutagenesis in the offspring. Translational Andrology and Urology. 2017;**6**(Suppl. 4):S761-S764. DOI: 10.21037/tau.2017.09.13

[121] Feng Z, Hu W, Amin S, Tang MS. Mutational spectrum and genotoxicity of the major lipid peroxidation product, trans-4-hydroxy-2-nonenal, induced DNA adducts in nucleotide excision repair-proficient and -deficient human cells. Biochemistry. 2003;**42**(25):7848-7854. DOI: 10.1021/bi034431g

[122] Meseguer M, Santiso R, Garrido N, García-Herrero S, Remohí J, Fernandez JL. Effect of sperm DNA fragmentation on pregnancy outcome depends on oocyte quality. Fertility and Sterility. 2011;**95**(1):124-128. DOI: 10.1016/j.fertnstert.2010.05.055

[123] Bernstein KA, Rothstein R. At loose ends: Resecting a double-strand break. Cell. 2009;**137**(5):807-810. DOI: 10.1016/j.cell.2009.05.007

[124] Price BD, D'Andrea AD. Chromatin remodeling at DNA double-strand breaks. Cell. 2013;**152**(6):1344-1354. DOI: 10.1016/j.cell.2013.02.011

[125] Alharbi M, Hamouche F, Phillips S, Kadoch JI, Zini A. Use of testicular sperm in couples with SCSA-defined high sperm DNA fragmentation and failed intracytoplasmic sperm injection using ejaculated sperm. Asian Journal of Andrology. 2020;**22**(4):348-353. DOI: 10.4103/aja.aja_99_19

[126] Arafa M, AlMalki A, AlBadr M, et al. ICSI outcome in patients with high DNA fragmentation: Testicular versus ejaculated spermatozoa. Andrologia. 2018;**50**(1):10.1111/and.12835. DOI: 10.1111/and.12835

[127] Bradley CK, McArthur SJ, Gee AJ, Weiss KA, Schmidt U, Toogood L. Intervention improves assisted conception intracytoplasmic sperm injection outcomes for patients with high levels of sperm DNA fragmentation: A retrospective analysis. Andrology. 2016;**4**(5):903-910. DOI: 10.1111/andr.12215

[128] Cheung S, Schlegel PN, Rosenwaks Z, Palermo GD. Revisiting aneuploidy profile of surgically retrieved spermatozoa by whole exome sequencing molecular karyotype. PLoS One. 2019;**14**(1):e0210079. DOI: 10.1371/journal.pone.0210079

[129] Esteves SC, Santi D, Simoni M. An update on clinical and surgical interventions to reduce sperm DNA fragmentation in infertile men. Andrology. 2020;**8**(1):53-81. DOI: 10.1111/andr.12724

[130] Herrero MB, Lusignan MF, Son WY, Sabbah M, Buckett W, Chan P. ICSI outcomes using testicular spermatozoa in non-azoospermic couples with recurrent ICSI failure and no previous live births.

Andrology. 2019;**7**(3):281-287. DOI: 10.1111/andr.12591

[131] Zhang J, Xue H, Qiu F, Zhong J, Su J. Testicular spermatozoon is superior to ejaculated spermatozoon for intracytoplasmic sperm injection to achieve pregnancy in infertile males with high sperm DNA damage: XXXX. Andrologia. 2019;**51**(2):e13175. DOI: 10.1111/and.13175

[132] Xie P, Keating D, Parrella A, et al. Sperm genomic integrity by TUNEL varies throughout the male genital tract. The Journal of Urology. 2020;**203**(4):802-808. DOI: 10.1097/JU.0000000000000659

[133] Hammoud I, Bailly M, Bergere M, et al. Testicular spermatozoa are of better quality than epididymal spermatozoa in patients with obstructive azoospermia. Urology. 2017;**103**:106-111. DOI: 10.1016/j.urology.2016.11.019

[134] Mehta A, Bolyakov A, Schlegel PN, Paduch DA. Higher pregnancy rates using testicular sperm in men with severe oligospermia. Fertility and Sterility. 2015;**104**(6):1382-1387. DOI: 10.1016/j.fertnstert.2015.08.008

[135] Muratori M, Tamburrino L, Marchiani S, Cambi M, Olivito B, Azzari C, et al. Investigation on the origin of sperm DNA fragmentation: Role of apoptosis, immaturity and oxidative stress. Molecular Medicine. 2015;**21**(1):109-122. DOI: 10.2119/molmed.2014.00158

[136] Moskovtsev SI, Jarvi K, Mullen JBM, Cadesky KI, Hannam T, Lo KC. Testicular spermatozoa have statistically significantly lower DNA damage compared with ejaculated spermatozoa in patients with unsuccessful oral antioxidant treatment. Fertility and Sterility. 2010;**93**(4):1142-1146. DOI: 10.1016/j.fertnstert.2008.11.005

[137] Aboulmaouahib S, Madkour A, Kaarouch I, Sefrioui O, Saadani B, Copin H, et al. Impact of alcohol and cigarette smoking consumption in male fertility potential: Looks at lipid peroxidation, enzymatic antioxidant activities and sperm DNA damage. Andrologia. 2018;**50**(3):e12926. DOI: 10.1111/and.12926

[138] Boeri L, Capogrosso P, Ventimiglia E, Pederzoli F, Cazzaniga W, Chierigo F, et al. Heavy cigarette smoking and alcohol consumption are associated with impaired sperm parameters in primary infertile men. Asian Journal of Andrology. 2019;**21**(5):478-485. DOI: 10.4103/aja.aja_110_18

[139] Verhaeghe F, Di Pizio P, Bichara C, Berby B, Rives A, Jumeau F, et al. Cannabis consumption might exert deleterious effects on sperm nuclear quality in infertile men. Reproductive Biomedicine Online. 2020;**40**(2):270-280. DOI: 10.1016/j.rbmo.2019.11.002

[140] Yatsenko AN, Turek PJ. Reproductive genetics and the aging male. Journal of Assisted Reproduction and Genetics. 2018;**35**(6):933-941. DOI: 10.1007/s10815-018-1148-y

[141] Evenson DP, Djira G, Kasperson K, Christianson J. Relationships between the age of 25,445 men attending infertility clinics and sperm chromatin structure assay (SCSA®) defined sperm DNA and chromatin integrity. Fertility and Sterility. 2020;**114**(2):311-320. DOI: 10.1016/j.fertnstert.2020.03.028

[142] Rosiak-Gill A, Gill K, Jakubik J, Fraczek M, Patorski L, Gaczarzewicz D, et al. Age-related changes in human sperm DNA integrity. Aging (Albany NY). 2019;**11**(15):5399-5411. DOI: 10.18632/aging.102120

[143] Morrison CD, Brannigan RE. Metabolic syndrome and infertility

in men. Best Practice & Research. Clinical Obstetrics & Gynaecology. 2015;**29**(4):507-515. DOI: 10.1016/j.bpobgyn.2014.10.006

[144] Le MT, Nguyen TTT, Nguyen TT, Van Nguyen T, Nguyen TAT, Nguyen QHV, et al. Does conventional freezing affect sperm DNA fragmentation? Clinical and Experimental Reproductive Medicine. 2019;**46**(2):67-75. DOI: 10.5653/cerm.2019.46.2.67

[145] Thomson LK, Fleming SD, Aitken RJ, De Iuliis GN, Zieschang JA, Clark AM. Cryopreservation-induced human sperm DNA damage is predominantly mediated by oxidative stress rather than apoptosis. Human Reproduction. 2009;**24**(9):2061-2070. DOI: 10.1093/humrep/dep214

[146] O'Neill HC, Nikoloska M, Ho H, Doshi A, Maalouf W. Improved cryopreservation of spermatozoa using vitrification: Comparison of cryoprotectants and a novel device for long-term storage. Journal of Assisted Reproduction and Genetics. 2019;**36**(8):1713-1720. DOI: 10.1007/s10815-019-01505-x

[147] Schulz M, Risopatrón J, Uribe P, Isachenko E, Isachenko V, Sánchez R. Human sperm vitrification: A scientific report. Andrology. 2020;**8**(6):1642-1650. DOI: 10.1111/andr.12847

[148] Amidi F, Pazhohan A, Shabani Nashtaei M, Khodarahmian M, Nekoonam S. The role of antioxidants in sperm freezing: A review. Cell and Tissue Banking. 2016;**17**(4):745-756. DOI: 10.1007/s10561-016-9566-5

[149] O'Flaherty C. Redox regulation of mammalian sperm capacitation. Asian Journal of Andrology. 2015;**17**(4):583-590

[150] Agarwal A, Prabakaran S, Allamaneni S. What an andrologist/urologist should know about free radicals and why. Urology. 2006;**67**(1):2-8

[151] Robinson L, Gallos ID, Conner SJ, et al. The effect of sperm DNA fragmentation on miscarriage rates: A systematic review and meta-analysis. Human Reproduction. 2012;**27**(10):2908-2917

[152] Shi T-Y, Chen G, Huang X, et al. Effects of reactive oxygen species from activated leucocytes on human sperm motility, viability and morphology: ROS, PMN, human semen, sperm quality. Andrologia. 2012;**44**(Suppl. 1):696-703

[153] de Castro LS, de Assis PM, Siqueira AFP, et al. Sperm oxidative stress is detrimental to embryo development: A dose-dependent study model and a new and more sensitive oxidative status evaluation. Oxidative Medicine and Cellular Longevity. 2016;**2016**:8213071

[154] Cocuzza M, Sikka SC, Athayde KS, Agarwal A. Clinical relevance of oxidative stress and sperm chromatin damage in male infertility: An evidence based analysis. International Brazilian Journal of Urology. 2007;**33**(5):603-621

[155] Lanzafame FM, La Vignera S, Vicari E, Calogero AE. Oxidative stress and medical antioxidant treatment in male infertility. Reproductive Biomedicine Online. 2009;**19**(5):638-659

[156] Saleh RA, Agarwal A. Oxidative stress and male infertility: From research bench to clinical practice. Journal of Andrology. 2002;**23**(6):737-752

[157] Bansal AK, Bilaspuri GS. Impacts of oxidative stress and antioxidants on semen functions. Veterinary Medicine International. 2010;**2010**:686137. DOI: 10.4061/2011/686137

[158] Niederberger C. Re: The role of sperm oxidative stress in male infertility and the significance of oral antioxidant therapy. The Journal of Urology. 2012;**187**(4):1377

[159] Padron OF, Brackett NL, Sharma RK, Lynne CM, Thomas AJ Jr, Agarwal A. Seminal reactive oxygen species and sperm motility and morphology in men with spinal cord injury. Fertility and Sterility. 1997;**67**(6):1115-1120. DOI: 10.1016/s0015-0282(97)81448-3

[160] de Lamirande E, Gagnon C. Impact of reactive oxygen species on spermatozoa: A balancing act between beneficial and detrimental effects. Human Reproduction. 1995;**10**(Suppl. 1): 15-21. DOI: 10.1093/humrep/10.suppl_1.15

[161] Agarwal A, Ahmad G, Sharma R. Reference values of reactive oxygen species in seminal ejaculates using chemiluminescence assay. Journal of Assisted Reproduction and Genetics. 2015;**32**(12):1721-1729. DOI: 10.1007/s10815-015-0584-1

[162] Dias TR. Measurement of reactive oxygen species in semen samples using Chemiluminescence. Methods in Molecular Biology. 2021;**2202**:103-109. DOI: 10.1007/978-1-0716-0896-8_9

[163] Vessey W, Perez-Miranda A, Macfarquhar R, Agarwal A, Homa S. Reactive oxygen species in human semen: Validation and qualification of a chemiluminescence assay. Fertility and Sterility. 2014;**102**(6):1576-83.e4. DOI: 10.1016/j.fertnstert.2014.09.009

[164] Kamkar N, Ramezanali F, Sabbaghian M. The relationship between sperm DNA fragmentation, free radicals and antioxidant capacity with idiopathic repeated pregnancy loss. Reproductive Biology. 2018;**18**(4):330-335. DOI: 10.1016/j.repbio.2018.11.002

[165] Bassiri F, Nasr-Esfahani MH, Forozanfar M, Tavalaee M. Relationship between sperm parameters with sperm function tests in infertile men with at least one failed cycle after intracytoplasmic sperm injection cycle. International Journal of Fertility and Sterility. 2020;**13**(4):324-329. DOI: 10.22074/ijfs.2020.5750

[166] Cilio S, Rienzo M, Villano G, Mirto BF, Giampaglia G, Capone F, et al. Beneficial effects of antioxidants in male infertility management: A narrative review. Oxygen. 2022;**2**(1):1-11. DOI: 10.3390/oxygen2010001

[167] Aziz N, Agarwal A, Lewis-Jones I, Sharma RK, Thomas AJ Jr. Novel associations between specific sperm morphological defects and leukocytospermia. Fertility and Sterility. 2004;**82**(3):621-627. DOI: 10.1016/j.fertnstert.2004.02.112

[168] Ricci G, Presani G, Guaschino S, Simeone R, Perticarari S. Leukocyte detection in human semen using flow cytometry. Human Reproduction. 2000;**15**(6):1329-1337. DOI: 10.1093/humrep/15.6.1329

[169] Brunner RJ, Demeter JH, Sindhwani P. Review of guidelines for the evaluation and treatment of leukocytospermia in male infertility. World Journal of Mens Health. 2019;**37**(2):128-137. DOI: 10.5534/wjmh.180078

[170] Jung JH, Kim MH, Kim J, Baik SK, Koh SB, Park HJ, et al. Treatment of leukocytospermia in male infertility: A systematic review. World Journal of Mens Health. 2016;**34**(3):165-172. DOI: 10.5534/wjmh.2016.34.3.165

[171] Szlauer R, Jungwirth A. Haematospermia: Diagnosis and treatment. Andrologia. 2008;**40**(2):120-124. DOI: 10.1111/j.1439-0272.2007.00821.x

[172] Khodamoradi K, Kuchakulla M, Narasimman M, Khosravizadeh Z, Ali A, Brackett N, et al. Laboratory and clinical management of leukocytospermia and hematospermia: A review. Therapeutic Advances in Reproductive Health. 2020;**14**:2633494120922511. DOI: 10.1177/2633494120922511

[173] Munkel Witz R, Krasnokutsky S, Lie J, Shah SM, Bayshtok J, Khan SA. Current perspectives on hematospermia: A review. Journal of Andrology. 1997;**18**(1):6-14

[174] Coppens L. Diagnosis and treatment of obstructive seminal vesicle pathology. Acta Urologica Belgica. 1997;**65**(2):11-19

[175] Rijsselaere T, Van Soom A, Maes D, Verberckmoes S, de Kruif A. Effect of blood admixture on in vitro survival of chilled and frozen-thawed canine spermatozoa. Theriogenology. 2004;**61**(7-8):1589-1602. DOI: 10.1016/j.theriogenology.2003.09.008

[176] Pu Y, Yang X, Guo Y, Zhu X, Yan L, Lu S. Sperm aneuploidy and recurrent pregnancy loss: A systematic review and meta-analysis. Cogent Biology. 2020;**6**(1):1759393. DOI: 10.1080/23312025.2020.1759393

[177] Fragouli E, Alfarawati S, Spath K, Jaroudi S, Sarasa J, Enciso M, et al. The origin and impact of embryonic aneuploidy. Human Genetics. 2013;**132**(9):1001-1013. DOI: 10.1007/s00439-013-1309-0

[178] Schuppe HC, Pilatz A, Hossain H, Diemer T, Wagenlehner F, Weidner W. Urogenital infection as a risk factor for male infertility. Dtsch Arztebl International. 2017;**114**(19):339-346. DOI: 10.3238/arztebl.2017.0339

[179] Dissanayake A. Significance of evaluating immature germ cells during semen analysis. International Journal of Infertility and Fetal Medicine. 2022;**13**(2):42-46. DOI: 10.5005/jp-journals-10016-1217

Chapter 3

Utilization of a Fertile Chip in Cases of Male Infertility

Sirin Aydin and Mehmet Eflatun Deniz

Abstract

Infertility is a significant reproductive health issue affecting 10–15% of couples of reproductive age worldwide. The male component adds 30–50% to IVF failure. In the examination of male infertility, sperm count, morphology, motility, and genomic integrity of sperm are crucial factors. Several strategies for generating morphologically and genetically superior sperms for use in IUI and IVF procedures or experimental research have been developed. Density gradient and swim-up approaches are two of the most commonly used applications. As this procedure needs centrifugation, it has been observed that it may have a negative impact on sperm viability, increase oxygen radicals, and result in sperm DNA fragmentation. Inadequacies in sperm extraction procedures may have unfavorable long-term consequences in terms of fertilization success, continuation of pregnancy, and embryo health. Microfluidic sperm preparation is an alternate method for decreasing DNA fragmentation at this stage, despite the fact that it has only been established recently. However, these innovative techniques have little clinical trials. According to studies, sperm sorting chips are user-friendly, inexpensive, and do not require many manual stages.

Keywords: male infertility, fertile chip, microfluidic sperm preparation, embryo, sperm quality

1. Introduction

Infertility affects 10–15% of couples worldwide [1]. The malefactor of infertility is a cause of infertility in 40–50% of infertile couples, and it coexists with female infertility [2, 3]. One of the common causes of male infertility is low sperm count owing to primary testicular failure. Nutritional problems, stress, and chronic inflammation decrease the quantity and quality of sperm. Low sperm count, low sperm motility, and structural differences in sperm all make it harder for sperm to fertilize an oocyte [4].

Evaluation of male infertility has historically been based on semen analysis, which has been classified in accordance with World Health Organization (WHO) guidelines including sperm volume, concentration, motility, and morphology [5]. However, roughly 15% of infertile patients followed for male factor parameters have normal sperm parameters [6]. Accepted as a novel indicator of sperm quality, sperm DNA damage plays a crucial role in fertilization, implantation, and transmission of paternal genetic information to progeny [7, 8]. Recent research has focused on the possible effects of sperm DNA damage, particularly in male infertility [9]. In addition, semen samples from infertile men have been found to contain extremely reactive oxygen radicals (ROS), including hydroxyl radicals (OH), superoxide anion (O2-), and hydrogen peroxide (H2O2) [10]. It has been shown that low DNA integrity, high ROS levels, and DNA fragmentation have a big effect on male infertility [10–12].

For this reason, high-level sperm analysis methods that evaluate DNA integrity, DNA fragmentation rates, and the number of reactive oxygen species (ROS) are currently under investigation [13]. Traditional methods for selecting sperm in assisted reproduction still use motility and morphology, ignoring important factors like DNA integrity, the number of ROS, membrane maturation, and the selection of non-apoptotic sperm [10]. In the studies, it is asserted that activities such as centrifugation, pipette mixing, and washing, which are commonly utilized in conventional methods, generate ROS formation, resulting in DNA damage and an increase in the DNA fragmentation rate [14, 15]. Also, using a centrifuge to choose sperm takes time, and technicians have different ways of evaluating the results [16, 17].

Natural sperm selection in the female genital tract is influenced by a series of anatomical barriers that begin with the cervix and uterus and terminate in the uterine tube, which is where fertilization takes place. These barriers begin with the cervix and uterus and continue until they reach the uterine tube [18]. Instead of centrifugation stages that can create chemical and reactive oxygen radicals, microfluidic fluid technologies imitate the natural sperm selection pathways in the female genital tract. Thus, it is stated that fewer oxygen radicals are produced, sperm DNA fragmentation is reduced, and sperm DNA integrity is enhanced. Also, research has shown that the sperm survival rate, the sperm total motility rate, and the sperm velocity rate are better than those of other methods [14, 15].

The "Fertile Chip®," a microfluidic liquid-based sperm selection technology, has been shown to select sperm with less DNA damage in a number of experiments now published in the scientific literature. Microinjection with sperm collected using these methods has been the subject of a small number of studies. This essay will focus on the evaluation of fertile chips to the male factor.

1.1 Assessment of male fertility

Male factor contributes to at least 50% of infertile couples and is the sole cause of infertility in 15–20% of couples [19] (**Table 1**). Sperm must complete normal spermatogenesis phases for conception. It includes maturation and capacitation, hyperactivation, attachment to the zona pellucida, acrosome reaction, sperm-oocyte membrane fusion, chromatin decondensation, and male–female pronucleus fusion [20]. Normal genetic structure and a normally functioning hormonal axis are essential for these processes to occur.

Due to a greater understanding of the male reproductive system and the significance of the male factor in infertility, the treatment of male infertility and its methodology has advanced rapidly over the past two decades. IUI can be utilized to achieve pregnancy in cases of minor male factor and IVF can be used in cases of more severe diseases [21].

Pituitary Hypothalamic Causes: • Isolated gonadotropin deficiency due to idiopathic causes' • Kallmann syndrome • Single gene mutations (e.g., GnRH receptor, FSH or transcription factor defects involving pituitary development) • Tumor of the hypothalamus and pituitary (e.g., Craniopharyngioma, macroadenoma) • Infiltrative conditions (sarcoidosis, histiocytosis, transfusion siderosis, hemochromatosis) • Hyperprolactinemia • Medicines (GnRH analog, androgens, estrogens, glucocorticoids, opiates) • Chronic disease or malnourishment • Infections (e.g., meningitis) • Obesity
Primary Gonadal Conditions • Klinefelter syndrome • Deletion of the Y chromosome • Cryptorchidism • Varicosele • Inoculations (e.g., Viral orchitis, Leprosy, Tuberculosis) • Medicines (e.g., alkylating agents, alcohol, antiandrogens, cimetidine) • Radioactivity and environmental toxins (e.g., temperature, smoking, metals, organic solvents, insecticides) • Chronic conditions (kidney failure, cirrhosis, cancer, sickle cell anemia, amyloidosis, vasculitis, celiac disease)
Sperm Transport Disorders • Epididymal obstruction or impairment • Congenital bilateral absence of vas deferens (secondary to CFTR mutation) • Infections causing obstruction of the vas deferens (e.g., gonorrhea, chlamydia, tuberculosis) • Vasectomy • Kartagener syndrome (primary ciliary dyskinesia) • Young syndrome • Ejaculatory dysfunction (e.g., spinal cord disease, autoimmune dysfunction)

Table 1.
Male infertility causes.

1.1.1 Spermatogenesis

Spermatogenesis is the process by which sperm are produced from primordial germ cells. Approximately 75 days are required for the maturation of spermatogonia into mature sperm. Every 16 days, a new cohort of spermatogonia enters the human spermatogenesis cycle [22].

Spermatogenesis is an intricate differentiation process that begins at birth with the transformation of spermatogonial stem cells [23]. It has three phases: mitotic proliferation of spermatogonia, meiosis of spermatocytes, and haploid differentiation of spermatids [24]. Mitosis is responsible for the multiplication of differentiating spermatogonia (with 46 chromosomes). After the proliferation phase, the prophase of the first meiosis commences, during which spermatocytes remain for an extended period, homologous chromosome pairs, synapses, and homologous recombinations are formed, and homologous recombinations occur [25]. Later, the spermatocytes separate into sister chromosomes and divide into two cells, resulting in the production of secondary spermatocytes. These cells also divide very rapidly, and the resulting haploid spermatids initiate the spermiogenesis stage of differentiation. During spermiogenesis, sperm-specific structures such as the flagellum and acrosome are formed. Additionally, the nucleus condenses and the majority of histones in the DNA structure are replaced with sperm-specific protamines, causing chromatin to become dense [26]. Spermation is the process by which spermatozoa released into the tubular lumen travel to the epididymis for final maturation and storage [27]. In the epididymis, spermatozoa gain progressive movement and continue to mature for approximately 10 days [28].

The epididymis stores sperm until ejaculation. Capacitation and hyperactivation occur in the female reproductive tract [29].

FSH and LH secreted by the pituitary and stimulated by the release of hypothalamic gonadotropin-releasing hormone provide hormonal control over spermatogenesis (GnRH). In the hypothalamus, pituitary, and testis axis, a negative feedback control system exists. High serum testosterone levels inhibit the release of GnRH and LH, but physiological testosterone levels do not inhibit the release of FSH. Inhibin B, produced by Sertoli cells in response to FSH stimulation, inhibits FSH secretion at the pituitary gland [30].

1.1.2 Causes of male infertility

Male infertility can be divided into 4 major categories [21]: Hypothalamic–pituitary disorders (pretesticular disorders, secondary hypogonadism), testicular disorders (primary spermatogenesis failure and primary hypogonadism), posttesticular defects (sperm transport disorders), and idiopathic (**Table 1**).

1.1.3 Anamnesis

Evaluation of the male partner should begin at the same time as the evaluation of the female partner, beginning with a thorough medical history. Furthermore, the anamnesis should contain the following; infertility evaluation, genitourinary history (trauma, genital infection, difficulty sustaining an erection or ejaculating), medical record (history of high fever, chronic illness, drug use, smoking and alcohol, operation history) and family history [31].

1.1.4 Physical examination

If a gynecologist is performing the infertility evaluation, the physical examination may be delayed if the initial evaluation of the male patient does not reveal an abnormal anamnesis or a problem with the semen analysis. However, abnormal sperm analysis or an abnormal medical history is a cause for a physical examination, and the patient should be evaluated by a urologist [32].

A thorough physical examination may reveal the absence of secondary sex characteristics, suggestive of hypogonadism, or the absence of the vas deferens, a cause of obstructive azoospermia. Although physical examination should not be performed prior to sperm analysis, it is essential when there is a possibility of a problem in the clinical history or when searching for reversible causes of potentially abnormal sperm analysis parameters [31].

1.1.5 Semen analysis

Semen analysis, in the evaluation of male infertility, is the most significant parameter that provides information about the functional status of the seminiferous tubules, epididymis, and accessory sex glands [33]. A period of sexual abstinence of two to five days is required in order to obtain an optimal sample of sperm. While semen volume and density decrease when fasting periods are shortened, sperm motility and morphology do not change, and when fasting periods are prolonged, semen volume and density increase along with an increase in dead, immobile, and morphologically abnormal sperm [34]. Sperm can be collected in a sample container by masturbation or by using condoms designed for sperm collection that do not contain sperm-toxic substances. Ideal sample collection would occur in the laboratory. If the sample is collected at home, it must be transported at room temperature or body temperature and examined within one hour. The delay in the review may affect certain parameters. For instance, after two hours, there is a progressive decrease in motility as the activity of free radicals increases.

Both macroscopically and microscopically, sperm are evaluated on the basis of the following factors:

1.1.6 Macroscopic evaluation

Coagulation, liquefaction time, color, appearance, viscosity, volume, and pH are the macroscopically evaluated parameters.

1.1.7 Microscopic evaluation

Sperm aggregation: It is the result of nonmotile sperm adhering to one another or to nonsperm cells in the environment.

Agglutination of sperm: It is the coexistence of motile sperm by adhering head-to-head, tail-to-tail, or in a mixed state. It is labeled as Grades 1 through 4.

Concentration of sperm: It is the quantity of sperm per milliliter is the sperm concentration. Using a Makler counting chamber, the total number of sperm in 10 medium-sized squares is recorded as millions per milliliter. The same count is repeated four times across ten frames, and the average is then calculated. Normal sperm has a lower reference value of 15×10^6 /ml [35]. While sperm concentrations below this value are associated with a poor prognosis for fertility, there is no conclusive evidence that concentrations above 15×10^6 /ml improve fertility prognosis [36]. According to some sources, the probability of conception rises until the concentration reaches 40 to 50×10^6 cells per milliliter, and then it remains constant [37, 38]. Severe oligozoospermia is diagnosed when the concentration of sperm is below 5×10^6/ml. In the case of severe oligozoospermia, endocrinological and genetic testing should be conducted.

Total sperm number: It is the total number of sperm in the ejaculate, and the lower reference value is 39×10^6. It is calculated by multiplying the sperm concentration by the volume. If no sperm cells are detected during the initial microscopic examination, the entire ejaculate is centrifuged at 3000 g for 15 minutes, and pellet drops are examined between the lamella and lamella. And if sperm cells are seen (cryptozoospermia), the total number, motility, and distinct morphological feature are recorded. A condition known as azoospermia occurs when no sperm cells can be found in the entire sperm pellet. At least two tests must demonstrate the absence of sperm.

Movement of sperm: Motility is the proportion of sperm that exhibit tail movement. After liquefaction, it must be completed within one hour.

According to WHO 2010 [39], a simple system for grading motility is recommended that distinguishes spermatozoa with progressive or nonprogressive motility from those that are immotile. The motility of each spermatozoon is graded as follows:

Progressive motility (PR): Spermatozoa moving actively, either linearly or in a large circle, regardless of speed.

Nonprogressive motility (NP): All other patterns of motility with an absence of progression, e.g. swimming in small circles, the flagellar force hardly displacing the head, or when only a flagellar beat can be observed.

Immotility (IM): No movement.

This system evaluates the proportion of sperm that fall into each category. According to the World Health Organization, a + b should exceed 40%, while an alone should surpass 32% [39]. Asthenospermia is a movement disorder characterized by a decrease in motility, forward movement, or both. In these patients, structural abnormalities of spermatozoa, long-term sexual abstinence, genital infections, anti-sperm antibodies, varicocele, partial ductal obstruction, and idiopathic factors may be to blame.

1.1.8 Sperm morphology

For the evaluation of sperm morphology, the sperm must be stained. The most common dyeing techniques are the Papanicolau method and the Diff-Quick method. WHO criteria and Kruger's strict criteria are the most common standards for evaluating sperm morphology [40]. In order for sperm to be considered normal, its head, neck, middle section, and tail must all be normal. The proportion of sperm with normal morphology should be 14% according to Kruger's strict criteria and > 4% according to the World Health Organization. Normal values in sperm analysis do not represent the bare minimum required for fertility. Aside from these characteristics, the male could be fertile. However, even individuals with normal sperm parameters may be infertile [41].

1.1.9 Sperm viability

Sperm viability is based on the examination of sperm cell membrane integrity, and sperm viability tests are particularly significant when the percentage of increasingly motile sperm is less than 40%. In the eosin-nigrosin or eosin-Y test, sperm with compromised membrane integrity absorb the dye and appear stained, whereas in the hypoosmotic swelling (HOS) test, sperm with intact membranes swell by absorbing the hypoosmolar fluid and their tails are curved. At least 200 sperm cells are required to determine sperm viability. The minimum acceptable reference value for sperm viability testing is 58%.

1.1.10 Nonsperm cells

In addition to sperm cells, the ejaculate contains epithelial cells of the genitourinary system, immature germinal cells, and leukocyte cells. Other cells than leukocytes are also referred to as round cells. The number of round cells and leukocytes in normal ejaculate should be 1×10^6 per milliliter. If an increase in round cells is seen, a leukocyte peroxidase test or leukocyte markers should be performed to determine whether these cells are leukocytes. None of the parameters of standard sperm analysis are specific for demonstrating the fertilization capacity of sperm, and standard sperm analysis may not be adequate for distinguishing definitively between fertile and infertile sperm. Consequently, sperm function tests are required [42].

1.1.10.1 Sperm function tests

WHO accepts sperm function tests as research tests that predict the in vitro fertilization potential of sperm [42].

Computer-assisted analysis of sperm: CASA (computer-assisted sperm analysis) can be used to evaluate sperm concentration, motility, and morphology, as well as the spiral movement pattern and hyperactivation sperm acquire during capacitation [43].

Acrosome response: The acrosome is a membrane-bound structure in the sperm's head region that contains proteolytic enzymes that are essential for penetrating the zona pellucida. One of these proteolytic enzymes is acrosine. Infertile men have a premature spontaneous acrosome reaction, which hinders zona pellucida penetration [44].

Zona pellucida (ZP): It plays a crucial role in the regulation of fertilization. The acrosome reaction is triggered by the binding of spermatozoa to the zona pellucida via the ZP3 receptor [45], which is the only physiological stimulus for the acrosome reaction. Sperm must recognize and bind to species-specific receptors in ZP for oocyte fertilization.

Both the "Hemizona assay" and the "competitive intact zona binding assay" are frequently used as zona pellucida attachment tests [43]. Due to the difficulty of locating human oocytes in both of these tests, they are not commonly used to assess male infertility.

Test for oocyte penetration in hamsters: It is used to demonstrate the success of in vivo and in vitro fertilization as a predictive test [46]. The test evaluates spermatozoal viability, acrosome reaction, ability to penetrate the oolemma, and oocyte fusion.

Test for hypo-osmolar swelling (HOST): Permeability to water is a crucial physiological characteristic of all cell membranes. Membranes permit the selective passage of liquids and molecules. The HOS test can evaluate the sperm membrane, which plays an important functional role during fertilization. There was a correlation between the number of swollen sperm in the sample of sperm and the number of sperm that successfully fertilized the hamster egg. The HOS test is predicated on the viability of spermatozoa under moderate hypoosmotic stress. Since dead spermatozoa lack intact membranes, they cannot swell. Classifying HOS-reactive cells from A to G based on the degree of swelling and tail curl. When 200 sperm are counted, the percentage is reported. Sperm with a HOS reaction of greater than 60% is considered normal. Less than 50% tail curl is considered abnormal. Acceptable is an intermediate value between 50 and 60%. HOS can be used as an additional sperm viability indicator and in the diagnosis of immotile cilia syndrome [43, 47].

Reactive oxygen radicals: Oxidative stress is one of the most important mediators in a variety of male infertility etiologies; it has many negative effects on sperm, including DNA damage. Oxidative stress occurs when levels of ROS and other free radicals are significantly elevated, when the delicate balance between oxidizing agents and antioxidants is upset, or when antioxidant levels drop significantly. Reducing oxidative stress is a possible strategy for treating male infertility. Seminal oxidative stress measurement is essential for identifying and monitoring patients who may benefit from treatment [48].

Mitochondrial activity tests: Spermatozoa obtain the energy necessary for flagellar movement from adenosine triphosphate (ATP) produced by mitochondria in the middle portion of spermatozoa. Spermatozoa require a sufficient amount of mitochondrial apparatus in the female genital tract in order to produce the necessary ATP during their journey to the oocyte. For the demonstration of the mitochondrial oxidoreductase enzyme, nitro blue tetrazolium and similar indicators are used. With these indicators, the middle portion of motile sperms with abundant mitochondria is prominently stained, whereas the middle portion of immobile sperms with low mitochondrial activity is either not stained at all or is stained less. Their staining revealed a statistically significant correlation between mitochondrial activities and sperm motility [43].

DNA damage tests: These are crucial for ensuring normal embryo development. The effect of disulfide cross-links between protamines, which provide chromatin condensation in the nucleus, partially preserves the integrity of sperm DNA. Sperm DNA damage can be caused by internal factors like protamine deficiency and mutations, or by external factors like heat, radiation, and gonadotoxins. The term "DNA fragmentation" refers to irreparable denatured or damaged sperm DNA. Various clinical tests for measuring sperm DNA fragmentation rates have been developed [19]. Over the years, an increasing number of sperm DNA integrity tests have been developed. The mechanism for evaluating DNA integrity in these tests varies. While some tests directly measure breaks in the DNA helix, others reveal abnormalities in sperm chromatin structure [48, 49]. DNA damage in male germ cells appears to be linked to poor sperm quality, impaired preimplantation development, an increased risk of miscarriage, and infertility [50].

1. **Nuclear chromatin decondensation test**: Although sperm contains half as much DNA as a typical eukaryotic cell, its volume is only one-thirtieth as large. Due to the reduction in volume, DNA packaging is a very complicated process. The chromatin of spermatozoa is highly condensed before fertilization. Fertilization requires appropriate nuclear chromatin decondensation and subsequent formation of pronuclei. Spermatozoa's highly condensed chromatin is due to the S-S bonds between histones. EDTA (ethylenediaminetetraacetic acid) and glutathione can induce dissociation between bonds in vitro. This method of inducing decondensation is indicative of the fertility of spermatozoa. More than 70% nuclear decondensation in sperm is considered normal [51].

2. **DNA fragmentation index**: DNA damage can be evaluated directly by DNA fragmentation using the TUNEL (terminal deoxynucleotidyl transferase-mediated deoxyuridine triphosphate) assay, SCSA (sperm chromatin structure assay), sperm chromatin distribution, or comet assay. The percentage of sperm with DNA fragmentation was negatively correlated with normal sperm morphology and motility. DNA fragmentation may be caused by advanced male age, genetic causes, environmental toxins, endocrine disorders, alcohol, tobacco use, and diet.

1.2 Assisted reproductive technology (ART)

The majority of assisted reproductive techniques facilitate conception in a laboratory to assist infertile couples in having children. Intrauterine insemination (IUI), in vitro fertilization (IVF), and intracytoplasmic sperm injection (ICSI) are the most common assisted reproductive technologies (ARTs) [52]. In preparation for ART, spermatozoa must be collected from the male. After collecting sperm and washing them using swim-up or density gradient centrifugation techniques, the motile sperm are selected. During the ovulation phase of IUI, spermatozoa are introduced into the uterus. Following stimulation of follicular development in the ovaries, primary oocytes are collected for IVF and ICSI. Multiple oocytes are extracted in order to produce multiple embryos for implantation. The use of sperm and oocyte to complete IVF or ICSI [39].

1.2.1 Intracytoplasmic injection of sperm (ICSI)

ICSI was developed primarily to facilitate fertilization in cases where sperm motility or morphology prevented spermatozoa from crossing the zona pellucida. This method involves injecting a spermatozoon directly into the cytoplasm of the oocyte to facilitate fertilization [53].

ICSI, on the other hand, is problematic because spermatozoa no longer face the obstacles they do during natural conception and are not subject to natural selection. For a successful pregnancy to occur, a viable spermatozoa with good DNA must be injected into the oocyte since natural selection is inhibited by this method [54]. Since there is no natural selection of sperm, selecting the appropriate sperm is crucial.

1.2.2 The importance of sperm selection in ICSI treatment

Despite decades of widespread use of ART to treat infertility, live birth rates remain relatively low [55]. According to the Centers for Disease Control and Prevention (CDC), it is unknown why so many insemination attempts fail to result in fertilization, while only a third of many ART cycles result in a live birth [56]. Infertile men have abnormal sperm parameters, including low sperm concentration, poor motility, abnormal morphology, and elevated sperm DNA damage levels. Low ROS concentrations are necessary for essential sperm functions such as capacitation, hyperactivation, and acrosome reaction, and excessive ROS production is typically regulated by antioxidants [57]. High levels of ROS and low levels of antioxidants can cause oxidative stress, which reduces sperm motility, DNA integrity, and viability. Reduced DNA integrity leads to decreased IVF pregnancy rates, an increase in preimplantation developmental abnormalities, and an increase in early pregnancy loss [57].

Very few of the millions of sperm that are poured into the vagina reach the oocyte. Naturally occurring in the female genital tract, this is a very precise and flawless elimination system. As sperm reach the vagina, vaginal mechanical stimulations support the sperm's swimming movement, directing them toward the uterus and tuba. In the storage area, sperm undergo a maturation process known as capacitation. The mature sperm move toward the oocyte via chemotaxis and thermotaxis following capacitation. Sperm penetrate cumulus cells as a result of chemotaxis, bind to sperm receptors in the oocyte, and initiates the acrosome reaction. Consequently, fertilization occurs [58].

Today, sperm selection techniques for ART bypass the barriers of natural selection and select sperm based primarily on motility and morphology, ignoring other important factors such as DNA integrity, ROS production, membrane maturation, and non-apoptotic sperm selection [18]. In addition, traditional sperm selection techniques such as density gradient centrifugation (DGS), conventional swimming (CSW), and direct swimming (DSW) generate high levels of ROS through the use of multiple centrifugation steps, resulting in DNA damage due to oxidative stress [59]. According to clinical data, a DNA fragmentation index above 30% reduces the likelihood of natural and artificial conception [60].

Additionally, while fertilized oocytes have DNA repair mechanisms, spermatozoa do not, so they cannot repair DNA breaks after spermatogenesis [60]. Therefore, in order to select sperm with normal DNA and fewer ROS and to increase ART success rates, it is necessary to develop new sperm selection techniques in addition to enhancing existing ones. To ensure that healthy sperm are selected, new sperm selection methods must closely mimic the natural selectivity of the female genital tract.

1.2.3 Conventional sperm selection techniques

Traditional methods for sperm selection involve multiple washing and centrifugation steps. Density gradient centrifugation (DGS), conventional swim-up (CSW), and direct swim-up are the most frequently employed conventional sperm selection techniques (DSW).

Density gradient centrifugation (DGS), conventional swim-up (CSW), and direct swim-up are the most frequently employed conventional sperm selection techniques (DSW).

- **Density gradient centrifugation (DGS) technique**: It enables the selection of high-quality sperm and their differentiation from other cell types and cell debris. As it is simpler to standardize than the swim-up technique, the results are more consistent. This method is used to retrieve sperm for IVF and ICSI. This technique involves the centrifugation of seminal plasma based on density gradients. Using density gradients containing colloidal silica-coated silane, this method separates cells based on their density. Furthermore, motile sperm swim through the gradient material and form a soft pellet at the tube's bottom. The most common simple two-stage discontinuous density gradient preparation method consists of an upper layer with a density of 40% (v/v) and a lower layer with a density of 80% (v/v). Using density gradient centrifugation to prepare sperm typically results in highly motile sperm free of cell debris, contaminating leukocytes, nongerm cells, and degenerative germ cells [39].

- **Direct swim-up (DSW) technique:** Sperm can be chosen based on their ability to swim from the seminal plasma into the culture medium. This technique is known as the "swim-up" method. Prior to employing this method, sperm should ideally not be diluted or centrifuged. Otherwise, sperm membranes may be susceptible to peroxidative damage [61]. Therefore, direct flotation is the preferred technique for separating motile sperm. Direct flotation can be accomplished by either spreading the culture medium on top of the liquefied sperm or by spreading the liquefied sperm as a layer beneath the culture medium. Next, motile sperm enter the culture medium. Although this method yields fewer sperm than washing, it is useful when the proportion of motile sperm in the sperm is low (e.g., for IVF and ICSI) because it selects sperm based on their motility [39].

- **Conventional swim-up technique (CSW):** Before incubation, sperm are precipitated in the conventional swim-up technique by centrifugation. Then, using a pipette, the 1 ml portion floating on the top is removed and utilized. It is a technique that relies solely on sperm motility. Asthenozoospermia and oligozoospermia may render it inappropriate. In cases of severe male infertility, its use is therefore restricted.

Although conventional methods are effective at selecting motile and morphologically normal sperm, they are insufficient for selecting sperm DNA integrity, membrane maturation, detailed structural characteristics, and non-apoptotic sperm [62].

1.2.4 Advanced sperm selection methodologies

Zeta Potential: Approximately between −16 mV and − 20 mV, the zeta potential of sperm is the electrical potential between the sperm membrane and its surroundings. Using a latex glove, the sample of washed sperm is pipetted into the positively charged centrifuge tube and gently mixed in the tube two to three times. After one minute of centrifugation, Sperm and other cells that do not adhere to the edge of the tube are removed (**Figure 1**). Since no electrophoresis equipment is required, the zeta method is inexpensive and simple to employ. Additionally, the Zeta treatment has been successfully applied to freeze-thawed sperm samples [63]. However, its effectiveness in oligozoospermic samples with a low sperm count is limited. When electrophoretic methods are compared to the DGS method, it has been observed that the sperms obtained have a high level of maturity, morphology, and DNA integrity, but their motility is low [63, 64].

MACS: Magnetic activated cell sorting system early apoptosis is characterized by the externalization of phosphatidylserine (PS), which is located on the outer surface of the sperm membrane. Utilizing a MACS, the selection of nonapoptotic sperm is achieved in this method [65]. Annexin V binds to paramagnetic microbeads that mark and separate apoptotic sperm in the event of PS externalization. A heterogeneous concentration of sperm cells is initially incubated with microbeads conjugated with Annexin V; however, only apoptotic sperm with externalized PS bind to these beads. The mixture of beads and sperm is passed through a MACS column equipped with a magnet. This magnet retains microbead-labeled cells in the interior of the colon and ensures their gradual removal by a steady flow of unmarked cells [66]. Due to the inability of MACS to remove leukocytes and germ cells, this technique is utilized in conjunction with DGS [67] (**Figure 2**). Recent ICSI studies comparing sperm samples prepared with or without MACS revealed no statistically significant differences in implantation, miscarriage, or live birth rates [68]. Before concluding that this technique is effective in ICSI procedures, it should be evaluated in studies with larger sample sizes, using a larger number of samples.

Hyaluronic acid adherence: Hyaluronic acid (HA) is the primary constituent of the cumulus oophorus' extracellular matrix. Binding sites for hyaluronic acid in the sperm plasma membrane indicate sperm maturity. There are two ways to select HA-bound sperm: physiological intracytoplasmic sperm injection (PICSI) and the sperm-slow procedure. Both methods require sperm washing or centrifugation. In order to select sperm, a product called "PICSI dish" with four HA-fixed compartments has been developed. A drop of the washed sperm is placed on the edge of the HA spot, and after 15 minutes, the HA-bound sperm are collected with an injection pipette and used for ICSI [69] (**Figure 3**). Additionally, HA binding is commonly

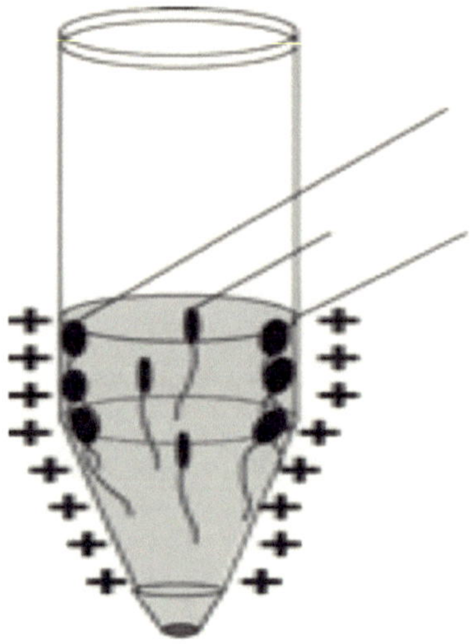

Figure 1.
Separation of sperm by zeta potential.

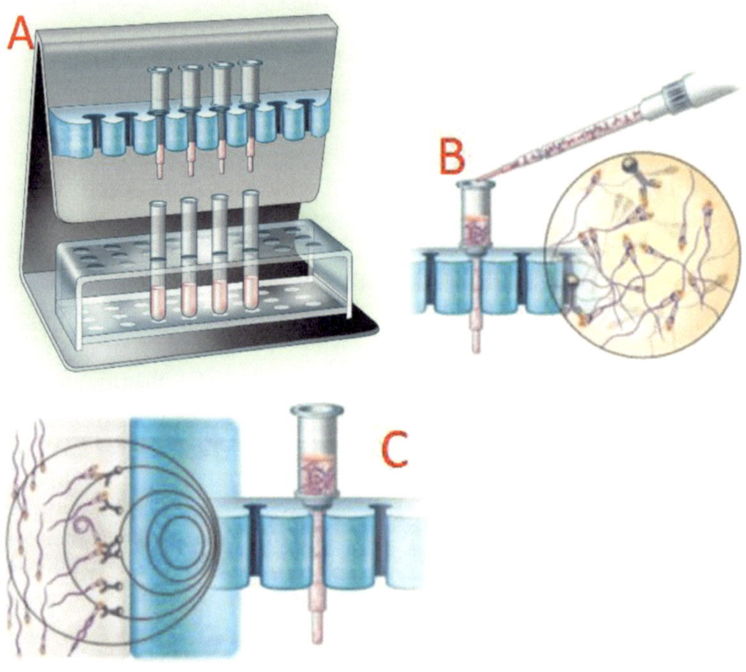

Figure 2.
Separation of sperm by MACS. Loading the tubes into the device (A), putting Annexin V-labeled apoptotic sperm and non-apoptotic sperm into the tubes (B), magnetic capture of Annexin V-bound apoptotic sperm and advancement of non-apoptotic sperm into the collection tube (C).

used to select mature sperm with a low frequency of chromosomal abnormalities. This increases the likelihood of genetic complications following ICSI. In a study of semen samples from men undergoing fertility treatment, it was discovered that

DOI: http://dx.doi.org/10.5772/intechopen.107108

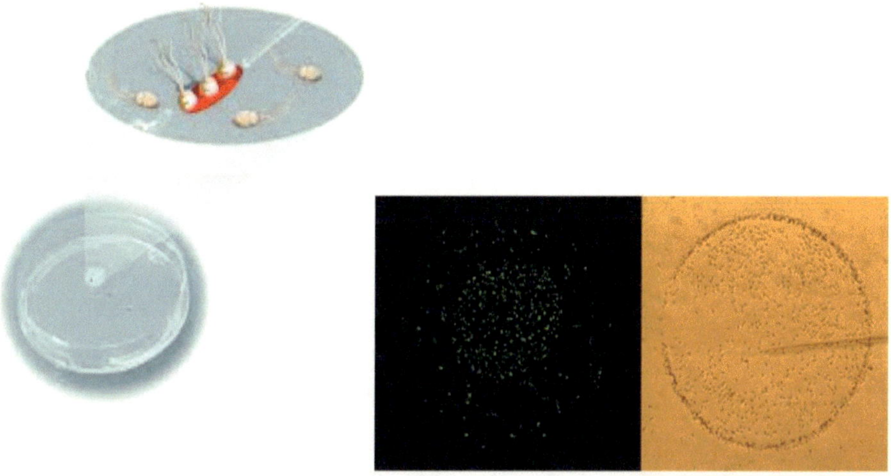

Figure 3.
Sperm appearance in the PICSI petri dish.

autosomal disomy, diploidy, and sex chromosome disomy were significantly lower in HA-linked sperm than in non-binding sperm [69].

Electrophoresis-based sperm selection: Electrophoresis (Microflow CS-10) is a technique that selects sperms based on their surface charge. Normally, mature sperm are negatively charged due to the presence of CD52 and glycosylated phosphatidylinositol on their surface. The electrophoresis device is a cassette in which a semen sample is placed, a voltage is applied, and morphologically normal, negatively charged sperm move across a 5 m polycarbonate membrane toward the positive electrode, leaving immature sperm and leukocytes behind [70]. DNA integrity, sperm morphology, and motility were not significantly different between DGS and electrophoresis. In addition, because there is no centrifugation step in sperm selection by electrophoresis, there is less oxidative DNA damage due to the decreased exposure to ROS [70] (**Figure 4**).

Morphological evaluation of motile sperm organelles (motile sperm organellar morphology examination; MSOME): Examining the morphology of sperm under high magnification microscopes allows for the morphological evaluation of motile sperm organelles-based sperm selection. MSOME is applied at up to 6300x magnification, whereas standard ICSI is performed at 600x magnification. In this technique, which was developed by Bartoov et al. the structural characteristics of sperm are investigated in depth. To determine the healthiest sperm, the Acrosomal region, Post-Acrosomal region, Neck, Mitochondria, Flagella, Tail, Vacuole areas, and the ratio of these vacuole areas to the head are calculated [71]. MSOME has been used in conjunction with standard ICSI procedures and is named after intracytoplasmic morphology-selected sperm injection (IMSI) (**Figure 5**). It plays a crucial role in sperm selection for men with severe infertility.

Birefringence: Birefringence of sperm is evaluated using an inverted microscope equipped with polarized lenses. Using double refraction, sperm with reactive acrosomes can be selected during ICSI without compromising motility or viability [72]. Sperm with birefringence can be selected for microinjection, and the quality of these sperms appears to be high. A significant positive correlation exists between the proportion of birefringent sperm and other sperm parameters, including concentration,

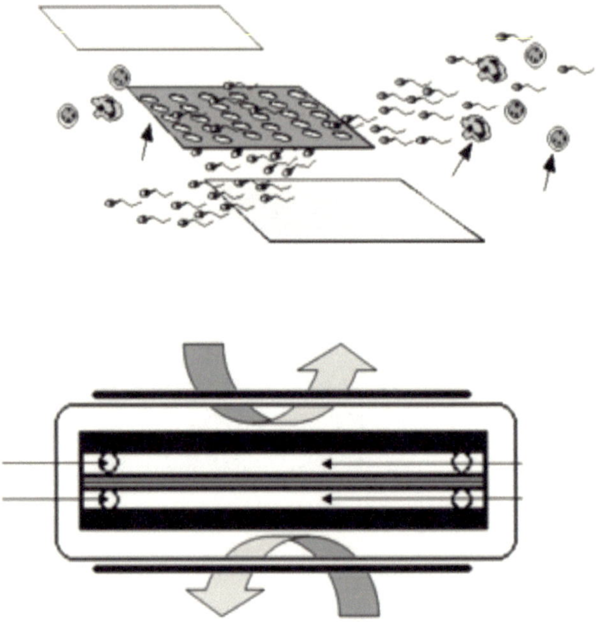

Figure 4.
Separation of sperm by electrophoretic method-MicroflowCS-10.

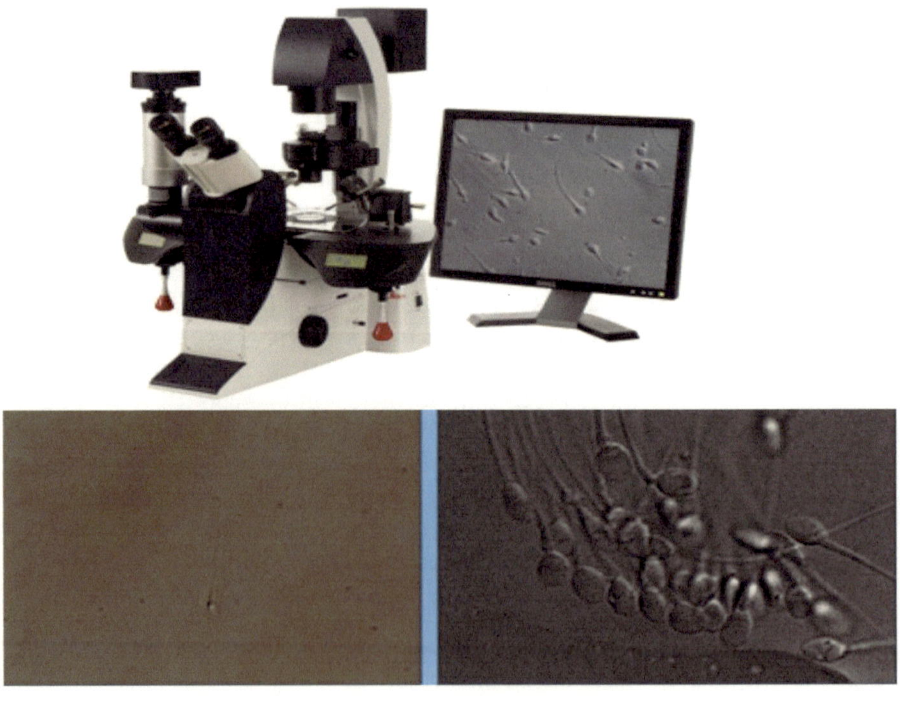

Figure 5.
Sperm selection for IMSI.

motility, and viability [72]. Similar to MSOME and IMSI, polarized microscopy for sperm selection requires additional equipment, time, and technical expertise. Comparing the microinjection method performed by evaluating sperm birefringence and routine ICSI, a high pregnancy rate and decreased miscarriage rate were observed with this new method in patients with heavy male factor [72].

Selection of sperm using a microfluidic liquid model: "Microfluidic channel system (spermchip)" is one of the methods developed for sperm selection that can prevent sperm losses and DNA damage caused by conventional sperm preparation methods. In developing this technique, the path followed by sperm during natural conception served as a model. This system includes a microchip with microchannels that mimics the intrauterine, cervical, and vaginal canal microenvironments of sperm. Microfluidic channels are formed in the microchip by a 1.5 mm thick combination of Polymethylmethacrylate (PMMA) and a 50-micron thick double-sided adhesive (DSA) film. The integration of a microchip-coupled device (CCD) into the chip enables the automatic recording of sperm movement within the microfluidic channel. Incorporating the integrated system into the microfluidic channel. The microfluidic channel medium was pre-filled with serum-supplemented human tubal fluid (HTF) medium. The sperm sample is pipetted into the column at the top

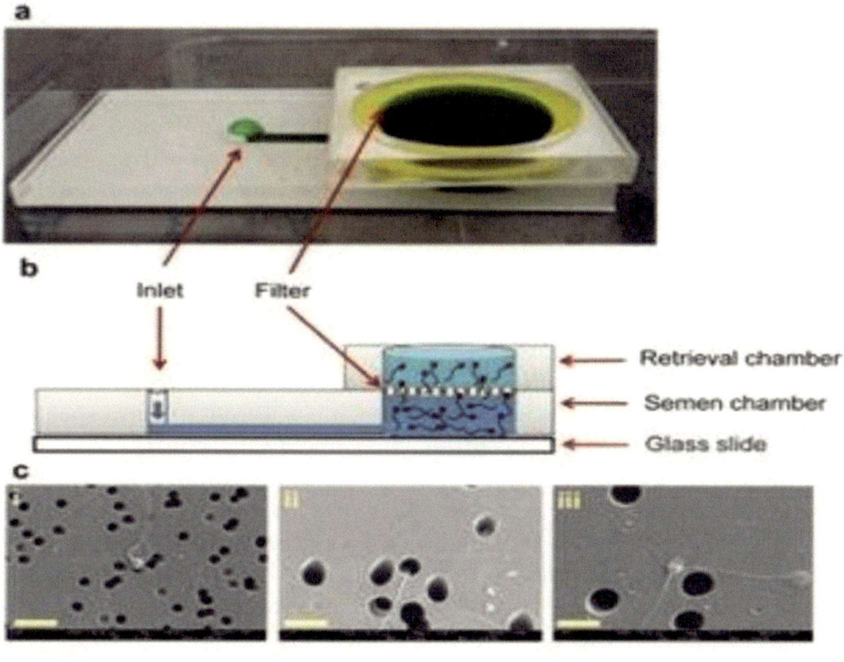

Figure 6.
Microfluidic channel system. Filtered motile sperm; semen sample; (a) the photo of the MSS showing inlet, filter and two PMMA chambers. The MSS was filled with color dye to enhance contrast; (b) the illustration demonstrates the MSS design and working principle. The MSS consists of one inlet for the injection of raw unprocessed semen sample and two PMMA chambers separated by nucleoporin track-etched membrane filter. The most healthy and motile sperm swim through the filter leaving unhealthy dead sperm in the bottom chamber; (c) SEM images of polycarbonate nuclepore track-etched membrane filters of different microspore diameters, i) 3 μm ii) 5 μm and iii) 8 μm. These images show the comparative size of various filter pores and sperm. The scale bar is 10 μm.

channel entrance using a pipette. Sperm are anticipated to swim from duct systems of a particular length.

ICSI involves the collection and use of floating sperm. Moreover, since the microchip can be placed on the integrated device (CCD), the sperm's shadow movement can be monitored and recorded [73]. (**Figure 6**). Microfluidic fluid technologies mimic the natural sperm selection pathways that take place in the female genital organs, rather than centrifugation steps that can generate ROS. Thus, it is stated that fewer oxygen radicals are formed, DNA fragmentation of sperms is lower and their DNA integrity is higher. In addition, studies have shown that sperm viability rate, sperm total motility rate, sperm velocity rates are higher than other methods [14, 15].

2. Discussion

Evaluation of male infertility requires a thorough examination of sperm. Significant determinants of the success of ART include sperm motility, morphology, viability, DNA integrity, apoptosis, and maturation. Recent research has revealed that the DNA integrity of sperm is essential for normal fertilization and embryo development. As a result, improved sperm selection techniques are used to identify higher-quality and healthier sperm for ICSI treatment. Although it has been established that the vast majority of these new sperm selection approaches outlined before can select for sperms with a greater DNA integrity and a lower DNA fragmentation rate, this is not the case for all of these techniques. Patients with male factor infertility who underwent IVF were studied in a prospective randomized controlled trial that compared the effects of microfluidic sperm selection technologies to the conventional swim-up strategy. Fertilization rates and embryo quality, which were among the key findings of this study, were comparable across the two groups, as evidenced by the results of this randomized controlled experiment. The study group had a greater rate of live births, implantation, and clinical pregnancy [73]. The fact that this study found statistically significant differences in the rates of implantation, pregnancy, clinical pregnancy, and live birth makes it an impressive piece of research. Despite having comparable numbers of grade 1 and 2 embryos, the control group had more grade 3 embryos. This may suggest that the Fertile Chip was used to select sperm of a higher quality, or that other parameters influencing embryo quality are not reflected in sperm morphology.

The microfluidic sperm sorting chip is simple to use, inexpensive, chemical-free, mechanical-free and perturbation-free, and it removes the centrifugation stage. At an ideal time point, the most motile and functional spermatozoa with the correct structure, high DNA integrity, and a low ROS level can be selectively passed via the microchannels of a microfluidic sperm sorting device, leaving behind the less motile or immotile spermatozoa [14].

The increase or decrease in DNA fragmentation levels observed in gradient technique applications, as well as the heterogeneity of the results reported in previous studies, may be attributable to initial cellular DNA fragmentation rates or centrifugation. In a 2018 study, Quinn et al. compared traditional sorting procedures to microfluidic chip approaches. DNA fragmentation rates utilizing the microchip method were much lower than those using the gradient method, according to the study's findings [74]. The primary purpose of IVF treatment, however, was not evaluated in this study. Yang et al. discovered a statistically significant difference in embryo implantation rate between infertile individuals with high sperm DNA fragmentation index

(DFI ≥15%) values and those with low (DFI < 15%) DFI-ICSI values ($p < 0.01$). There were no significant differences in fertilization rates, embryo quality, or blastocyst development [75]. Despite the lack of a statistically significant difference in embryo quality, the difference in implantation rate suggests that morphological parameters and DFI alone are insufficient to evaluate embryo quality.

When sperm separation was performed using the microfluidic platform, a small cohort of couples undergoing ICSI achieved pregnancy rates of 58.8% and implantation rates of 34.5%, according to a study by Parella et al. In the same study, it was believed that this was because the use of microfluidic sperm selection increased the likelihood of producing euploid embryos [76].

Using density gradient selection and microfluidic sperm sorting, Parella et al. evaluated a novel method for choosing spermatozoa with intact chromatin. This work demonstrates that microfluidic selection produces spermatozoa with high genomic integrity and increases the possibility of producing euploid embryos [77].

Green et al. explored if sperm DNA fragmentation (SDF) in the ICSI sample affects the results of euploid blastocyst transfer. According to the findings of this study, SDF levels on the day of ICSI were not associated with embryological or clinical outcomes following euploid blastocyst transfer.

Increased SDF levels are associated with lower sperm concentration and number of motile sperm [78]. Given that the transferred embryos in this study were euploid embryos with good DNA integrity, it was not anticipated that we would assess the effect of DFI. As preimplantation genetic diagnosis (PGD) is a more invasive operation, and for individuals who cannot undergo PGD for budgetary reasons, the microfluidic technology can be used to pick a more capable embryo. With a sperm DFI > 20%, the clinical pregnancy rate of IVF-ET was significantly reduced, while with a sperm DFI > 30%, the rate of available embryos decreased significantly and the biochemical pregnancy rate increased dramatically, according to a study report published in the current scientific literature. There was no correlation between sperm DFI and fertilization, embryo cleavage, or high-quality embryo rates in IVF-ET. A high DFI reduced the pregnancy rate without impairing embryo quality [79]. By simulating the natural pathways that choose healthy spermatozoa traveling via the cervix, uterine cavity, and fallopian tubes, microfluidic selection may be useful in selecting higher-quality spermatozoa.

In the current literature, one study examined the effects of using microfluidic chips vs. gradient-density centrifugation for sperm selection in ICSI cycles in male infertility patients. According to the findings of this study, there were no statistically significant differences between the groups in terms of CPR and continued PR, although they were significantly higher in the group using microfluidic sperm sorting chips for male infertility [80]. In couples with a total motile sperm count between 1 and 5 million, the rise in pregnancy rate was more substantial ($p < 0.01$). Nonetheless, this was a retrospective study in which the spermatozoa of the study group had very poor morphology and the groups were not homogenous.

Guler et al. have conducted a prospective, randomized, controlled study evaluating the impact of density gradient centrifugation and microfluidic chip sperm preparation techniques on embryo development in astheno-teratozoospermia patient populations. Although the density gradient group had a higher sperm concentration, the microfluidic chip group had much greater motility (progressive and total). On the third day, there were no significant differences in fertilization rates or proportions of grade 1 and grade 2 embryos, as determined by the research. In addition, whereas the proportions of poor, fair, and good blastocysts on day 5 did not differ significantly, the microfluidic chip group had a much higher proportion of exceptional blastocysts (indicating high-quality embryos). The microfluidic chip sperm preparation produced sperm with greater motility and higher quality blastocysts on day 5, in patients with asthenoteratozoospermia [81].

3. Conclusion

The different procedures presented in this chapter for human sperm selection have advantages and disadvantages, and as described, several of these strategies have produced inconsistent results, leaving their therapeutic usefulness uncertain. Among these processes, standard sperm separation techniques (swim-up and DGC) are the most commonly utilized in ART laboratories, despite the uncertainty surrounding their deleterious effects on sperm cells. Due to the "excellent" characteristics of selected sperm, however, microscopy-based selection approaches are becoming increasingly popular. However, microscopy-based approaches and some of the other mentioned technologies are too costly or technically sophisticated to be utilized in ordinary ART settings.

The optimal sperm sorting process for ART should efficiently separate healthy, motile, and morphologically normal sperm that are capable of fertilizing oocytes. In contrast to conventional sperm-separating methods, which require many centrifugation steps to retrieve sperm cells, the optimal sperm sorting strategy should not use centrifugation. In fact, it has been demonstrated that sample centrifugation induces sperm cell ROS generation and DNA fragmentation. Importantly, the process must be non-invasive, as the same sperm extracted based on one or more functional features must be utilized for fertilization. In addition, the embryologist must select the appropriate sperm selection procedure based on the infertile status of the patient, such as oligospermia or obstructive azoospermia, as well as sample quality. Therefore, it is quite difficult to choose a single strategy from those described in this review. As a result, several laboratories combine multiple approaches to improve the quality and quantity of picked sperm. Insufficient randomized controlled studies and meta-analyses exist to aid the embryologist in making a decision. In this regard, lab-on-chip systems offer a number of practical benefits, including the ability to sort sperm through improved automated methods and reduce sperm losses caused by complex protocols and multiple transfers. Studies demonstrated that chips for sperm sorting are simple to use, economical, do not require several manual stages, and are not dependent on embryologist skill, hence eliminating human error and permitting standardization of sperm separation for assisted reproductive technology (ART) treatments.

Considering the above-mentioned promising results, such labs-on chips are expected to soon become more commonly used in infertility treatment centers around the world.

DOI: http://dx.doi.org/10.5772/intechopen.107108

Author details

Sirin Aydin[1*] and Mehmet Eflatun Deniz[2]

1 Dr. Turgut Noyan Application and Research Center, Baskent University Adana, Turkey

2 Department of Urology, City Hospital, Adana, Turkey

*Address all correspondence to: dr.sirinaydinn@gmail.com

References

[1] Gnoth C, Godehardt E, Frank-Herrmann P, Friol K, Tigges J, Freundl G. Definition and prevalence of subfertility and infertility. Human Reproduction. 2005;**20**:1144-1147

[2] Saleh RA, Agarwal A, Nelson DR, Nada EA, ElTonsy MH, et al. Increased sperm nuclear DNA damage in normozoospermic infertile men: A prospective study. Fertility and Sterility. 2002;**78**:313-318

[3] Nallella KP, Sharma RK, Aziz N, Agarwal A. Significance of sperm characteristics in the evaluation of male infertility. Fertility and Sterility. 2006;**85**:629-634

[4] Frey K. Male reproductive health and infertility. Primary Care. 2010;**37**:643-652

[5] World Health Organization. WHO Laboratory Manual for the Examination and Processing for Human Semen. 5th ed. Switzerland: WHO Press; 2010. pp. 223-225

[6] Agarwal A, Allamaneni SS. Sperm DNA damage assessment: A test whose time has come. Fertility and Sterility. 2005;**84**:850-853

[7] Lin MH, Kuo-Kuang Lee R, Li SH, Lu CH, Sun FJ, et al. Sperm chromatin structure assay parameters are not related to fertilization rates, embryo quality, and pregnancy rates in in vitro fertilization and intracytoplasmic sperm injection, but might be related to spontaneous abortion rates. Fertility and Sterility. 2008;**90**:352-359

[8] Lewis SE, Agbaje I, Alvarez J. Sperm DNA tests as useful adjuncts to semen analysis. Systems Biology in Reproductive Medicine. 2008;**54**:111-125

[9] Sakkas D, Alvarez JG. Sperm DNA fragmentation: Mechanisms of origin, impact on reproductive outcome, and analysis. Fertility and Sterility. 2010;**93**:1027-1036

[10] Rappa KL, Rodriguez HF, Hakkarainen GC, RaymondM A, Mutter GL, Waseem A. Sperm processing for advanced reproductive technologies: Where are we today? Biotechnology Advances. 2016;**34**:578-582. DOI: 10.1016/j.biotechadv.2016.01.007

[11] Coughlan C, Clarke H, Cutting R, Saxton J, Waite S, et al. Sperm DNA fragmentation, recurrent implantation failure and recurrent miscarriage. Asian Journal of Andrology. 2015;**17**:681-685

[12] Collins JA, Barnhart KT, Schlegel PN. Do sperm DNA integrity tests predict pregnancy with in vitro fertilization? Fertility and Sterility. 2008;**89**:823-831

[13] Rappa KL, Rodriguez HF, Hakkarainen GC, Anchan RM, Mutter GL, Asghar W. Sperm processing for advanced reproductive technologies: Where are we today? Biotechnology Advances. 2016;**34**:582-587. DOI: 10.1016/j.biotechadv.2016.01.007

[14] Asghar W, Velasco V, Kingsley JL, Shoukat MS, Shafiee H, Anchan RM, et al. Selection of functional human sperm with higher DNA integrity and fewer reactive oxygen species. Advanced Healthcare Materials. 2014;**3**(10):1671-1679

[15] Zhang X, Khimji I, Gurkan UA, Safaee H, Catalano PN, Keles HO, et al. Lensless imaging for simultaneous microfluidic sperm monitoring and sorting. Lab on a Chip. 2011;**11**(15):2535-2540

[16] Ko Y-J, Maeng J-H, Lee B-C, Lee S, Hwang SY, Ahn Y. Separation of

progressive motile sperm from mouse semen using on-chip chemotaxis. Analytical Sciences. 2012;**28**:27

[17] Tasoglu S, Safaee H, Zhang X, Kingsley JL, Catalano PN, Gurkan UA, et al. Exhaustion of racing sperm in nature-mimicking microfluidic channels during sorting. Small. 2013;**9**:3374

[18] Henkel R. Sperm preparation: State-of-the-art--physiological aspects and application of advanced sperm preparation methods. Asian Journal of Andrology. 2012;**14**:260

[19] Practice Committee of American Society for Reproductive Medicine. Diagnostic evaluation of the infertile male: A committee opinion. Fertility and Sterility. 2012;**98**(2):294-301

[20] Sharlip ID et al. Best practice policies for male infertility. Fertility and Sterility. 2002;**77**(5):873-882

[21] Fritz MA, Speroff L. Clinical Gynaecologic Endocrinology and Infertility. 8th ed. Philadelphia: Lippincott Williams & Wilkins; 2011

[22] Amann RP. The cycle of the seminiferous epithelium in humans: A need to revisit? Journal of Andrology. 2008;**29**:469-487

[23] Kanatsu-Shinohara M, Shinohara T. Spermatogonial stem cell self-renewal and development. Annual Review of Cell and Developmental Biology. 2013;**29**:163-187

[24] American Society for Reproductive Medicine. MicroRNAs and spermatogenesis. Fertility and Sterility. 2014;**101**:1552-1562

[25] Miller MP, Amon A, Unal E, Meiosis I. When chromosomes undergo extreme makeover. Current Opinion in Cell Biology. 2013;**25**:687-696

[26] Rathke C, Baarends WM, Awe S, Renkawitz-Pohl R. Chromatin dynamics during spermiogenesis. Biochimica et Biophysica Acta. 2014;**1839**:155-168

[27] Guyonnet B, Dacheux F, Dacheux J-L, Gatti J-L. The epididymal transcriptome and proteome provide some insights into new epididymal regulations. Journal of Andrology. 2011;**32**:651-664

[28] Hinrichsen MJ, Blaquier JA. Evidence supporting the existence of sperm maturation in the human epididymis. Journal of Reproduction and Fertility. 1980;**60**:291

[29] Samplaski MK et al. New generation of diagnostic tests for infertility: Review of specialized semen tests. International Journal of Urology. 2010;**17**(10):839-847

[30] Mawhinney M, Mariotti A. Physiology, pathology and pharmacology of the male reproductive system. Periodontology 2000. 2013;**61**(1):232-251

[31] McLaren JF. Infertility evaluation. Obstetrics and Gynecology Clinics of North America. 2012;**39**(4):453-463

[32] Collins JA, Burrows EA, Wilan AR. The prognosis for live birth among untreated infertile couples. Fertility and Sterility. 1995;**64**:22-28

[33] Esteves SC. Clinical relevance of routine semen analysis and controversies surrounding the 2010 World Health Organization criteria for semen examination. International Braz J Urol. 2014;**40**(4):443-453

[34] Pellestor F, Girardet A, Andreo B. Effect of long abstinence periods on human sperm quality. International Journal of Fertility and Menopausal Studies. 1993;**39**(5):278-282

[35] Cooper TG, Noonan E, von Eckardstein S, Auger J, Baker HW, Behre HM, et al. World Health Organization reference values for human semen characteristics. Human Reproduction Update. 2010;**16**:231

[36] Weissman A, Howles CM, Shoham Z, editors. Textbook of Assisted Reproductive Techniques. 5th ed. Vol. 1. Laboratory Perspectives. CRC Press; 2018. DOI: 10.1201/9781351228237

[37] Guzick DS, Overstreet JW, Factor-Litvak P, Brazil CK, Nakajima ST, Coutifaris C, et al. Sperm morphology, motility, and concentration in fertile and infertile men. The New England Journal of Medicine. 2001;**345**:1388

[38] Bonde JP, Ernst E, Jensen TK, Hjollund NH, Kolstad H, Henriksen TB, et al. Relation between semen quality and fertility: A population-based study of 430 first-pregnancy planners. Lancet. 1998;**352**:1172

[39] World Health Organization. Department of Reproductive Health and Research. World Health Organization Laboratory Manual for the Examination and Processing of Human Semen. 5th ed. Geneva, Switzerland: World Health Organization; 2010

[40] Ombelet W et al. Results of a questionnaire on sperm morphology assessment. Human Reproduction. 1997;**12**(5):1015-1020

[41] K A. Erkek infertilitesi. Temel Üroloji 2007. 3: p. 967-1012

[42] Boitrelle F, Robin G, Marcelli F, Albert M, Leroy-Martin B, Dewailly D, et al. A predictive score for testicular sperm extraction quality and surgical ICSI outcome in non-obstructive azoospermia: A retrospective study. Human Reproduction. 2011;**26**(12):3215-3221

[43] Talwar P, Hayatnagarkar S. Sperm function test. Journal of Human Reproductive Sciences. 2015;**8**(2):61-69

[44] Speroff L, Frıtz MA. The Clinical Gynecologic Endocrinology and Infertility. 7th ed. Philadelphia: Lippincott Williams & Wilkins; 2005

[45] Oehninger S et al. Hemizona assay and its impact on the identification and treatment of human sperm dysfunctions. Andrologia. 1992;**24**(6):307-321

[46] Barrett CLR, Canale D, Cooper TG, de Jonge C, Fraser LR, et al. Consensus workshop on advanced diagnostic andrology techniques ESHRE (European Society of Human Reproduction and Embryology) andrology special interest group. Human Reproduction. 1996;**11**:1463

[47] Stanger JD et al. Hypo-osmotic swelling test identifies individual spermatozoa with minimal DNA fragmentation. Reproductive Biomedicine Online. 2010;**21**(4):474-484

[48] Agarwal A et al. Oxidation-reduction potential of semen: What is its role in the treatment of male infertility? Therapeutic Advances in Urology. 2016;**8**(5):302-318

[49] Schulte RT et al. Sperm DNA damage in male infertility: Etiologies, assays, and outcomes. Journal of Assisted Reproduction and Genetics. 2010;**27**(1):3-12

[50] Lewis SE, Aitken RJ. DNA damage to spermatozoa has impacts on fertilization and pregnancy. Cell and Tissue Research. 2005;**322**(1):33-41

[51] Palermo GD et al. Perspectives on the assessment of human sperm chromatin integrity. Fertility and Sterility. 2014;**102**(6):1508-1517

[52] Boivin J, Bunting L, Collins JA, Nygren KG. International estimates of infertility prevalence and

treatment-seeking: Potential need and demand for infertility medical care. Human Reproduction. 2007;**22**:2800-2800

[53] Palermo G, Joris H, Devroey P, Van Steirteghem AC. Pregnancies after intracytoplasmic injection of single spermatozoon into an oocyte. The Lancet. 1992;**340**:17-18

[54] Schultz RM, Williams CJ. The science of ART. Science. 2002;**296**:2188-2190

[55] Wright VC, Chang J, Jeng G, Macaluso M. Assisted reproductive technology surveillance—United States, 2005. MMWR Surveillance Summaries. 2008;**57**:1-23

[56] Jamieson DJ, Boulet SL, Chang J, Crawford S, Kissin D, et al. Centers for Disease Control and Prevention. American Society for Reproductive Medicine. Society for Assisted Reproductive Technology. Assisted Reproductive Technology Fertility Clinic Success Rates Report. Atlanta (GA); 2012

[57] Wright C, Milne S, Leeson H. Sperm DNA damage caused by oxidative stress: Modifiable clinical, lifestyle and nutritional factors in male infertility. Reproductive Biomedicine. 2014;**28**:684-703

[58] Eisenbach M, Giojalas LC. Sperm guidance in mammals—An unpaved road to the egg. Nature Reviews Molecular Cell Biology. 2006;**7**(4):276-285

[59] Aitken R, Bronson R, Smith T, De Iuliis GN. The source and significance of DNA damage in human spermatozoa; a commentary on diagnostic strategies and straw man fallacies. Molecular Human Reproduction. Aug 2013;**19**(8):475-485. DOI: 10.1093/molehr/gat025. Epub 2013 Apr 1. PMID: 23548339

[60] González-Marín C, Gosálvez J, Roy R. Types, causes, detection and repair of DNA fragmentation in animal and human sperm cells. International Journal of Molecular Sciences. 2012;**13**(11):14026-14052

[61] Aitken RJ, Clarkson JS. Significance of reactive oxygen species and antioxidants in defining the efficacy of sperm preparation techniques. Journal of Andrology. 1988;**6**:367-376

[62] Foong SC, Fleetham JA. O'Keane JA, Scott SG, tough SC, Greene CA, a prospective randomized trial of conventional in vitro fertilization versus intracytoplasmic sperm injection in unexplained infertility. Journal of Assisted Reproduction and Genetics. 2006;**23**(3):137-140

[63] Kam TL, Jacobson JD, Patton WC, Corselli JU, Chan PJ. Retention of membrane charge attributes by cryopreserved-thawed sperm and zeta selection. Journal of Assisted Reproduction and Genetics. 2007;**24**:429-434

[64] Razavi SH, Nasr-EsfahaniMH DMR, Shayesteh M, Tavalaee M. Evaluation of zeta and HA-binding methods for selection of spermatozoa with normal morphology, protamine content and DNA integrity. Andrologia. 2010;**42**:13-19

[65] Grunewald S, Paasch U, Glander HJ. Enrichment of non-apoptotic human spermatozoa after cryopreservation by immunomagnetic cell sorting. Cell and Tissue Banking. 2001;**2**:127-133

[66] Manz R, Assenmacher M, Pfluger E, Miltenyi S, Radbruch A. Analysis and sorting of live cells according to secreted molecules, relocated to a cellsurface affinity matrix. Proceedings of the National Academy of Sciences of the United States of America. 1995;**92**:1921-1925

[67] Said TM, Grunewald S, Paasch U, Glander H-J, Baumann T, Kriegel C, et al. Advantage of combining magnetic cell separation with sperm preparation techniques. Reproductive Biomedicine Online. 2005a;**10**:740-746

[68] Romany L, Garrido N, Motato Y, Aparicio B, Remohí J, Meseguer M. Removal of annexin V–positive sperm cells for intracytoplasmic sperm injection in ovum donation cycles does not improve reproductive outcome: A controlled and randomized trial in unselected males. Fertility and Sterility. Dec 2014;**102**(6):1567-75.e1. DOI: 10.1016/j.fertnstert.2014.09.001. Epub 2014 Oct 11. PMID: 25305728

[69] Jakab A, Sakkas D, Delpiano E, Cayli S, Kovanci E, Ward D, et al. Intracytoplasmic sperm injection: A novel selection method for sperm with normal frequency of chromosomal aneuploidies. Fertility and Sterility. 2005;**84**:1665-1673

[70] Fleming S, Ilad R, Griffin AG, Wu Y, Ong K, Smith H, et al. Prospective controlled trial of an electrophoretic method of sperm preparation for assisted reproduction: Comparison with density gradient centrifugation. Human Reproduction. 2008;**23**:2646-2651

[71] Bartoov B, Berkovitz A, Eltes F, Kogosowski A, Menezo Y, Barak Y. Real-time fine morphology of motile human sperm cells is associated with IVF-ICSI outcome. Journal of Andrology. 2002;**23**(1):1-8

[72] Gianaroli L, Magli MC, Collodel G, Moretti E, Ferraretti AP, Baccetti B. Sperm head's birefringence: A new criterion for sperm selection. Fertility and Sterility. 2008;**90**:104-112

[73] Aydın Ş, Bulgan Kılıçdağ E, Çağlar Aytaç P, Çok T, Şimşek E, Haydardedeoğlu B. Prospective randomized controlled study of a microfluidic chip technology for sperm selection in male infertility patients. Andrologia. Jul 2022;**54**(6):e14415. DOI: 10.1111/and.14415. Epub 2022 Mar 8. PMID: 35263457

[74] Quinn MM, Jalalian L, Ribeiro S, Ona K, Demirci U, Cedars MI, et al. Microfluidic sorting selects sperm for clinical use with reduced DNA damage compared to density gradient centrifugation with swim-up in split semen samples. Human Reproduction. 2018;**33**(8):1388-1393. DOI: 10.1093/humre p/dey239

[75] Yang SJ, Li T, Liu W, Li SJ, Xie N, Zhang C, et al. Pre-implantation genetic screening in intracytoplasmic sperm injection for infertile patients with high sperm DNA fragmentation index. Zhonghua Nan Ke Xue. Jan 2018;**24**(1):39-44. Chinese. PMID: 30157358

[76] Parrella A, Choi D, Keating D, Rosenwaks Z, Palermo G. A microfluidic device for selecting the most progressively motile spermatozoa yields a higher rate of euploid embryos. Fertility and Sterility. 2018;**110**(4):e342. DOI: 10.1016/j.fertnstert.2018.07.955

[77] Parrella A, Keating D, Cheung S, Xie P, Stewart JD, Rosenwaks Z, et al. A treatment approach for couples with disrupted sperm DNA integrity and recurrent ART failure. Journal of Assisted Reproduction and Genetics. 2019;**36**(10):2057-2066. DOI: 10.1007/s1081 5-019-01543-5

[78] Green KA, Patounakis G, Dougherty MP, Werner MD, Scott RT, Franasiak JM. Sperm DNA fragmentation on the day of fertilization is not associated with embryologic or clinical outcomes after IVF/ICSI. Journal of

Assisted Reproduction and Genetics. 2020;**37**(1):71-76. DOI: 10.1007/s10815-019-01632-5

[79] Luo Q-X, Liao Y-B, Huang C-P, Guo J-H, Liang X-D. Correlation of sperm DNA fragmentation index with age and semen parameters and its influence on the outcomes of IVF-ET. Zhonghua Nan Ke Xue = National Journal of Andrology. 2020;**26**(8):708-712

[80] Ozcan P, Takmaz T, Yazici MGK, Alagoz OA, Yesiladali M, Sevket O, et al. Does the use of microfluidic sperm sorting for the sperm selection improve in vitro fertilization success rates in male factor infertility? The Journal of Obstetrics and Gynaecology Research. 2021;**47**(1):382-388

[81] Guler C, Melil S, Ozekici U, Donmez Cakil Y, Selam B, Cincik M. Sperm selection and embryo development: A comparison of the density gradient centrifugation and microfluidic Chip sperm preparation methods in patients with Astheno-Teratozoospermia. Life (Basel). 2021;**11**(9):933

Section 3

In vitro Maturation, Oocyte Cryopreservation and Quality Management

Chapter 4

In vitro Maturation (IVM) Perspectives

Bassim Alsadi

Abstract

The basic concept of in vitro maturation (IVM) of oocytes in practice clinic consists of the collection of immature oocytes from small antral follicles before spontaneous ovulation and then left to mature in vitro. IVM is based on the observations of Pincus and Enzmann in 1935 and Edwards in 1965, which highlighted the spontaneous nuclear maturation of the follicles when they were removed from their ovarian context and matured in vitro, and these first discoveries of in vitro folliculogenesis laid the foundations for the present research on the technique of in vitro maturation. In vitro folliculogenesis represents not only the possibility of extending the availability of female gametes in terms of the number of fertilizable oocytes but also a model within which to understand the complex mechanisms that regulate the synergistic development between the follicle and the female gamete. Deeper understanding of the complex orchestration of maturation, nuclear and cytoplasmic, of the oocyte based on research of bases on animal oocytes allowed the clinical application of the IVM technique to begin in reproductive medicine.

Keywords: In vitro maturation, oocyte maturation, infertility, antral follicles, folliculogenesis, nuclear and cytoplasmic maturation, polycystic ovary syndrome (PCOS)

1. Introduction

The in vitro maturation method (IVM) is a new approach to the treatment of infertility. The aim is to reduce the cost of drugs in IVF procedures and the risk of severe forms of OHSS. In order to establish the optimal protocol, historically, the method had undergone a different transformation, starting with the rejection of the use of gonadotropins for stimulation to a method with minimal application of gonadotropins. In recent years, the application of this method has decreased, but IVM will find its place and remain one of the main methods of infertility treatment.

The benefits of IVM in clinical practice have been widely recognized in, first of all, the lack of the use of gonadotropins for controlled ovarian stimulation and consequently the absence of the risk of ovarian hyperstimulation syndrome especially in women with polycystic ovary syndrome (PCOS).

In vitro folliculogenesis represents not only the possibility of extending the availability of female gametes in terms of the number of fertilizable oocytes but also a model within which to understand the complex mechanisms that regulate the synergistic development between the follicle and the female gamete.

Deeper understanding of the complex orchestration of the nuclear and cytoplasmic maturation of the oocyte based on the basic research in animal oocytes allowed us to begin the clinical application of the IVM technique in human reproductive medicine.

The most promising technique to avoid ovarian hyperstimulation syndrome (in women with PCOS and non-PCOS) is to bypass the entire controlled ovarian stimulation phase by culturing immature oocytes to produce fertilizable eggs in a process called in vitro maturation.

However, in vitro maturation is not yet fully optimized universally in various medically assisted reproduction centers.

The mature human oocyte is the key ingredient for fertility, highly specialized in the process of oogenesis, which includes growth, differentiation, and maturation of the female gamete.

There are multiple differences between in vivo maturation and in vitro maturation of oocytes. Unlike oocytes matured in vivo, the oocyte cumulus complex (CCO) is typically recovered from medium antral follicle dimensions that have not reached complete "oocyte capacity," the mechanism that describes the changes that occur in the oocyte of the dominant follicles before the LH hormone peak that allows the oocyte to achieve full development competence [1, 2].

In the IVM technique, the oocytes are inevitably retrieved from the follicles in various stages of development, ranging from antral to atresic follicles, and grown in optimal conditions. By understanding the recovery meiotic division as well as through increased optimization of culture media with specific formulation for the oocytes maturation in vitro, we will be able to develop IVM techniques in optimal conditions, not only to enhance the competence for the development of oocytes but also to improve the results in terms of an increase in the fertilization and implanting rates.

The growth and quality of the oocytes depend on the normal development and its differentiation process. However, the egg itself also carries out a direct function in the follicular environment, for example, by preventing early luteinization, by regulating both the secretion of the cumulus oophorus cells and the cumulus matrix. Another direct function of the oocyte includes the expression of LH hormone receptors on the cells of the cumulus and granulosa cells. The oocyte-cumulus complex is aspirated from the small antral follicles for the IVM technique with the aim of replacing intrafollicular conditions.

For the success of IVM, there are various factors that influence the competence for the development of the oocyte in vitro, which include the choice of culture medium, additives such as serum, various growth factors, as well as the somatic cells that make up and surround the oocyte. The various culture media were originally proposed for somatic cells, and for this, there is a clinical need for formulation of specific culture media for the in vitro maturation of human oocytes.

2. Oocytes maturation

The maturation of oocytes is a complex process involving the nuclear maturation (the progression of the meiotic cycle) and cytoplasmic maturation.

In vitro studies have provided information about the importance of substances that affect the maturation of oocytes and its inhibition such as cAMP, growth factors, gonadotropins, purines, and steroids.

The development of the oocytes is gradually acquired during their prolonged period of growth in which the oocytes remain arrested in the same phase of first meiosis but undergo a noticeable increase in volume and alterations in cellular behavior; this is indicated by an intense metabolic activity, which, in turn, is reflected in marked biosynthetic changes and ultrastructural variations of oocytes. It is around this time that many of the macromolecules essential for further development, both before and after ovulation, get produced and accumulate within the oocyte; in addition, the rate of protein synthesis and total protein increase in parallel with the expansion of cell volume.

IVM differs from in vivo oocyte maturation in three fundamental ways.

Firstly, the cumulus-oocyte complex is usually collected from small or medium-sized antral follicles (6–12 mm of diameter), which have not completed their final maturation or capacitation of oocytes and, therefore, do not have the necessary organization for cytoplasmic maturation to support early embryogenesis [1, 2].

Secondly, the mechanical removal of the oocyte-cumulus complex from the follicle would lead to the loss of the natural environment of meiotic inhibition with the resulting spontaneous or "premature" meiotic maturation in vitro. In this way, nuclear maturation occurs before the cytoplasm has reached full maturity.

Thirdly, the population of small antral follicles collected from the oocyte-cumulus complex for IVM is very heterogeneous regarding their stages of developments and atresia.

The oocyte acquires an increasingly greater competence in a gradual and progressive manner as it passes through the various stages of folliculogenesis, from the moment in which the oocyte begins to grow through the differentiation of the somatic cells that surround the oocytes.

For this reason, it is important that the egg cell is adequately protected from the action of all chemical or physical agents able to damage it and compromise its development [3, 4]. This primary role is played by the follicular cells surrounding the female gamete, creating around it a microenvironment suitable for correct maturation [5, 6].

The oocytes are arrested in the prophase of the first meiosis during the prenatal life for several years until sexual maturity is reached, and the follicular growth is completed by the actions of gonadotropins [7]. However, the oocytes will be able to resume meiosis spontaneously when they are removed from the follicles [8]. This shows the presence of inhibitory molecules in the follicle that keep the oocytes in arrested meiotic.

In addition, several possible inhibitory molecules such as intracellular 3′,5′- cyclic adenosine monophosphate [cAMP], Hypoxanthine, steroid hormones, and several other factors derived from the granulosa cells have a role in keeping the oocytes meiotic arrest [9, 10].

A sophisticated complex of numerous intercellular interactions, including growth factors, cAMP, and gap junction between oocytes and granulosa cells, are involved in the arrest process in the first phase of meiosis in vivo.

3. Nuclear maturation

Nuclear maturation typically includes the period between recovery of the meiosis of an oocyte, which was arrested in prophase I, and the passage to metaphase II (MII) stage when the oocyte undergoes a new arrest pending fertilization.

Morphologically, these events are represented by the rupture of the germinal vesicles (GV) and asymmetric cytoplasmic division of the oocyte subsequent to the extrusion of the first polar body (PB). The germinal vesicle (GV) is the nucleus of the oocyte.

4. Cytoplasmic maturation

Cytoplasmic maturation can be defined as the process in which the female gamete passes from an incompetent evolutionary cell to a state of functional capacity of addressing and supporting the events of fertilization and early embryonic development, and it was first described by Delage in 1901 to clarify that the concept of cytoplasmic maturation was not necessarily synchronous with nuclear maturation [4].

Assisting at the microscopic level, the process of cytoplasmic maturation is more difficult compared to nuclear maturation, which is a relatively evaluable process at the microscopic level.

Cytoplasmic maturation involves the accumulation of mRNA and proteins and post-translational modifications that are necessary to achieve a competence in the development of the oocyte. In addition, a number of cytoplasmic organs (Golgi complexes, mitochondria, endoplasmic reticulum) proliferate in ooplasm as a result of their peripheral dislocation, which is regulated from a system of microtubules [4].

5. Role of gonadotropins in meiotic recovery

The signals involved in the resumption of meiosis in the oocyte are little known, but two experimental in vitro models provided the framework for a large part of our understanding of this process.

In 1935, Pincus and Enzmann observed that mammalian oocytes spontaneously resumed meiosis when removed from the follicular environment.

This observation led to the hypothesis that follicle cells sent inhibitory signals to the oocyte to maintain meiotic arrest.

Other studies have shown that LH promotes the maturation of the oocytes indirectly through the activation of granulosa cells [11, 12].

In vivo, meiosis resumes in response to a pre-ovulatory luteinizing LH hormone increase; in this way, the primary oocyte completes the first meiotic division and stops at the level of II° metaphase with the formation of two haploid cells:

- a cell that preserves almost all of the oocyte's cytoplasm, called secondary oocyte
- a cell with very little cytoplasm, called the 1st polar globe.

6. Cellular communication and gap junction

The oocyte and follicular cells are intimately associated and are in communication across a vast network of gap junctions and are composed of membrane protein structures called connexins. Several types of different connexins have been located in the ovarian follicle [13].

Gap junctions play an important role in maintaining the oocyte in meiotic arrest by transferring inhibitory molecules such as cAMP, which are generated from somatic follicular cells [14].

Recently, it has been supposed that heterologous gap junctions play a role in the regulation of oocyte chromatin configuration [15].

The communication between the oocyte and the granulosa cells is possible through the presence of the connexins (Cx 43). Experimental evidence has shown that in mice with deficiency of the connexin 37 gene, there is no formation of Graafian follicles, the ovulatory process fails, they develop many inappropriate corpora lutea, and also the growth of the oocyte is arrested earlier before it reaches maturation competences. This shows that the intercellular communication via gap junctions regulates and coordinates critically the complex mechanism of cellular interactions for the maturation of oocytes [16, 17].

The second mechanism of communication between oocyte and granulosa cells is mediated by paracrine factors (**Figure 1**), which play a fundamental role in directing the growth and differentiation of ovarian follicles. Paracrine factors secreted by the oocyte are essential for the expansion of cumulus cells and to keep their own phenotype [19].

Most of the studies concerning paracrine factors have focused on some members of the transforming growth factor β (TGFβ) superfamily, such as Growth Differentiation Factor 9 (GDF9), Bone Morphogenetic Protein 15 (BMP15), and others. The great interest in these paracrine factors is mainly due to the fact that an alteration of the expression of their respective genes greatly impairs ovarian function and fertility [18–20].

Studies carried out on knockout mice have shown that deletions at the level of such factors involved in the proliferation of granulosa cells, in particular of GDF9,

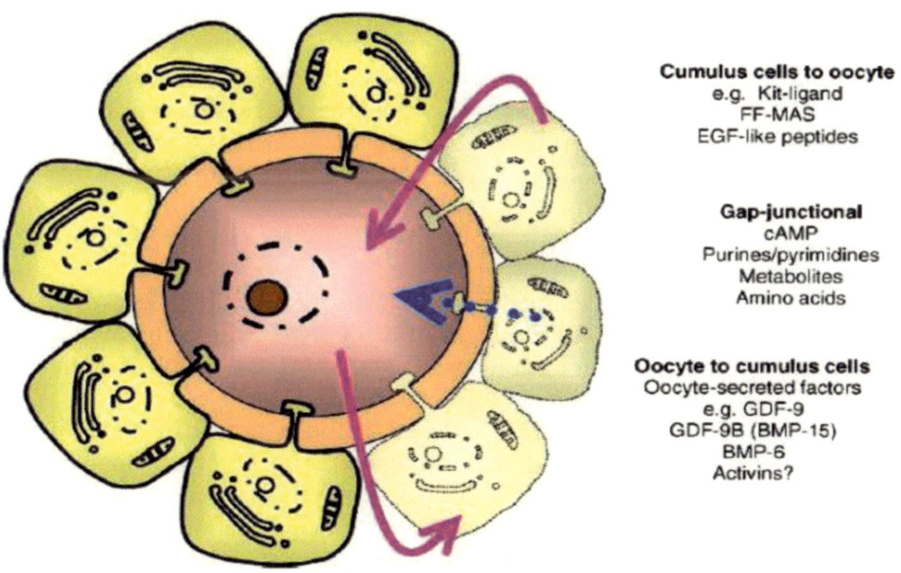

Figure 1.
Communication between oocyte and somatic cells is essential for the growth and development of both the female gamete and the follicle. This bi-directional communication axis is mediated by paracrine factors (solid arrows) and by the exchange of small molecules via gap junctions (dashed arrow) [18].

induce the production of a sterile phenotype in which the development of the follicles is arrested, obtaining a single layer of cells that delimit a large oocyte [21]. This demonstrates how granulosa cells need GDF9 for their own proliferation.

The feedback communication between oocyte and somatic cells is also needed to coordinate the resumption of meiosis by the female gamete and the ovulation process. Immature or non-competent oocytes have been shown not to interact in appropriate manner in this communication system and do not progress to ovulation [22, 23].

Although several studies have highlighted important aspects of the relationship between oocyte and somatic cells, much remains to be investigated regarding the cellular communication pathways that are selectively activated. Since this bidirectional communication arrangement seems to be a prerequisite to ensuring proper oocyte development, it is important to know and study the molecular basis of such events.

7. The role of the cyclic AMP (cAMP)

The cyclic adenosine monophosphate (cAMP) is the second messenger for the transduction of the signal of gonadotropins. The FSH and LH hormones exert their biological function, activating membrane receptors of target cells and, consequently, activating adenyl cyclase, which leads to the production of cyclic AMP, which is one of most important intracellular signaling molecules that is responsible for the maintenance of meiotic arrest in the oocytes.

Resumption of meiosis occurs after a drop in cyclic AMP levels; the cAMP acts as a regulator of gap junction communication [24].

Phosphodiesterases (PDEs) are important regulators and play a critical role in the maturation of oocytes and their meiotic recovery. In mammals, the Phosphodiesterases (PDE) constitute a large family of various isoenzymes and are classified into 11 subtypes, PDE1–PDE11. Their regulation is cell-tissue specific.

The mechanisms by which cAMP maintains meiotic arrest are related to the diffusion of cAMP from somatic cells (granulosa and cumulus cells) to the oocyte and the increase in the intra-oocyte level of cAMP, preventing the maturation of oocytes [25].

The precise mechanism by which the intracellular concentrations of cAMP may produce a stimulation or an inhibitory response in the oocyte during the meiosis is not entirely clear.

As previously discussed, high levels of cAMP keep the oocyte in the meiotic arrest, and this is supported by in vitro studies.

Adding substances to the culture media able to maintain a high level of intracellular cAMP or agents that prevent the degradation of cAMP will maintain meiotic arrest of oocytes. The stimulatory or inhibitory effect of cAMP is dependent on the levels of cAMP in the different compartments of the follicle.

The mammalian oocyte acquires a series of competencies during the follicular development, involving chromatin remodeling occurring in the germinal vesicles (GV). The chromatin configuration in the germinal vesicles is correlated with increased competence in the development of oocytes in different mammalian species in which diffuse chromatin condenses into a perinuclear ring.

Ovarian folliculogenesis is regulated by a delicate balance between several intraovarian factors. An imbalance or any dysfunction between these various factors causes abnormal folliculogenesis and, consequently, directly compromises the competence of oocyte development.

It appears that the interactions between hormones and growth factors produced locally in the follicular microenvironment are highly organized, and the timing and extent of these interactions are pivotal to establishing the intrafollicular cascade of the ovarian follicle development.

Albuz et al. [26] evaluated the role of cyclic AMP modulators added to pre-IVM of bovine or mouse cumulus-oocyte complexes (COCs) and observed an almost 100-fold increase in COCs' cyclic AMP levels. With this technique, they simulated the physiological maturation of the oocytes, giving the definition of "simulated physiological maturation of the oocytes" (SPOM). SPOM imitates oocyte maturation in vivo and has benefits for IVM, which can be used in IVM protocols to optimize clinical outcomes [26].

8. Epidermal growth factor (EGF)

Epidermal growth factor (EGF) is a growth factor that plays an important role in the regulation of cell proliferation and differentiation [27]. In the human oocyte, EGF is found in the follicular microenvironment (**Figure 2**) regulating the development and maturation of oocytes [27–29].

In vitro studies show that exposure of the cumulus-oocyte complex (CCO) to the growth factor EGF stimulates the expansion of cumulus cells (CC) and improves nuclear and cytoplasmic maturation of oocytes from metaphase I (MI) to metaphase

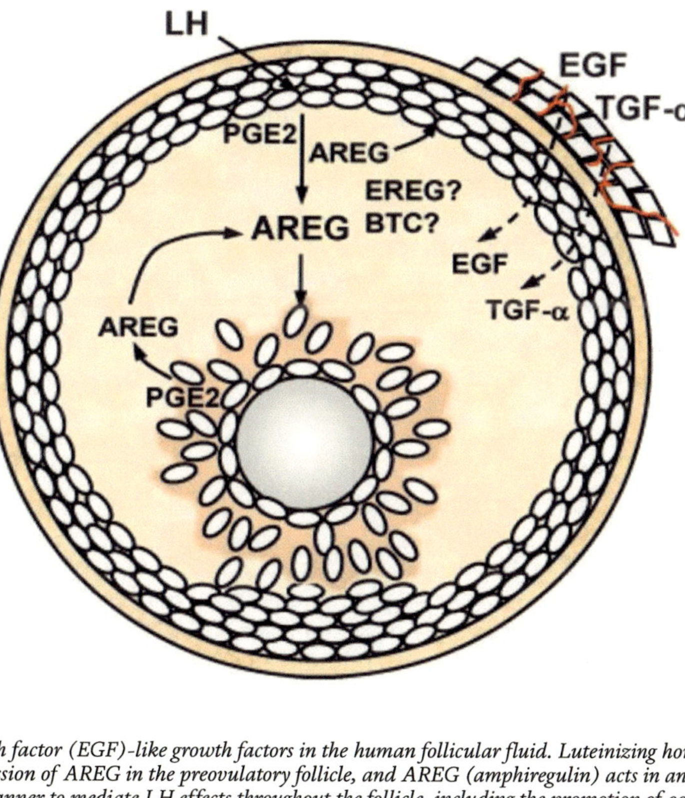

Figure 2.
Epidermal growth factor (EGF)-like growth factors in the human follicular fluid. Luteinizing hormone (LH) induces the expression of AREG in the preovulatory follicle, and AREG (amphiregulin) acts in an autocrine and paracrine manner to mediate LH effects throughout the follicle, including the promotion of oocyte meiotic resumption and cumulus expansion [27].

II (MII) both in human oocytes and in other mammals, facilitating the fertilization and embryonic development [30].

Other studies suggest that EGF levels in the follicular microenvironment have an inverse correlation with oocyte maturation [27, 31, 32].

In women with polycystic ovary syndrome (PCOS), EGF levels in the follicular microenvironment are higher compared to non-PCOS women, and this may suggest the role of the EGF factor in the maintenance of the PCOS phenotype [33, 34].

The EGF inhibits estrogen synthesis in granulosa cells and is involved in the maintenance of the PCOS phenotype with the arrest of follicle growth in PCOS women [34].

Therefore, it is assumed that an alteration of the regulation of EGF synthesis and/or its action mediated through its specific receptor (EGF-R) can cause anovulatory infertility in women with polycystic ovary syndrome [28].

The correlation between high levels of EGF growth factor in the follicular microenvironment and the quality and competence of the oocytes is yet to be clarified.

In addition, other various factors called EGF-like factors have been identified such as amphiregulin, epiregulin, and betacellulin in the follicular microenvironment [35, 36]; however, the specific physiological function of the various EGF-like factors in PCOS patients remains unknown.

9. Fibroblast growth factor (FGF)

Fibroblast growth factors (FGFs) are a group of polypeptides that play a fundamental role in cell growth, development, tissue repair, and cell transformation. They are expressed in the granulosa (GC) and theca cells of growing follicles and are considered physiological regulators of FSH action [34, 37].

Recent studies have revealed high levels of fibroblast growth factor (FGF) in the follicular microenvironment and serum of polycystic ovary syndrome patients (PCOS) versus non-PCOS patients, leading to an inverse correlation of oocyte maturity; this contributes to alterations in the intrafollicular environment with consequent arrest of follicular development in patients with polycystic ovary syndrome [34, 37].

Therefore, the alterations of FGF in the follicular microenvironment and in the serum remain controversial, and the impact of FGF on the maturation of oocytes and the embryonic development requires further elucidation in PCOS patients.

10. Transforming growth factor-β family (TGF-β family)

Among the many growth factors in the intrafollicular microenvironment, the various members of the TGF-β family play an important biological role in the growth of follicle and oocyte development. These members of the TGF-β family include: anti-Mullerian hormone, activin, follistatin, inhibin, and growth differentiation factor-9 (GDF-9).

Under different physiological conditions, the various TGF-β family factors can promote or block the growth of the ovarian follicle and/or the differentiation of the granulosa-oocyte complex that is related to the pathogenesis of PCOS [38–40].

11. FF meiosis-activating sterol (follicle fluid meiosis-activating sterol)

FF meiosis-activating sterol (FF-MAS) is an endogenous signaling molecule present in the follicular microenvironment of the oocyte and is an intermediate metabolite in cholesterol biosynthesis [41].

Many in vitro studies show that FF-MAS exposure can promote nuclear and cytoplasmic maturation of the oocyte [42] and improve the fertilization rate [41, 43, 44].

Recent in vitro studies have showed that FF-MAS improves the quality of oocytes retrieved from women with PCOS to undergo the IVM technique [41, 45].

12. Growth differentiation factor-9 and bone morphogenetic protein-15 (GDF-9/BMP-15)

Growth differentiation factor-9 and bone morphogenetic protein-15 (GDF-9/BMP-15) are members of the transforming growth factor beta (TGF-β) superfamily and are highly expressed in oocytes during their development and growth [46, 47].

BMP-15 and GDF-9 have a fundamental role in regulating the functions of cumulus cells (CC) through the process of mitosis, proliferation, apoptosis, and the signal transduction mechanism [38, 46, 47].

Data from in vitro experiments on animal models show that coincubation of cumulus cells(CC) with either BMP-15 or GDF-9 greatly promotes the maturation of oocytes and improves the production of blastocytes [6].

An altered expression of BMP-15 or GDF-9 during folliculogenesis can be related to female infertility [46, 48, 49] and an increase in correlations with the pathogenesis of polycystic ovary syndrome (PCOS) [46, 48, 50, 51].

A correlation was observed between a high BMP-15 level in the follicular fluid and an improvement in oocyte quality, higher rates of fertilization, and embryonic development in women who underwent to IVF, suggesting that BMP-15 can be a good indicator of the maturity of the oocyte and its potential for fertilization [52].

GDF-9 expression in cumulus cells is lower in patients with PCOS and can lead to premature luteinization and decreased oocyte development [34, 53].

The decreased expression of GDF-9 in cumulus cells (CC) can also be related to the high rate of miscarriage in women with polycystic ovary syndrome syndrome [51].

The expression of BMP-15 and GDF-9 in oocytes and cumulus cells (CC) may provide valuable support for the regulation of the follicular microenvironment during the maturation process of the oocytes.

A recent study has demonstrated that the expression of GDF-9 and BMP-15 tends to be higher in PCOS patients when compared with a control group and therefore may be involved in follicular dysplasia in PCOS [51].

Further studies on the role of BMP-15 or GDF-9 in folliculogenesis will be essential in understanding those factors involved in the regulation of the pathogenesis of PCOS and help to improve in vitro oocyte maturation (IVM) in women with PCOS.

13. Optimizing in vitro maturation (IVM) in clinical practice and outcomes

It is actually not surprising that current in vitro culture systems fail to support the differentiation of oocytes with their maximum potential development. In fact, only some of the follicular characteristics are maintained in vitro by culture of the intact cumulus-oocyte complex (CCO) with the supplementation of certain growth factors in the culture media (**Figure 3**). In addition, the supports by the granulosa cells, the follicular fluid, the basal lamina, and theca cells are missing altogether in the phase of oocytes in vitro maturation. A strategy aimed to maintain meiotic arrest in vitro can allow events that take place in the cumulus-oocyte complex (COC) to progress further. Even with this strategy, however, the oocyte cannot remain under the influence of cumulus cells for as long as it would be in vivo, in addition to the interaction from other follicular compartments that are still missing.

New approaches that more closely mirror the follicular conditions are essential.

Recently, a two-stage approach, the first phase of which includes the in vitro prematuration stage (pre-IVM) and the second phase includes prolongation of the in vitro maturation (extended-IVM) combined with the use of FSH and drugs that arrest meiosis, has shown better egg development in vitro [26]. In this way, a phase of prematuration of immature oocytes could be beneficial to enable the biochemical processes that accompany the cytoplasmic rearrangements to develop in a more physiological way (**Figure 4**). The possible strategy could be to adopt the in vitro follicle coculture system using specific pharmacological agents that act on the metabolism of the cAMP, on the synthesis protein, and the inhibition of phosphodiesterase.

Egg retrieval during IVM has similar aspects to the conventional IVF technique, but smaller diameter needle and lower suction pressures are used generally to recover intact cells of the cumulus complex from small follicles. The diameter of the

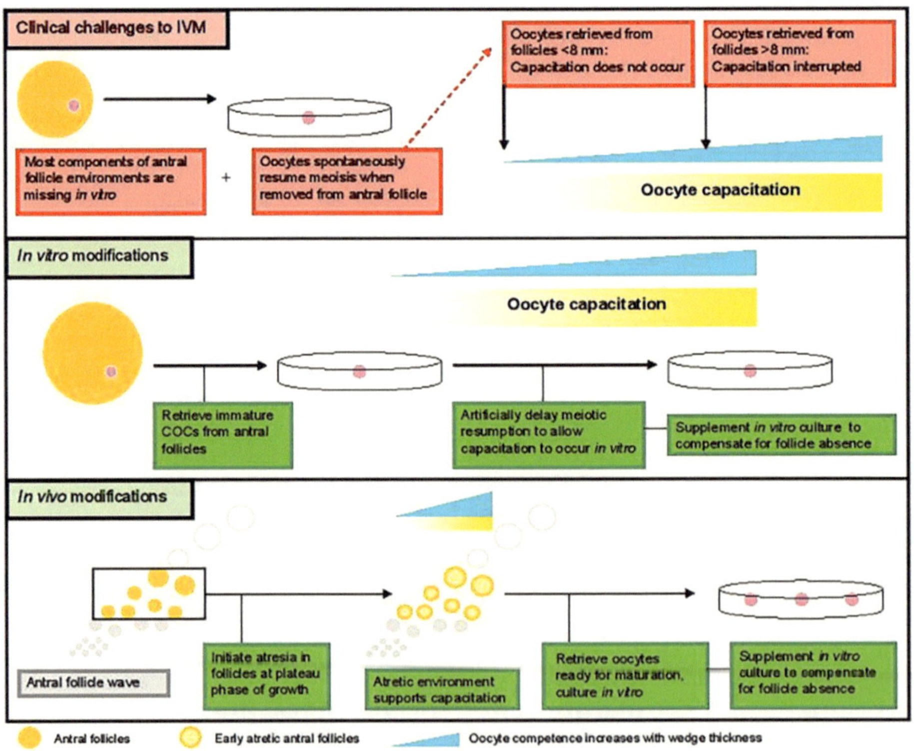

Figure 3.
The absence of the antral follicle environment remains an obstacle to in vitro maturation (IVM) success and other clinical assisted reproductive technology (ART) protocols [54].

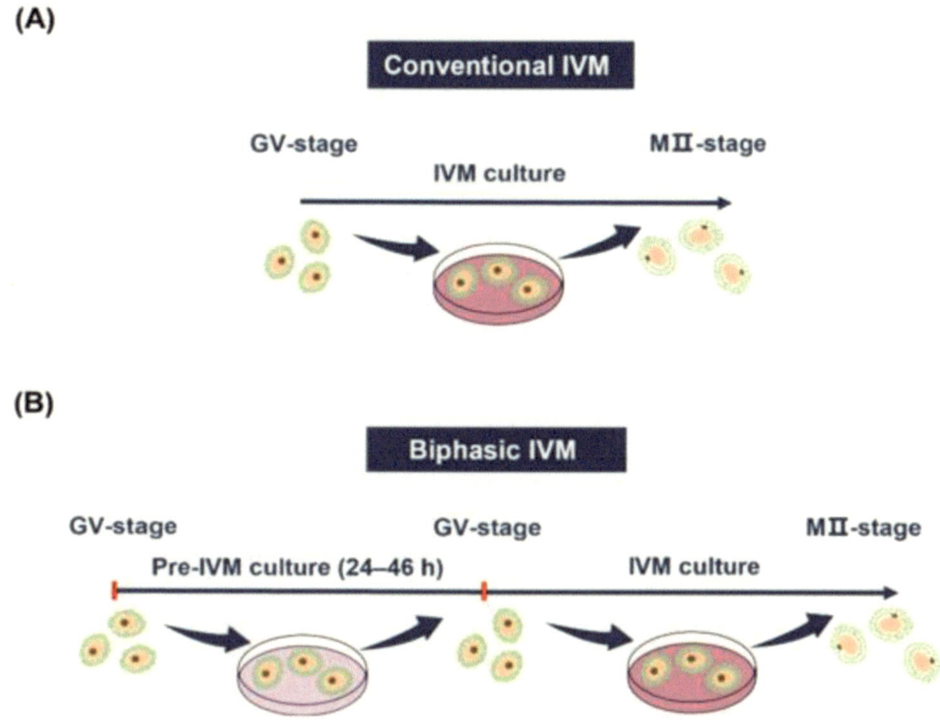

Figure 4.
Conventional and biphasic IVM culture systems. (A) Conventional IVM system, only includes IVM culture phase. (B) Biphasic IVM system, includes a pre-IVM culture phase before IVM culture. The pre-IVM culture inhibits resumption of meiosis in immature oocytes and provides time for acquiring developmental potential. MII, metaphase II [55].

aspiration needle involved varies from 17 to 20 gauge, and the aspiration pressure is around 80 mmHg to avoid traumatizing the cumulus complex cells and denuding the oocyte.

During the oocyte retrieval in the IVF, the follicle curetting technique is frequently practiced, which consists of the rapid and delicate rotation of the needle clockwise and counterclockwise inside the follicle after the complete aspiration of the follicular liquid, with the advantage of an increased likelihood of aspirating all oocytes and a reduced risk of ovarian hyperstimulation syndrome (OHSS) secondary to the removal of more granulosa cells. This technique may enhance the oocyte yield by 22% [56].

IVM has attracted attention in clinical practice for its safety, repeatability, cost-effectiveness, and almost no risk of OHSS along with acceptable clinical pregnancy rates and live-birth rates [57].

Siristatidis et al. in a systematic review and meta-analysis reviewed IVM in patients with and without PCOS and concluded that IVM was an effective treatment option when offered to infertile women with PCOS [58].

Edwards conducted several studies [59–61] on the in vitro maturation of the human oocyte (IVM), and the first techniques of human IVF were based on the use of IVM. IVM is considered the progenitor of the current in vitro fertilization treatment [57, 62].

The collection of mature oocytes from preovulatory follicles in women with normal cycles became possible after the introduction of laparoscopy into gynecological practice in the 1970s [63] and with the advent of in vitro fertilization and the successful birth of Louise Brown; IVF with controlled ovarian stimulation has become a common practice.

Although the primary indication of IVM was in patients with polycystic ovarian syndrome (PCOS), IVM has much broader indications including poor ovarian reserve and repeated IVF failures [64]. IVM can also be used in cases of resistant ovary syndrome and fertility preservation [65–67].

Other potential indications of IVM may be in normo–ovulatory patients, patients with previous failed IVF attempts and a history of OHSS (ovarian hyperstimation syndrome), emergency oocyte retrieval due to malignant tumors in patients who are candidates for ovarian chemotoxic therapy, poor responders, and IVM for rescue IVF cycles.

In vitro maturation of immature oocytes from unstimulated ovaries with mature follicular fluid could be used successfully in an oocyte donation program after IVF in which Cha et al. reported the first IVM birth from immature oocytes egg donors [68].

In vitro maturation and developmental proficiency of oocytes retrieved from patients with untreated polycystic ovaries resulted in the first IVM from the mother's own immature oocytes in 1994 [69]. Over 5000 babies have been born since then with IVM technique [70].

Seok et al. studied the predictive role of the anti-Müllerian hormone (AMH) on IVM selection in PCOS patients and concluded that AMH was a valuable factor in predicting clinical outcomes in such patients who preferred IVM as the treatment of choice [71].

Other predictive factors in IVM have been investigated and evidenced that Estradiol, FSH concentration, and AFC (antral follicular counts) were found to be predictive factors in the decision on whether to initiate IVM, and endometrial thickness and leading follicle size were predictive factors for the timing of the retrieval of immature oocytes [72].

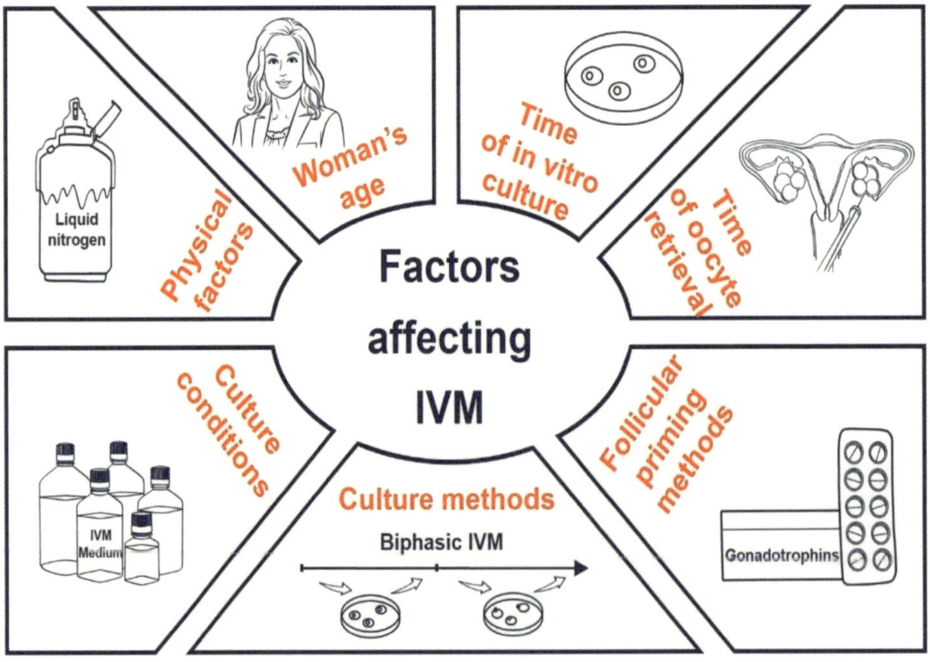

Figure 5.
Factors influencing the IVM of human oocytes [74].

IVM offers a possibility in cancer patients with a desire to preserve their fertility by retrieving immature oocytes in the luteal phase, which can be successfully matured in vitro; therefore, if there is insufficient time for a conventional retrieval of the follicular phase oocytes in a stimulated/unstimulated cycle prior to chemotherapy, a luteal phase retrieval could be considered as an option [73].

Factors influencing IVM of human oocyte are shown in **Figure 5**: the application of a biphasic IVM culture system, culture medium conditions, different protein sources, womens' age, criopreservation, and different follicular priming methods. Prospective RCT studies in the future may put in place their specific roles and implications in IVM and the possibility for increasing the successful outcome rate of IVM.

14. Conclusion

In the reproductive system of mammals, the development of oocytes takes place within the highly specialized microenvironment of an ovarian follicle. The follicle has the task of facilitating the complex and the delicate process of oogenesis.

Egg differentiation ultimately depends on the cooperation and coordination of the function of the antral follicle as a whole. By understanding the differentiation of the oocyte, we must clarify the functions of the compartments of the antral follicles as well as their relationship to each other.

Further efforts must continue to reveal how the components of the follicular microenvironment drive egg differentiation.

The ability of the oocyte to modulate its development is codependent between interaction between the oocytes and their respective follicles which presents a further obstacle to in vitro culture of oocytes.

The state of the art of the IVM technique attempts to replicate the essential components of the follicular microenvironment for the benefit of oocytes in vitro but must also try to understand how, when, and why the oocyte induces changes to this follicular microenvironment.

Although nuclear and cytoplasmic maturation of oocytes can proceed independently of each other, both processes must be coordinated in order to ensure the competence of oocyte development. Therefore, maintaining the transzonal connections between the granulosa cells and oocyte for a continuous exchange of substances and regulatory factors between the two cell compartments.

Maintaining the oocyte in a state of meiotic arrest using both coculture with pharmacological agents and providing growth factors and hormone supplements to support the completion of cytoplasmic maturation of the oocyte could theoretically lead to an improvement in development of the oocyte.

Knowledge of the molecular mechanisms of oocyte maturation are still Insufficient, and the culture media currently in use are not capable of supporting the complex paracrine events of in vitro maturation.

One possible strategy to improve oocyte-development competence in the IVM technique is to align meiotic and cytoplasmic maturation by delaying spontaneous meiotic recovery. It is speculated that this may provide the time for cytoplasmic changes (e.g., storage of mRNA and proteins, morphological changes, ultrastructural remodeling) and could improve the synchronization of immature oocytes.

The ovaries host various local growth factors involved in folliculogenesis, and the physiological significance of autocrine/paracrine regulation, the integrated effects of their action, and their implication in reproduction medicine remain to be established.

Oocyte quality is a key factor in female fertility, yet we have a poor understanding of what constitutes oocyte quality and the mechanisms that govern it. The ovarian follicular microenvironment through the granulosa cells (GC) and the cumulus cells (CC) is responsible for the growth and gradual acquisition of competence in the development of the oocyte; however, the communications between the oocyte, granulosa cells (GC), and cumulus cells (CC) are bidirectional, with the oocyte secreting growth factors acting locally to direct the differentiation and function of the cumulus cells (CC).

The ability of oocytes to regulate their own microenvironment constitutes one important component of oocyte quality, and improving our knowledge of the oocyte-cumulus cell (CC) interactions will improve IVM efficiency and thus provide new options for infertility treatment.

Establishing a global registry for all births with the IVM technique would be desirable for the long-term and follow-up of perinatal and postnatal outcomes.

By evaluating the cellular structures of the oocytes (such as the reticulum endoplasmic, the mitochondrion, and the Golgi apparatus), the sensitivities of the reserves of calcium, chromosome dynamics, and apoptosis during embryogenesis are essential topics for the structural study of the oocyte and its optimization of the IVM technique in clinical practice.

Overall, current efforts are focused on understanding the complex interaction between the oocyte and cumulus cells in an attempt to overcome the artifacts and to develop a system of in vitro maturation that is capable of supporting oocyte developmental competence.

Author details

Bassim Alsadi
Rome University, Rome, Italy

*Address all correspondence to: balsadi@hotmail.com

References

[1] Hyttel P, Fair T, Callesen H, Greve T. Oocyte growth, capacitation and final maturation in cattle. Theriogenology. 1997;**47**:23-32

[2] Hendriksen PJ, Vos PL, Steenweg WN, Bevers MM, Dieleman SJ. Bovine follicular development and its effect on the *in vitro* competence of oocytes. Theriogenology. 2000;**53**:11-20

[3] Eppig JJ, Schultz RM, O'Brien M, Chesnel F. Relationship between the developmental programs controlling nuclear and cytoplasmic maturation of mouse oocytes. Developmental Biology. 1994;**164**:1-9

[4] Eppig JJ. Coordination of nuclear and cytoplasmic oocyte maturation in eutherian mammals. Reproduction, Fertility, and Development. 1996;**8**:485-489

[5] Hussein TS, Froiland DA, Amato F, Thompson JG, Gilchrist RB. Oocytes prevent cumulus cell apoptosis by maintaining a morphogenic paracrine gradient of bone morphogenetic proteins. Journal of Cell Science. 2005;**118**:5257-5268

[6] Hussein TS, Thompson JG, Gilchrist RB. Oocyte-secreted factors enhance oocyte developmental competence. Developmental Biology. 2006;**296**:514-521

[7] Tsafriri A, Pomerantz SH. Oocyte maturation inhibitor. Clinics in Endocrinology and Metabolism. 1986;**15**:157-170

[8] Pincus G, Enzmann E. The comparative behaviour of mammalian eggs in vivo and in vitro. The Journal of Experimental Medicine. 1935;**62**:665-675

[9] Cho WK, Stern S, Biggers JD. Inhibitory effect of dibutyryl cAMP on mouse oocyte maturation in vitro. The Journal of Experimental Zoology. 1974;**187**:383-386

[10] Thomas RE, Armstrong DT, Gilchrist RB. Differential effects of specific phosphodiesterase isoenzyme inhibitors on bovine oocyte meiotic maturation. Developmental Biology. 2002;**244**:215-225

[11] Tsafriri A, Lindner HR, Zor U, Lampbrecht SA. In vitro induction of meiotic division in follicle-enclosed rat oocytes by LH, cyclic AMP and prostaglandin E2. Journal of Reproduction and Fertility. 1972;**31**:39-50

[12] Tsafriri A, Dekel N. Molecular mechanisms in ovulation. In: Findlay JK, editor. Molecular Biology Female Reproductive System. San Diego: Academic Press; 1994. pp. 207-258

[13] Kidder GM, Mhawi AA. Gap junctions and ovarian folliculogenesis. Reproduction. 2002;**123**:613-620

[14] Dekel N, Lawrence TS, Gilula NB, Beers WH. Modulation of cell-to-cell communication in the cumulus-oocyte complex and the regulation of oocyte maturation by LH. Developmental Biology. 1981;**86**:356-362

[15] Luciano AM, Franciosi F, Modina SC, Lodde V. Gap junction-mediated communications regulate chromatin remodeling during bovine oocyte growth and differentiation through cAMP-dependent mechanism(s). Biology of Reproduction. 2011;**85**(6):1252-1259

[16] Bruzzone R, White TW, Paul DL. Connections with connexins: The

molecular basis of direct intercellular signalling. European Journal of Biochemistry. 1996;**238**:1-27

[17] Bukovsky A, Svetikova M, Caudle MR. Oogenesis in cultures derived from adult human ovaries. Reproductive Biology and Endocrinology. 2005;**3**(1):17

[18] Gilchrist RB, Ritter LJ, Armstrong DT. Oocyte-somatic cell interactions during follicle development in mammals. Animal Reproduction Science. 2004;**82-83**:431-446

[19] Simon AM, Goodenough DA, Li E, Paul DL. Female infertility in mice lacking connexin 37. Nature. 1997, 1997;**385**:525-529

[20] Yeo CX, Gilchrist RB, Lane M. Disruption of Bi-directional oocyte-cumulus paracrine signaling during In vitro maturation reduces subsequent mouse oocyte developmental competence. Biology of Reproduction. 2009;**80**(5):1072-1080

[21] Dong J, Albertini DF, Nishimori K, Kumar TR, Lu N, Matzuk MM. Growth differentiation factor-9 is required during early ovarian folliculogenesis. Nature. 1996;**383**:531-535

[22] Albertini DF, Sanfins A, Combelles CM. Origins and manifestations of oocyte maturation competencies. Reproductive Biomedicine Online. 2003;**6**:410-415

[23] Plancha C, Sanfins A, Rodrigues P, et al. Cell polarity during folliculogenesis and ogenesis. Reproductive Biomedicine Online. 2005;**10**:478-484

[24] Dekel N, Beers WH. Development of the rat oocyte in vitro: Inhibition and induction of maturation in the presence or absence of the cumulus oophorus. Developmental Biology. 1980;**75**:247-254

[25] Anderson E, Albertini DF. Gap junctions between the oocyte and companion follicle cells in the mammalian ovary. The Journal of Cell Biology. 1976;**71**:680-686

[26] Albuz FK, Sasseville M, Lane M, Armstrong DT, Thompson JG, Gilchrist RB. Simulated physiological oocyte maturation (SPOM): A novel *in vitro* maturation system that substantially improves embryo yield and pregnancy outcomes. Human Reproduction. 2010;**25**(12):2999-3011

[27] Hsieh M, Zamah AM, Conti M. Epidermal growth factor-like growth factors in the follicular fluid: Role in oocyte development and maturation. Seminars in Reproductive Medicine. 2009;**27**:52-61

[28] Almahbobi G, Misajon A, Hutchinson P, Lolatgis N, Trounson AO. Hyperexpression of epidermal growth factor receptors in granulosa cells from women with polycystic ovary syndrome. Fertility and Sterility. 1998;**70**:750-758

[29] Jamnongjit M, Gill A, Hammes SR. Epidermal growth factor receptor signaling is required for normal ovarian steroidogenesis and oocyte maturation. PNAS. 2005;**102**:16257-16262

[30] De La Fuente R, O'Brien MJ, Eppig JJ. Epidermal growth factor enhances preimplantation developmental competence of maturing mouse oocytes. Human Reproduction. 1999;**14**:3060-3068

[31] Das K, Phipps WR, Hensleigh HC, Tagatz GE. Epidermal growth factor in human follicular fluid stimulates mouse oocyte maturation in vitro. Fertility and Sterility. 1992;**57**:895-901

[32] Ozornek MH, Bielfeld P, Krussel JS, Hirchenhain J, Jeyendran RS,

Koldovsky U. Epidermal growth factor and leukemia inhibitory factor levels in follicular fluid. Association with in vitro fertilization outcome. The Journal of Reproductive Medicine. 1999;**44**:367-369

[33] Volpe A, Coukos G, D'Ambrogio G, Artini PG, Genazzani AR. Follicular fluid steroid and epidermal growth factor content, and in vitro estrogen release by granulosa - luteal cells from patients with polycystic ovaries in an IVF/ET program. European Journal of Obstetrics, Gynecology, and Reproductive Biology. 1991;**42**:195-199

[34] Artini PG, Monteleone P, Toldin MRP, Matteucci C, Ruggiero M, Cela V, et al. Growth factors and folliculogenesis in polycystic ovary patients. Expert Review of Endocrinology and Metabolism. 2007;**2**:215-223

[35] Shimada M, Hernandez-Gonzalez I, Gonzalez-Robayna I, Richards JS. Paracrine and autocrine regulation of epidermal growth factor-like factors in cumulus oocyte complexes and granulosa cells: Key roles for prostaglandin synthase 2 and progesterone receptor. Molecular Endocrinology. 2006;**20**:1352-1365

[36] Tse AC, Ge W. Differential regulation of betacellulin and heparin-binding EGF-like growth factor in cultured zebrafish ovarian follicle cells by EGF family ligands. Comparative Biochemistry and Physiology. Part A, Molecular & Integrative Physiology. 2009;**153**:13-17

[37] Artini PG, Monti M, Matteucci C, Valentino V, Cristello F, Genazzani AR. Vascular endothelial growth factor and basic fibroblast growth factor in polycystic ovary syndrome during controlled ovarian hyperstimulation. Gynecological Endocrinology. 2006;**22**:465-470

[38] Van der Spuy ZM, Dyer SJ. The pathogenesis of infertility and early pregnancy loss in polycystic ovary syndrome in Arulkumaran S (editor). Clinics in Obstetrics and Gynaecology. 2004;**18**(5):755-771

[39] Diamanti-Kandarakis E. Polycystic ovarian sysndrome: Pathophysiology, molecular aspects and clinical implications. Expert Reviews in Molecular Medicine. 2008;**10**:e3

[40] Dumesic DA, Abbott DH. Implications of polycystic ovary syndrome on oocyte development. Seminar Reprod Med. 2008;**26**:53-61

[41] Grondahl C. Oocyte maturation. Danish Medical Bulletin. 2008;**55**:1-16

[42] Tsafriri A, Motola S. Are steroids dispensable for meiotic resumption in mammals? Trends in Endocrinology and Metabolism. 2007;**18**:321-327

[43] Bivens CIM, Lindenthal BL, Brien MJO, Wigglesworth K, Blume T, Grondahl C, et al. A synthetic analogue of meiosis-activating sterol (FF-MAS) is a potent agonist promoting meiotic maturation and preimplantation development of mouse oocytes maturing in vitro. Human Reproduction. 2004;**19**:2340-2344

[44] Faerge I, Strejcek F, Laurincik J, Rath D, Niemann H, Schellander K, et al. The effect of FF-MAS on porcine cumulus–oocyte complex maturation, fertilization and pronuclear formation in vitro. Zygote. 2006;**14**:189-199

[45] Chian RC, Buckett WM, Tulandi T, Tan SL. Prospective randomized study of human chorionic gonadotrophin priming before immature oocyte retrieval from unstimulated women with polycystic ovarian syndrome. Human Reproduction. 2000;**15**:165-170

[46] Gilchrist RB, Lane M, Thompson JG. Oocyte-secreted factors: Regulators of cumulus cell function and oocyte quality function and oocyte quality. Human Reproduction Update. 2008;**14**:159-177

[47] Chen YJ, Sy Z, Qiao J, Liu P, Lian Y, Zheng XY. Expression of bone morphogenetic protein-15 in human oocyte and cumulus granulosa cells primed with recombinant follicle stimulating hormone followed by human chorionic gonadotropin. Fertility and Sterility. 2009;**92**:2045-2046

[48] Teixeira Filho FL, Baracat EC, Lee TH, Suh CS, Matsui M, Chang RJ, et al. Aberrant expression of growth differentiation factor-9 in oocytes of women with polycystic ovary syndrome. The Journal of Clinical Endocrinology and Metabolism. 2002;**87**:1337-1344

[49] Shimasaki S, Moore RK, Otsuka F, Erickson GF. The bone morphogenetic protein system in mammalian reproduction. Endocrine Reviews. 2004;**25**:72-101

[50] Franks S, Robberts R, Hardy K. Gonadotrophin regimens and oocyte quality in women with polycystic ovaries. Reproductive Biomedicine Online. 2002;**6**:181-184

[51] Zhao SY, Qiao J, Chen YJ, Liu P, Li J, Yan J. Expression of growth differentiation factor-9 and bone morphogenetic protein-15 in oocytes and cumulus granulosa cells of patients with polycystic ovary syndrome. Fertility and Sterility. 2010;**94**:261-267

[52] Wu YT, Tang L, Cai J, Lu XE, Xu J, Zhu XM, et al. High bone morphogenetic protein-15 level in follicular fluid is associated with high quality oocyte and subsequent embryonic development. Human Reproduction. 2007;**22**:1526-1531

[53] Takebayashi K, Takakura K, Wang H, Kimura F, Kasahara K, Noda Y. Mutation analysis of the growth differentiation factor-9 and -9B genes in patients with premature ovarian failure and polycystic ovary syndrome. Fertility and Sterility. 2000;**74**:976-979

[54] Hennet ML, Combelles CM. The antral follicle: A microenvironment for oocyte differentiation. The International Journal of Developmental Biology. 2012;**56**:819-831

[55] Yang H, Kolben T, Meister S, Paul C, van Dorp J, Eren S, et al. Factors influencing the In vitro maturation (IVM) of human oocyte. Biomedicine. 1904;**2021**:9

[56] Dahl SK, Cannon S, Aubuchon M, Williams DB, Robins JC, Thomas MA. Follicle curetting at the time of oocyte retrieval increased the oocyte yield. Journal of Assisted Reproduction and Genetics. 2009;**26**:336-339

[57] Yang ZY, Chian RC. Development of in vitro maturation techniques for clinical applications. Fertility and Sterility. 2017;**108**:577-584

[58] Siristatidis C, Sergentanis TN, Vogiatzi P, Kanavidis P, Chrelias C, Papantoniou N, et al. In vitro maturation in women with vs. without polycystic ovarian syndrome: A systematic review and meta-analysis. PLoS One. 2015;**10**:e0134696

[59] Edwards RG. Maturation in vitro of human ovarian oocytes. Lancet. 1965;**286**:926-929

[60] Edwards RG, Donahue RP, Baramki TA, Jones HW Jr. Preliminary attempts to fertilize human oocytes matured in vitro. American Journal of Obstetrics and Gynecology. 1966;**96**:192-200

[61] Edwards RG, Bavister BD, Steptoe PC. Early stages of fertilization in vitro of human oocytes matured in vitro. Nature. 1969;**221**:632-635

[62] De Vos M, Smitz J, Thompson JG, Gilchrist RB. The definition of IVM is clear-variations need defining. Human Reproduction. 2016;**31**:2411-2415

[63] Steptoe PC, Edwards RG. Laparoscopic recovery of preovulatory human oocytes after priming of ovaries with gonadotrophins. Lancet. 1970;**1**:683-689

[64] Walls ML, Ryan JP, Keelan JA, Hart R. In vitro maturation is associated with increased early embryo arrest without impairing morphokinetic development of useable embryos progressing to blastocysts. Human Reproduction. 2015;**30**:1842-1849

[65] Lim KS, Chae SJ, Choo CW, Ku YH, Lee HJ, Hur CY, et al. In vitro maturation: Clinical applications. Clinical and Experimental Reproductive Medicine. 2013;**40**:143-147

[66] Chang EM, Song HS, Lee DR, Lee WS, Yoon TK. In vitro maturation of human oocytes: Its role in infertility treatment and new possibilities. Clinical and Experimental Reproductive Medicine. 2014;**41**:41-46

[67] Li Y, Pan P, Yuan P, Qiu Q, Yang D. Successful live birth in a woman with resistant ovary syndrome following in vitro maturation of oocytes. Journal of Ovarian Research. 2016;**9**:54

[68] Cha KY, Koo JJ, Ko JJ, Choi DH, Han SY, Yoon TK. Pregnancy after in vitro fertilization of human follicular oocytes collected from nonstimulated cycle, their culture in vitro and their transfer in adonor oocyte program. Fertility and Sterility. 1991;**55**:109-113

[69] Trounson A, Wood C, Kausche A. In vitro maturation and the fertilization and developmental competence of oocytes recovered from untreated polycystic ovarian patients. Fertility and Sterility. 1994;**62**:353-362

[70] Sauerbrun-Cutler MT, Vega M, Keltz M, McGovern PG. In vitro maturation and its role in clinical assisted reproductive technology. Obstetrical & Gynecological Survey. 2015;**70**:45-57

[71] Seok HH, Song H, Lyu SW, Kim YS, Lee DR, Lee WS, et al. Application of serum anti-Mullerian hormone levels in selecting patients with polycystic ovary syndrome for in mitro maturation treatment. Clinical and Experimental Reproductive Medicine. 2016;**43**:126-132

[72] Fadini R, Dal Canto MB, Mignini Renzini M, Brambillasca F, Comi R, Fumagalli D, et al. Effect of different gonadotrophin priming on IVM of oocytes from women with normal ovaries: A prospective randomized study. Reproductive Biomedicine Online. 2009;**19**:343-351

[73] Demirtas E, Elizur SE, Holzer H, Gidoni Y, Son WY, Chian RC, et al. Immature oocyte retrieval in the luteal phase to preserve fertility in cancer patients. Reproductive Biomedicine Online. 2008;**17**:520-523

[74] Yang H, Kolben T, Meister S, Paul C, van Dorp J, Eren S, et al. Factors influencing the In vitro maturation (IVM) of human oocyte. Biomedicine. 2021;**9**(12):1904

Chapter 5

The Role of Oocyte Cryopreservation in Assisted Reproduction

Timothy J. Gelety

Abstract

Oocyte cryopreservation (OC) has progressed rapidly from an experimental procedure with limited success to a clinically accepted procedure, in large part due to significant improvements in the techniques and widespread laboratory adaptation of vitrification. With significant improvements in clinical outcome, elective oocyte cryopreservation has gained in popularity as a means of overcoming diminishing ovarian reserve associated with aging. With clinical pregnancy rates equal to utilizing retrieved oocytes, oocyte cryopreservation is being increasingly utilized as an adjunct to standard IVF and now plays a significant role in egg donation with the establishment of egg banks analogous to sperm banks. Continuing research and clinical experience will be instrumental in defining the role of OC going forward.

Keywords: oocyte cryopreservation, Vitrification, elective oocyte cryopreservation, decreased ovarian reserve, egg donation, egg banking

1. Introduction

The Nobel Prize winning work of RG Edwards lead to the first successful pregnancy resulting from in vitro fertilization (IVF) and the birth of Louise Brown in England in 1978 [1]. Numerous improvements in the technique of controlled ovarian hyperstimulation (COH), as well as laboratory fertilization and culture technique, subsequently resulted in rapid improvement in pregnancy success and worldwide clinical acceptance. Although the cryopreservation of mammalian embryos was originally described as early as 1947 [2], the first successful live births from cryopreserved/thawed embryos following IVF were reported in 1983 by Alan Trounson's group [3]. Cryopreservation of embryos following IVF quickly gained clinical acceptance by increasing overall pregnancy success and decreasing the need for additional procedures.

Cryopreservation of unfertilized human oocytes for the purpose of fertility preservation has always been an attractive alternative to cryopreservation and storage of human embryos, posing fewer ethical, moral, religious and legal problems. However, initial attempts at oocyte cryopreservation based on the laboratory success of cryopreservation of fertilized embryos was disappointing, resulting in only a handful of successful live births by 1987 [4].

Unfertilized oocyte cryopreservation had been vexed with the technical problems of potential meiotic spindle disruption, possibly resulting in aneuploidy when traditional slow freezing utilizing cryoprotectants was used [5]. In addition, although acceptable rates of freeze–thaw survival were observed, poor fertilization with IVF was common, as was polyspermic fertilization [6]. These problems were found to be a result of changes in the zona pellucida associated with cryopreservation [7]. As such, the procedure did not attain initial widespread clinical acceptance and was relegated to being considered an experimental procedure for many years.

The hurdle of cryopreservation of mature unfertilized human oocytes was overcome by the use of ultra-rapid freezing or "vitrification". Significant improvement in fertilization of cryopreserved-thawed oocytes was the result of the widespread clinical application of intracytoplamsic sperm injection (ICSI), where a single sperm is injected through the zona pelucida into the ooplasm, overcoming the problems of poor fertilization and potential polyspermic fertilization. As a result, many live-births have been achieved over the last 25 years, and the safety and efficacy of the procedure was confirmed [8, 9]. Of interest, following thousands of live-births world wide, the procedure was deemed no longer "experimental" in 2012 by the American Society for Reproductive Medicine (ASRM), leading to widespread clinical acceptance of the procedure [10].

Oocyte cryopreservation has long been suggested as a means of fertility preservation in young women wishing to delay childbearing into their fourth and fifth decades. Likewise, fertility preservation is paramount in young women faced with potentially sterilizing procedures such as chemotherapy or radiation treatment, as well as surgery associated with modern oncology treatments. Cryopreservation of mature unfertilized oocytes can also be a valuable adjunct in IVF, particularly when sperm for fertilization is not available on the day of oocyte retrieval. Finally, oocyte cryopreservation has the potential to play a significant role in oocyte donation: adding convenience as well as screening and expanded donor selection choices, analogous to sperm donation using commercial sperm banks.

2. Vitrification

Fertilized cleavage or blastocyst stage embryos contain a diploid chromosomal complement encased within the nucleus of each cell. Cryopreservation of embryos was done originally via slow freezing using cryoprotectants that were required to avoid damage associated with cooling to sub-zero temperatures. Cryoprotectants, either permeating such as propanediol (PROH), glycerol, or dimethysulfoxide (DMSO) or non-permeating such as sucrose, were utilized to displace intracellular water and avoid cellular damage from intracellular ice formation. Seeding, to induce ice formation outside the specimen, was followed by more rapid cooling to −196 degrees Celsius and storage in liquid nitrogen [11].

In 1985, Rall and Fahey introduced the process of vitrification for the cryopreservation of mammalian embryos [12]. Using higher concentrations of cryoprotectant and rapid cooling results in vitrification (glass formation), thereby avoiding intracellular ice formation. Trounson subsequently described ultrarapid freezing techniques in human embryos [5]. The potential toxicity of cryoprotectants at higher concentrations at room temperature requires their addition at lower temperatures, but the rapid exposure to low temperatures obviates the need for costly programmed biological freezing equipment. Significant advances in the techniques of vitrification have resulted in widespread clinical acceptance [13].

Unlike embryos, immature human oocytes, which are arrested in the diplotene stage of the first meiotic prophase, are recruited by gonadotropin stimulation at the beginning of the follicular phase at which time they experience significant antral growth or atresia. Developing antral follicles morphologically exhibit the germinal vesicle (GV) by light microscopy which contains the chromosomal complement. The oocyte resumes meiosis in response to the midcycle luetenizing hormone (LH) surge, as evidenced morphologically by extrusion of the first polar body which can be seen beneath the zona pellucida (ZP). The mature oocyte therefore demonstrates evidence of germinal vesicle breakdown (GVBD) which is associated with the appearance of the spindle apparatus and the presence of the first polar body, but remains arrested in the second meiotic metaphase (MII). With fertilization, meiosis is completed and the second polar body is extruded. The polar body contains the discarded haploid chromosomal complement of the oocyte, which is visible beneath the zona pelucida followed by formation of 2 pronuclei (2pn), visible morphologically on light microscopy.

Because MII oocytes contain chromosomes which are still attached to microtubular spindle, there were concerns regarding disassembly of the meiotic spindle and dispersal of the polar pericentriolar material upon freezing and thawing that could result in an increase in chromosomal aneuploidy. Early studies of murine oocyte ultrastructure using transmission electron microscopy (TEM) have shown little adverse effect on the meiotic spindle structure following freezing/thawing either with slow cooling or ultrarapid cooling [14]. Likewise, reports of cytogenetic evaluation following oocyte freezing/thawing followed by IVF have been reassuring in both mouse and in human [8, 9], suggesting no significant increase in meiotic nondisjunction resulting in aneuploidy.

Although early reports by Chen [15] suggested excellent survival following cryopreservation of mature oocytes, with the first successful pregnancy in humans reported in 1986, poor fertilization following freezing and thawing limited the clinical success of the procedure. Poor fertilization of previously cryopreserved mature oocytes as well as problems with polyspermic fertilization have suggested changes to the ZP, such as hardening of the zona, possibly resulting from premature cortical granule release associated with changes to the oolema as a consequence of freezing and thawing. TEM evaluations of cryopreserved/thawed oocytes have shown no evidence of premature cortical granule release [6], however using TEM studies in mammalian oocyte have revealed cracks in the ZP following freezing and thawing. This suggests that physical changes in the glycoprotein architecture of the ZP may be the cause of "hardening," preventing normal fertilization or conversely for polyspermic fertilization.

Intracytoplasmic Sperm Injection (ICSI), in which a single viable spermatozoa is injected through the ZP into the oolema, was developed as treatment for severe male factor infertility and resulted in the first live births in 1992 [16]. The development of the technique followed earlier attempts at zona drilling and sub-zonal insertion of sperm to enhance fertilization, which were also plagued by polyspermic fertilization. Extensive experience with ICSI has demonstrated excellent fertilization rates, often higher than seen with standard IVF [17] and obviates the problem of polyspermic fertilization through the injection of a single sperm. Based on these results, ICSI was subsequently found to provide high rates of normal fertilization in previously cryopreserved oocytes [18], resulting in the first live birth in 1997 [19].

2.1 Fertility preservation prior to cancer treatment

Over the past 50 years; significant advances in cancer therapies, and in particular chemotherapy, has resulted in major improvement in long-term patient survival [20]. Chemotherapy and radiation therapy as well as gonadectomy can decrease the reserve of viable oocytes, resulting in immediate or premature ovarian failure (POF). The type of chemo/radiotherapy, duration, cumulative dose and patient age, have all been shown to predict POF [21]. As survival for cancer patients continues to improve, counseling prior to potential iatrogenic infertility due to planned oncology therapy in reproductive age patients has become a clinical necessity regarding the available options for fertility preservation prior to treatment [20].

For long term cancer survivors who have experienced POF due to gonadotoxic therapies or even gonadectomy, options for having children include adoption or oocyte donation. For reproductive age women in a stable committed relationship, standard IVF utilizing COH followed by fertilization using her partner's sperm and cryopreservation and storage of resulting embryos is a reasonable option for women wishing to preserve the chance of having their own biologic offspring. COH and egg retrieval can be accomplished in a relatively short time period (14–21 days), allowing time to schedule prior to starting chemotherapy, radiation therapy, or surgery, and can even be accomplished successfully after early potential gonadotoxic therapy has begun [22]. Cryopreservation of embryos offers a predictable likelihood of pregnancy success based on the age of the patient as well as the number and the quality of embryos stored. Although data on live birth rates from stored embryos prior to cancer therapy are limited, patients can be counseled based on live birth rates following use of cryopreserved embryos from the general infertility population [20].

Oocyte cryopreservation has the advantage of not requiring a partner for single women facing cancer therapy and has fewer ethical, moral, religious and legal problems than the current widespread cryopreservation of embryos. Mature oocyte cryopreservation also requires COH using gonadotropin therapy, followed by out-patient surgical oocyte retrieval and cryopreservation. Like cryopreservation of embryos, information on the pregnancy success rates following fertilization of mature oocytes from cancer patients is limited. It is clear that the age of the patient at vitrification and the number of oocytes stored are predictors of pregnancy success [23]. Live birth rates from donor and infertile patients can be a guide to counseling cancer patients however, with live birth rates as high as 46.8% reported for women less than 35 years of age [20].

For prepubertal and adolescent women facing cancer treatment, gonadotropin therapy and egg retrieval are not reasonable options for obtaining multiple mature oocytes for cryopreservation. However, ovarian biopsy, in which ovarian cortical tissue containing several hundreds or thousands of immature oocytes can be obtained for cryopreservation, is an option. Laparoscopic Ovarian Biopsy (LOB) has been shown to be a safe and effective method for obtaining ovarian tissue for cryopreservation [24]. It can be performed at the time of general anesthesia for lymph node biopsy or central line placement, immediately prior to planned cancer therapies. Histologic evaluation from ovarian biopsies performed in pre-pubertal or adolescent females have shown viable immature oocytes, even after initiation of conservative chemotherapy [24]. This allows for obtaining ovarian tissue for cryopreservation prior to more complete myeloablative therapies such as total body irradiation used in preparation for bone marrow transplantation (BMT) [24].

Due to the complexity and limited success of in vitro maturation, frozen thawed immature human oocytes, like those found in cryopreserved ovarian tissue, require in vivo maturation [25]. This involves reimplantation of autologous cryo-thawed ovarian tissue back into the patient, survival of the autologous graft, and normal maturation of oocytes which can be harvested and used in conjunction with standard IVF to achieve pregnancy and live-births [26].

Two competing strategies have been championed. Oktay and others have pursued reimplantation of the previously cryopreserved-thawed ovarian tissue into the forearm [27].

This is analogous to the procedure used for preserving parathyroid gland function following total thyroidectomy. Technical problems related to monitoring the tissue, poor graft survival, and difficulty retrieving mature eggs, have limited the widespread acceptance of this procedure over the years.

An alternative option involves re-implantation of the cryo-thawed tissue into the remaining ovary or the ovarian bed as originally described by Gosden et al. in 1994 [25]. This approach has the advantage of superior graft survival, likely due to the excellent blood supply and high oxygen tension, ease of monitoring, and ease of oocyte retrieval which is unchanged from standard IVF and widely accessible to clinicians performing egg retrieval.

Concerns have been raised regarding the theoretic risk of reintroducing malignant cells or tissue, resulting in relapse of the original cancer or disease which prompted the cryopreservation of the ovarian tissue [28]. It is important to evaluate thawed ovarian tissue prior to autotransplantation and to involve pathology and oncology specialists in the consideration of its use. With proper screening, the risk appears small, with no reported recurrences [29]. With continued experience, overall the data on safety and efficacy, as well as reproductive outcomes, has by 2019 lead to ovarian tissue cryopreservation to be considered an established medical procedure [30, 31].

3. Planned oocyte cryopreservation

With improvements in vitrification of mature oocytes, as well as significantly improved fertilization using ICSI, the pregnancy rates using cryopreserved oocytes were found to be comparable to those found using fresh oocytes with IVF [32]. More importantly, studies of the health of babies born following the use of oocyte cryopreservation have shown no increase in congenital abnormalities [8, 9]. With these reassuring clinical results, OC was no longer considered experimental by the ASRM in 2012 [10].

The success of oocyte cryopreservation has led to increased interest in cryopreserving oocytes to extend the reproductive capacity in otherwise healthy women wishing to delay childbearing. Although the ASRM initially declined to recommend OC for the "sole purpose of circumventing reproductive aging in healthy women," intense interest and an undeniable increase in efficacy lead the organization to publish a risk/benefit "fact sheet" regarding OC by 2014, followed by a stronger supportive endorsement for the procedure by 2018 [33].

The rate of first birth to women age 35–39, as well as age 40–44, continues to increase in the U.S. [34]. Increasing emphasis on education, later age at marriage, access to effective contraception and opportunity for career advancement are among many of the reasons for this trend. However, with increasing maternal age, fertility decreases dramatically beginning at 35, due to decreasing oocyte quantity and quality, resulting in increasing chromosomal abnormalities seen in failure to conceive, miscarriage and birth defects [35].

Egg donation, using higher quality eggs from young healthy donors, has historically been the treatment of choice for women wishing to conceive in their fourth and fifth decades of life. OC performed at a younger age, prior to decreasing ovarian reserve, allows for having a child using a woman's own genetic material later in life. Because a woman's age, number and quality of oocytes strongly determine the chance of pregnancy, OC cryopreservation is likely to be most successful for younger women [23]. By the age of 38, research suggests that 25–30 oocytes may be required to provide a reasonable chance of pregnancy success [36]. The cost of the procedure must be considered, as well as the cost of long term storage, particularly in young women. In addition, the possibility of achieving pregnancy naturally or with standard fertility treatments, should be taken into consideration when considering planned OC [37]. Due to the fact that at age 20–30, the time of maximal career advancement also corresponds a woman's to optimal fertility, the available option for OC has prompted several large corporations to cover the costs associated with the procedure [38], providing additional incentive for career advancement and delayed childbirth.

3.1 In vitro fertilization and oocyte cryopreservation

The success and ready availability of OC has also resulted in increasing use of the technique as an adjunct to standard IVF procedures. On the day of egg retrieval, typically a fresh semen sample is required to prepare viable spermatozoa for either standard insemination or for ICSI to accomplish fertilization of multiple mature oocytes retrieved following COH. In cases of severe oligo-asthenospermia, several samples may be cryopreserved and "banked" to ensure adequate numbers of viable spermatozoa on the day of oocyte retrieval. In cases of obstructive azoospermia, surgical extraction of spermatozoa from the epididymis or testis is typically performed prior to the planned oocyte retrieval and cryopreserved, or the planned procedure for sperm retrieval can be scheduled on the same day to obtain a fresh specimen.

In clinical practice, there are cases when fresh sperm cannot be obtained on the day of egg retrieval, either because the male partner is unexpectedly unavailable or unable to provide a sample. Also, thawing of severely oligo-asthenic semen samples may yield insufficient viable spermatozoa to fertilize any or all of the mature oocytes retrieved, particularly in cases when several dozen oocytes are obtained following COH. Likewise, planned surgical extraction procedures can be unexpectedly delayed due to surgical scheduling requirements or fail to yield viable spermatozoa sufficient for fertilization. In these cases, cryopreservation of the unfertilized mature oocytes can be performed until such time adequate viable spermatozoa are available to accomplish IVF without compromising the success of the procedure.

Other common clinical situations can arise when insufficient viable mature oocytes are obtained at the time of egg retrieval, particularly in older patients or those with significantly decreased ovarian reserve. In these cases, additional cycles of COH and egg retrieval can be performed to increase the overall number of oocytes used in IVF and in particular when genetic screening using preimplantation genetic screening (PGS) is used [39], increasing the overall pregnancy success. In addition, for patients wishing to limit or avoid freezing embryos, supernumary mature oocytes retrieved following COH can be cryopreserved [40]. As seen for other indications for oocyte cryopreservation, pregnancy rates following transfer of fresh embryos in such cycles and embryos from previously cryopreserved "sister oocytes" from the same cycle are similar [41], suggesting no significant decrease in oocyte or embryo quality.

4. Oocyte donation

The clinical problem of infertility due to inadequate number or quality of oocytes available to produce a healthy pregnancy was overcome by the introduction of oocyte donation in 1984 [42]. Patients with diminished ovarian reserve due to advanced age, POF, or gonadectomy for cancer or benign disease could conceive a pregnancy with her partner, carry the pregnancy to term and deliver a healthy child using donated oocytes from a young, healthy woman, fertilized by the patient's husband's sperm, and the resulting embryos transferred to her uterus.

Options for obtaining oocytes include "known donors," such as family members including younger sisters, cousins or same-sex partners. Alternatively, anonymous donors, analogous to sperm donors, which are chosen by matching physical characteristics such as height, weight, hair color, eye color, ethnic background, etc., can be used. Anonymous donors must be carefully screened for the absence of infectious or heritable disease which could adversely affect the health of the offspring.

Sperm donors have the advantage of providing semen samples, which can be easily cryopreserved and banked, allowing for quarantine against potential infectious agents with long incubation periods and rapid availability of a wide selection of potential donors. Unlike sperm donors, oocyte donors initially require selection of a potential donor who would undergo COH using gonadotropin treatment and ultrasound monitoring followed by oocyte retrieval and insemination of the fresh mature oocytes using the patient's partner's fresh or previously banked semen sample.

Although thorough screening of a potential oocyte donor for health, infectious disease risk factors and family history of potential genetic disease is similar to semen donors, actual screening for infectious disease is required within 3 days of oocyte retrieval by the U.S. Food and Drug Administration (FDA), compared with a 6 week quarantine period required for banked semen samples. Cryopreservation of oocytes from healthy young donors allows for similar quarantining and "banking", with ready availability of healthy, screened oocytes which can be chosen by matching the donor's physical traits, as has been in use for sperm donors for many decades. However, concerns with respect to commercialization and marketing as well as cost effectiveness and accurate reporting of pregnancy outcomes remain.

Because commercial "egg banks" are not required to report clinical outcomes per cycle start, including pregnancy, miscarriage and live birth rates, as required by law under the auspices of the Society for Assisted Reproductive Technology (SART) to the centers of disease control (CDC), caution should be exercised when interpreting the pregnancy success rates advertised by such commercial enterprises as they compete for patients seeking donor eggs [43]. Known factors influencing pregnancy success using previously cryopreserved mature oocytes include younger age of the donor [44]. Also, donors who have had previous pregnancy success in fresh cycles are associated with a higher live birth rate using cryopreserved oocytes [45].

It is also clear that as the number of donor oocytes thawed increases, there is an associated increase in the cumulative live birth rate [45]. This raises the question of cost-effectiveness of utilizing commercial egg banks and their pricing structure in terms of the cost per oocyte. Considering the rate of fertilization, embryo cleavage, blastocyst formation, implantation and miscarriage, the chance of live birth has been estimated at 8% per thawed oocyte [46]. This must be compared with the multiple oocytes and embryos obtained through conventional egg donation, which may yield multiple embryos for transfer, as well as for cryopreservation of supernumary embryos for additional attempts at pregnancy, which can increase the overall cumulative probability of successful live birth.

5. Summary

The clinical success of IVF has resulted in the rapid development and adoption of innovations including COH, embryo cryopreservation, ICSI and oocyte donation, which have been successful in overcoming infertility from multiple etiologies resulting in the birth of more than 1 million children as of 2012 [47]. By 2018, 40 years after the birth of Louise Brown, more than 8 million children have been born, worldwide [48]. Due to significant technical challenges, largely overcome by rapid improvements in vitrification and fertilization, the innovation of clinically successful oocyte cryopreservation has been much more recent, having been approved for widespread use only since 2012 [10].

The principal application of the technology remains preserving fertility potential, both for medically necessary and elective indications. Cryopreservation of unfertilized eggs has the advantage of significantly fewer ethical, moral, religious and potentially legal problems when compared with the cryopreservation and potential long-term storage of embryos. The clinical utility of OC is also clear as an adjunct to fertility treatment using IVF as well as having a significant potential role in oocyte donation. As with all important emerging innovations in the field of assisted reproductive technology, continuing research and clinical experience will be instrumental in defining the role of OC going forward.

Author details

Timothy J. Gelety
The Arizona Center for Reproductive Endocrinology and Infertility, Tucson, Arizona, USA

*Address all correspondence to: tgelety@infertility-azctr.tuccoxmail.com

References

[1] Steptoe PC, Edwards RG. Birth after reimplantation of a human embryo. Lancet. 1978;**21**:366

[2] Chang MC. Normal development of fertilized rabbit ova stored low temperature for several days. Nature. 1947;**159**:602

[3] Trounson AO, Mohr L. Human pregnancy following cryopreservation, thawing and transfer of an eight-cell embryo. Nature. 1983;**305**:707

[4] Van Steirteghem AC, Van den Abbeel E. World results of human embryo cryopreservation. In: Mashiach S, Ben-Rafael Z, Laufer N, Schenker JG, editors. Advances in Assisted Reproductive Technologies. New York: Plenum Press; 1990. pp. 601-610

[5] Trounson AO. Preservation of human eggs and embryos. Fertility and Sterility. 1986;**46**:1

[6] Sathananthan AH, Trounson A, Freeman L, Brady T. The effects of cooling human oocytes. Human Reproduction. 1988;**3**:968-977

[7] Johnson MH, Pickering SJ, George MA. The influence of cooling of the properties of the zona pellucida of the mouse oocyte. Human Reproduction. 1988;**3**:383-387

[8] Tur-Kaspa I, Gal M, Horwitz A. Genetics and health of children born from cryopreserved oocytes. Fertility and Sterility. 2007;**88**:514

[9] Noyes N. Over 900 oocyte cryopreservation babies born with no apparent increase in congenital abnormalities. Repro Biomed Online. 2009;**18**:769-776

[10] The Practice Committees of the American Society for Reproductive Medicine. Mature oocyte cryopreservation: A guideline. Fertility and Sterility. 2013;**99**:37-43

[11] Gelety TG, Surrey ES. Cryopreservation of embryos and oocytes: An update. Current Opinion in Obstetrics & Gynecology. 1993;**5**(5):606-614

[12] Rall WF, Fahy GM. Ice-free cryopreservation of mouse embryos at – 196 degees by vitrification. Nature. 1985;**313**:573-575

[13] Trounson AO, Sjoblom P. Cleavage and development of human embryos in vitro after ultrarapid freezing and thawing. Fertility and Sterility. 1988;**50**:373

[14] Aigner S, Van de Elst J, Siebrzenhrubi E, Wildt L, Van Steirteghem AC. The influence of slow and ultrarapid freezing on the organization of the meoitic spindle of the mouse oocyte. Human Reproduction. 1992;**7**:857-864

[15] Chen C. Pregnancy after human oocyte cryopreservation. Lancet. 1986;**327**:884-886

[16] Palermo G, Joris H, Devroey P, Van Steirteghem AC. Pregnancies after intracytoplasmic injection of single spermatozoon into an oocyte. Lancet. 1992;**340**:17-18

[17] Tournaye H, Verheyen G, Albano C, Camus M, Van Landuyt L, Devroey P, et al. Intracytoplasmic sperm injection versus in vitro fertilization: A randomized controlled trial and a meta-analysis of the literature. Fertility and Sterility. 2002;**78**:1030-1037

[18] Gook DA, Schiewe MC, Osborn SM, Asch RH, Jansen RPS, Johnston WIH. Intracytoplasmic sperm injection and embryo development of human oocytes cryopreserved using 1,2 propanediol. Human Reproduction. 1995;**10**:2637-2641

[19] Porcu E, Ciotti PM, Fabbri R, Magrini O, Seracchioli R, Flamingni C. Birth of a healthy female after intracytoplasmic sperm injection of cryopreserved human oocytes. Fertility and Sterility. 1997;**68**:724-726

[20] Practice Committee of the American Society for Reproductive Medicine. Fertility preservation in patients undergoing gonadotoxic therapy or gonadectomy: A committee opinion. Fertility and Sterility. 2019;**112**:1022-1032

[21] Blumenfeld Z, Avivi I, Ritter M, Rowe JM. Preservation of fertility and ovarian function and minimizing chemotherapy-induced gonadotoxicity in young women. Journal of the Society for Gynecologic Investigation. 1999;**6**:229-239

[22] Cakmak H, Katz A, Cedars MI, Rosen MP. Effective method for emergency fertility preservation: Random-start controlled ovarian stimulation. Fertility and Sterility. 2013;**100**:1673-1680

[23] Doyle JO, Richter KS, Lim J, Stillman RJ, Graham JR, Tucker MJ. Successful elective and medically indicated oocyte vitrification and warming for autologous in vitro fertilization with predicted birth probabilities for fertility preservation according to number of cryopreserved oocytes and age at retrieval. Fertility and Sterility. 2016;**105**:459-466

[24] Gelety T, McReynolds S, Wu B, Graham M. Laparoscopic ovarian biopsy (LOB) for ovarian tissue cryopreservation (OTC). In: Proceedings of the 12th World Congress of In Vitro Fertilization and Molecular Reproduction. Bologna, Italy: Monduzzi Editore; 2002. pp. 141-146

[25] Gosden RG, Baird DT, Wade JC, Webb R. Restoration of fertility to oophorectomized sheep by ovarian autografts stored at −196 degrees C. Human Reproduction. 1994;**9**:597-603

[26] Donnez J, Dolmans MM, Demylle D, Jadoul P, Pirard C, Squiffler J. Live-birth after orthtopic transplantation of cryopreserved ovarian tissue. Lancet. 2004;**364**:1405-1410

[27] Oktay K, Economos K, Kan M, Rucinski J, Veeck L, Rosenwaks Z. Endocrine function and oocyte retrieval after autologous transplantation of ovarian cortical strips to the forearm. JAMA. 2001;**286**:1490-1493

[28] Meirow, Hardan I, Dor J, Fridman E, Elizur S, Ra'anani H, et al. Searching for evidence of disease and malignant contamination in ovarian tissue stored from hematologic cancer patients. Human Reproduction. 2008;**23**:1007-1013

[29] Meirow D, Ra'anani H, Shapira M, Brenghausen M, Chaim SD, Aviel-Ronen S, et al. Transplantations of frozen-thawed ovarian tissue demonstrate high reproductive performance and the need to revise restrictive criteria. Fertility and Sterility. 2016;**106**:467-476

[30] Forman EJ, Xinying L, Ferry KM, Scott K, Treff NR, Scott RT. Oocyte vitrification does not increase the risk of embryonic aneuploidy or diminish the implantation potential of blastocysts created after intracytoplasmic sperm injection: A novel, paired randomized controlled trial using DNA fingerprinting. Fertility and Sterility. 2012;**98**:644-649

[31] The Practice Committee of the American Society for Reproductive Medicine. Evidence-based outcomes after oocyte cryopreservation for donor oocyte in vitro fertilization and planned oocyte cryopreservation: A guideline. Fertility and Sterility. 2021;**116**:36-47

[32] Crawford S, Boulet SL, Kawwass JF, Jamieson DJ, Kissin DM. Cryopreserved oocyte versus fresh oocyte reproductive technology cycles; United States 2013. Fertility and Sterility. 2017;**107**:110-118

[33] The Ethics Committee of the American Society for Reproductive Medicine. Fertility preservation and reproduction in patients facing gonadotoxic therapies: An ethics committee opinion. Fertility and Sterility. 2018;**110**:380-386

[34] Martin JA, Hamilton BE, Osterman MJK. Births in the United States, 2020. NCHS Data Brief. 2021;**418**:1-8

[35] Munne S, Alikani M, Tomkin G, Grifo J, Cohen J. Embryo morphology, developmental rates and maternal age are correlated with chromosomal abnormalities. Fertility and Sterility. 1995;**64**:382-391

[36] Nagy ZP, Anderson RE, Feinberg EC, Hayward B, Mahony MC. The human oocyte preservation experience (HOPE) registry: Evaluation of cryopreservation techniques and oocyte source on outcomes. Reproductive Biology and Endocrinology. 2017;**15**:10

[37] Goldman RH, Racowsky C, Farland RV, Munné S, Ribustello L, Fox JH. Predicting the likelihood of live birth for elective oocyte cryopreservation: A counseling tool for physicians and patients. Human Reproduction. 2017;**32**:853-859

[38] Arielle YS, Mullin C, Hershlag A, Singer T, Goldman RH. Employer-based insurance coverage dramatically increases utilization of planned oocyte cryopreservation. Fertility and Sterility. 2019;**112**:e137-e138

[39] Chamayou S, Sicali M, Alecci C, Ragolia C, Liprino A, Nibali D, et al. The accumulation of vitrified oocytes is a strategy to increase the number of euploid available blastocysts for transfer after preimplantation genetic testing. Journal of Assisted Reproduction and Genetics. 2017;**34**:479-486

[40] Herrero L, Pareja S, Aragones M, Cobo A, Bronet F, Garcia-Velasco JA. Oocyte versus embryo vitrification for delayed embryo transfer: An observational study. Reproductive Biomedicine Online. 2014;**29**:567-572

[41] Rienzi L, Romano S, Albricci L, Maggiuli R, Capalbo A, Baroni E, et al. Embryo development of fresh 'versus' vitrified metaphase II oocytes after ICSI: A prospective randomized sibling-oocyte study. Human Reproduction. 2010;**25**:66-73

[42] Lutjen P, Trounson A, Leeton J, Findlay J, Wood C, Renou P. The establishment and maintenance of pregnancy using in vitro fertilization and embryo donation in a patient with primary ovarian failure. Nature. 1984;**307**:174

[43] American Society for Reproductive Medicine. Planned oocyte cryopreservation for women seeking to preserve future reproductive potential: An ethics committee opinion. Fertility and Sterility. 2018;**110**:1022-1028

[44] Trokoudes KM, Pavlides C, Zhang X. Comparison outcome of fresh and vitrified donor oocytes in an egg-sharing donation program. Fertility and Sterility. 2011;**95**:1996-2000

[45] Cobo A, Garrido N, Pellicer A, Remohi J. Six years' experience in ovum donation using vitrified oocytes: Report of cumulative outcomes, impact of storage time, and development of a predictive model for oocyte survival rate. Fertility and Sterility. 2015;**104**:1426-34. e1-e8

[46] Potdar N, Gelbaya TA, Nardo LG. Oocyte vitrification in the 21st century and post-warming fertility outcomes: A systematic review and meta-analysis. Reproductive Biomedicine Online. 2014;**29**:159-176

[47] Adamson GD, Tabangin M, Macaluso M, de Mouzon J. The number of babies born globally after treatment assisted reproductive technologies (ART). Fertility and Sterility. 2013;**100**:1807

[48] Fauser B. Towards the global coverage of a unified registry of IVF outcomes. RBMO. 2019;**38**:133-137

Chapter 6

Quality Management System in Medical Assisted Reproductive Technology (MART)

Delia Hutanu and Ioana Rugescu

Abstract

A quality management system (QMS) refers to an organization's broader approach to minimize deficiencies and errors, to meet regulatory compliance standards, and to satisfy a specified set of inherent characteristics during the health care services provided to patients. According to the European directives and recommendations (European Commission, 2006a, c, 2012; Council of Europe, 2013), working in compliance with a QMS is mandatory. The requirements cover the organization, management, personnel, equipment and materials, facilitics/premises, documentation, records, and quality review. The IVF clinics should consider total quality management (TQM) as an option, especially in these days when escalating regulatory scrutiny increases the pressure for professional accreditation. TQM is an integrative philosophy of management for continuously improving the quality of services and processes and includes quality assurance (QA), quality control (QC), quality improvement (QI), and risk assessment and risk management. QMS must become an essential topic for those who are working in MART.

Keywords: quality management system, total quality management

1. Introduction

Medical assisted reproductive technology (MART) represents the sum of medical procedures used by healthcare providers in order to help infertile patients to achieve a pregnancy. It is a complex process, and the success depends on various factors such as patient-related and some other not patient-related. The present chapter focuses on the quality management system involved in assisted reproductive facilities. Taking into account all European directives and recommendations, as well as the national laws/regulations, the present material wants to summarize the present status of the quality management system.

2. Quality management system

A quality management system (QMS) refers to an organization's broader approach to minimizing deficiencies and errors, meeting regulatory compliance standards, and satisfying a specified set of inherent characteristics during the health care services provided to patients.

According to the European directives and recommendations (European Commission, 2006a, c, 2012; Council of Europe, 2013), working in compliance with a QMS is mandatory. The requirements cover the organization, management, personnel, equipment and materials, facilities/premises, documentation, records, and quality review. Moreover, in vitro fertilization (IVF) clinics should consider total quality management (TQM) as an option, especially in these days when escalating regulatory scrutiny increases the pressure for professional accreditation. TQM is an integrative philosophy of management for continuously improving the quality of services and processes and includes quality assurance (QA), quality control (QC), quality improvement (QI), and even risk assessment and risk management. QMS must become the essential topic for those who are working in MART.

In the following pages, this chapter will bring together the most important information and tools that will allow the reader to start, implement, and maintain a QMS in his own unit, searched in literature, guidelines, and several consensuses. This chapter is intended to be a condensed pill of quality management information that will treat the reader's acute need for information on this topic.

The concept of "quality" has been defined over time in many ways and viewed from many angles and points of view, probably precisely because it has been and continues to be a topic of great importance and relevance. Any organization that respects itself and wants to be part of modern accreditation schemes has the entire activity based on the principles of a quality system. In 1979, Crosby defined five stages in the development of a quality management system and Garven in 1988 proposed a four-stage development model, so there it has been more than four decades since organizations are focused on good quality products or services. As a definition, although it seems simplistic, quality management; means coordinated activities to lead and control an organization in the field of quality.

2.1 Quality management principles

As an approach initially, eight principles were proposed as follows:

1. Process-based approach

2. Leadership

3. Staff involvement

4. Customer/patient orientation

5. Management approach as a system

6. Fact-based approach to decision making

7. Continuous improvement of performance

8. Mutually beneficial relationships with suppliers

In medically assisted human reproduction units, but especially in terms of testing, processing, cryopreservation, storage, distribution of reproductive cells and reproductive tissues in embryology and/or andrology laboratories it is imperative that the organization be based on ISO 9000 standards principles and other relational standards. In particular, the embryology part is especially important for the risk management and the minimization of errors.

As a result of the MART activity expansion and also taking into account the globalization that is taking place in the healthcare services sector, quality and risk management have become a necessity. In this context, in order to provide medical services that are intended to have the expected result in conditions of maximum safety, it was necessary that all licensed IVF units that offer such services operate in accordance with international standards, such as ISO 9001 [1], thus reflecting the current awareness of these services not only from a medical point of view but also from a commercial point of view.

The structure and organization of a licensed IVF unit may vary depending on a several number of factors, such as its size, and various types of organizational structures have been described in the literature by Dale, 1998; Heller and Hindle, 2003 [2, 3].

2.2 Legislation, certification, accreditation/licensing

Even if may vary from country to country, legislation, certification, and accreditation/licensing are often confused with each other or are seen as points of view in the management of an IVF unit, in fact, they are completely different concepts and all three work together for an integrated management system.

Legislation or the legislative requirements that an organization (IVF unit) must comply with in order to have permission to offer healthcare services. Compliance with legislative requirements is verified by an individual inspection of the unit and is confirmed by licensing/accreditation.

Generally, the legislative requirements are of the restrictive indicative type and provide precise indications regarding what an organization must comply with in accordance with the legislation in force.

The accreditation/licensing is the set of requirements and the process by which an organization must meet and is identified as complying, in order to be licensed / accredited and that they must maintain throughout the license/accreditation period. In EU member states, usually, this accreditation/licensing is issued by the Health Ministry and/or National Competent Authority. In other countries, the process may vary.

In addition, there is a certification that can be defined as a process by which an organization is identified as complying with and meeting certain criteria. In the case of IVF units, the ISO 9000 standards family applies (ISO 9001: 1994, ISO 9002: 1994, ISO 9003: 1994) with revised editions, for example, ISO 9001: 2002.

It is also possible to consider ISO 19011: 2002, as well as ISO 15189: 2003, and last but not least the ISO 17025: 2005 standard. The certification system implemented by ESHRE (European Society for Assisted Human Reproduction and Embryology-ARTCC) can also be considered. Regarding the legislative requirements for EU member states, the European Directives for Tissues and Cells and their implementation in the member state's national legislation must be taken into account. From this point of view, in the case of IVF clinics, we must consider the following:

- EUTCD Directive 2004 23 EC
- EUTCD Directive 2006 17 EC
- EUTCD Directive 2006 86 EC

In October 2020, the commission adopted its work program for 2021. The work program includes the revision of EU directives for tissues and cells. This revision comes after an evaluation of available translations of the preceding of the legislation, published in October 2019, confirming that the legislation had improved the safety and quality of blood, tissues, and cells used for transfusion, transplantation, or medically assisted reproduction. The evaluation also highlighted a number of gaps and shortcomings, which will be addressed to ensure the framework is up-to-date, fit for purpose, and future-proof. The initiative aims at updating the legislation in the direction of a more flexible alignment with scientific and technological developments tackling the re- emergence of communicable diseases, including lessons learned from the COVID-19 pandemic focusing on the increasing commercialization and globalization of the sector removing from legislation many technical provisions, which will allow a faster update of standards possibly merging the basic acts into a single instrument. The revision is planned to be adopted in the second quarter of 2022. The legal basis is provided by Article 168(4)(a) of the treaty on the functioning of the European Union [4].

Although the field of medically assisted human reproduction is very well known, quality management is much more used and implemented in embryology laboratories and it is based on monitoring cellular activity in terms of monitoring parameters in the workspace, equipment, etc.

It is well known that as a result of the action of some physic-chemical agents, the embryos are greatly affected, so that for correct implementation of a quality system all the parameters that can bring/produce changes regarding the embryonic development must be monitored.

Within an efficient quality management system, it is known that the performance indicators of the system play an important role, in our case the performance indicators of the activity.

In the quality management of an IFV unit, it is very important to be aware of the proactive tools in terms of risk management and to use these tools in a designed system in order to optimize the processes.

If we discuss the embryology or andrology laboratories, we must also standardize as much as possible the evaluation of oocytes, sperm, and embryos because they are considered to be essential components in the qualitative monitoring of the laboratory's processes.

Quality management is summarized as:

1. Quality control
2. Quality assurance
3. Quality improvement

From the point of view of risk management, the most important aspects to consider are:

1. Elimination of risk

2. Avoiding risks

3. Risk minimization

4. Risk transfer

5. Accepting risk

Regarding the management system:

1. Schematic of the processes

2. Analysis systems

3. Indicators and reference criteria

At this point, risk management is considered to be an integral part of proactive quality management [5, 6].

2.3 Indicators and benchmarks

Indicators: (we cannot control something we cannot measure).
That is why the indicators must be:

- Reliable- in order to measure something useful that is defining for the process to be monitored;

- Robust- in order to minimize foreign effects in the idea of measuring only the process to which it refers;

Routine data collection should not be difficult without a lot of extra work.

In order to optimize the activity and the results, it must be taken into account that the whole process is governed by the biology of gametes and embryos; therefore, it must ensure optimal conditions for gametes and embryos; protect gametes and embryos from physiological stress; and protect gametes and embryos from adverse external factors.

Cellular stress is a high-energy consumer and can also lead to altered gene expression and/or, for example, imprinting. Suboptimal embryonic culture may lead to irreparable changes that may affect the future conception product.

Another important step in quality management is the recognition of all the factors of influence that affect the processes in the embryology/andrology laboratories.

Possible sources of influence can be derived from the patient but also derived from clinical processes: ovarian stimulation, ovarian puncture during oocyte pick-up, embryo transfer, and luteal support.

The environmental design and construction of space, design of the workflow, equipment, work circuit, and air can influence the procedures. Among other factors that can have an influence on the process are: temperature, Co_2/pH, equipment calibration, and faulty operation.

The materials used in the IVF lab should be suitable for use, not to be embryo or cytotoxic, to be manufactured by a certified manufacturer in terms of quality (CE marking), or to be validated. All the methods used during the process have to be appropriate for the purpose, correctly chosen, SOP (documented), and lastly, the staff of the facility should be trained and skilled.

From the point of view of the sources of influence, the optimization of the system in the (embryology/andrology laboratories) for each component of the process must take into account the following:

1. Identify processes accurately.

2. Identifying the necessary pro factors to ensure the operability of the processes in optimal parameters.

3. Ensuring all of them as well as optimal control of these factors.

4. Identifying all the factors that can negatively influence the processes.

5. Ensuring that all possible interference is controlled, minimized and, if possible, eliminated.

6. Monitoring all processes and outcomes.

2.4 Key point indicators in IVF laboratory

Another important step for an efficient quality management system is the selection of key indicators for the medically assisted human reproduction process. In this case, the Vienna consensus on performance indicators in medically assisted human reproduction laboratories must be taken into account.

Performance indicators (PIs) are objective measures for assessing critical areas (patient safety, efficacy, fairness, patient fairness, timeliness, and effectiveness of medical treatments). In the activity of medically assisted human reproduction, quality indicators are needed for the systematic monitoring and evaluation of its contribution to patient care (ISO15189-2012), and it is a vital element in the quality management system (QMS) [6].

Any performance indicator must be reliable and robust, and the collection of data for tracking the indicator should be straightforward. In addition, the biological or technical process that we want to monitor must be defined with certainty. Key performance indicators (KPIs) are indicators that are considered essential for evaluating the introduction of a technique or process; setting minimum standards of competence; monitoring ongoing performance in a quality management system (for quality control (IQC), external quality assurance (EQA)); and benchmarking and quality improvement.

In general, the results of a series of key performance indicators (KPIs) will provide you with an adequate overview of the most important steps in the medically assisted human reproduction process [7].

The requirement for defining a process within quality management are:

1. Defining the process to be monitored,

2. Measuring only the desired process.

3. Minimization of external influences.

KPI	Competency	Benchmark
ICSI damage rate	≤10	≤5
ICSI normal fertilization rate	≥65	≥80
IVF normal fertilization rate	≥60	≥75
Failed fertilization rate IVF	<5	<5
Cleavage rate	≥95	≥99
Day 2 embryo development rate	≥50	≥80
Day 3 embryo development rate	≥45	≥70
Blastocyst development rate	≥40	≥60
Successful biopsy rate	≥90	≥95
Blastocyst cryosurvival rate	≥90	≥99
Implantation rate (cleavage stage)	≥25	≥35
Implantation rate (blastocyst stage)	≥35	≥60

Table 1.
KPIs in IVF lab.

In accordance with Vienna consensus [8], for a high-quality management system, three types of indicators have been identified that can be monitored:

a. Benchmarks - refer to the input indicators for assisted human reproduction activity and represent the connection between clinical and laboratory indicators.

b. Performance Indicators - this data should be documented and stored even if it is not currently reported in the control charts.

c. Key performance indicators - refer to the basic activity of the laboratory and always appear in the control diagrams (**Table 1**).

Considering the cryopreservation, the Alpha consensus on cryopreservation key performance indicators and benchmarks divided these into the following categories:

1. Cryopreserved oocytes KPI

2. Cryopreserved zygotes KPI

3. Cryopreserved embryos KPI

4. Cryopreserved blastocysts KPI

2.4.1 Oocytes

2.4.1.1 Morphological survival

This KPI was defined as the proportion of morphologically intact oocytes, based on the intention to inject, at the time of ICSI. Oocytes with oolemma or abnormal ooplasm at the time of ICSI should not be excluded (**Table 2**).

KPI		Competency	Benchmark
Morphological survival	Freezing	⩾50%	75%
	Vitrification	70%	85%

Table 2.
KPIS for morphological survival of cryopreserved oocytes.

As this KPI may be affected by the number of cases and/or the experience of the practitioner, different values have been assigned to achieve competence for both slow freezing and vitrification. Competency values are those that should be achieved by any practitioner, while reference intervals are aspirational targets.

2.4.1.2 Fertilization rate

The fertilization rate indicator was defined as the proportion of oocytes with two pronuclei at the time of fertilization verification (17 ± 1 h after insemination). The fertilization rate should be no more than 10% lower than that for the fresh oocyte in the center.

2.4.1.3 Embryonic development rate

The embryonic development rate indicator is defined as the proportion of embryos in the developmental stage that reach the stage of development specifically for the time of observation (2-cell stage at 26 ± 1 h after ICSI, 4-cells stage at 44 ± 1 h after insemination, 8-cells stage at 68 ± 1 h after insemination, morula stage at 92 ± 2 h after insemination, and the blastocyst stage at 116 ± 2 h after insemination).

The rate of embryonic development for embryos from vitrified oocytes should be the same as for the comparable population of fresh embryos from the bank of reproductive cells and tissues. For embryos from cryopreserved by slow freezing oocytes, some developmental delays may occur, but no more than 10–30% lower than that for the fresh embryos at the center.

2.4.1.4 Implantation rate

The implantation rate indicator was defined as the proportion of ultrasound-confirmed pregnancies with fetal heartbeat relative to the number of embryos transferred. The implantation rate for embryos from cryopreserved oocytes should be at most 10–30% lower than a comparable population of fresh embryos from the laboratory.

2.4.2 Zygotes

For zygotes produced by ICSI, the observations made during the ICSI procedure regarding the oocyte quality should always be recorded. This would allow a possible further analysis of the prevalence of oolemma/ooplasm abnormalities that could have been caused by the cryopreservation procedure.

2.4.2.1 Morphological survival rate

This KPI was defined as the proportion of morphologically intact zygotes immediately after thawing/devitrification compared to the number of morphologically preserved zygotes. A morphologically intact zygote is one that is similar in appearance to a fresh zygote. The same survival rate should be achieved by slow freezing as well as vitrification.

2.4.2.2 Cleavage rate

This KPI was defined as the proportion of thawed/devitrified zygotes that divide to form a cleavage embryo. The rate of division should be the same as for the comparable population of fresh embryos in the bank of reproductive cells and tissues.

2.4.2.3 Embryonic development rate

The embryonic development rate indicator is defined as the proportion of embryos in the developmental stage that reach the stage of development specifically for the time of observation.

2.4.2.4 Implantation rate

The implantation rate indicator was defined as the proportion of fetal ultrasound-confirmed pregnancies with fetal heart rate relative to the number of embryos transferred. The implantation rate for embryos from cryopreserved zygotes should be no more than 10–30% lower than that for the comparable population of fresh embryos at the center (**Table 3**).

2.4.3 Embryos

For the KPI calculation, the embryos selected for cryopreservation should meet the criteria for an optimal embryo at the cleavage stage.

2.4.3.1 Indicators - post-freezing survival rate from a morphological point of view

The KPIs that assess the post-freezing survival rate for embryos are based on the proportion of thawed/devitrified embryos with 100% and ⩾50% of the total intact embryos. For the first category, embryos thawed with 100% of the total intact embryos, the competence value is 40% and the benchmark is 55%, and for the devitrified embryos, the competence value is 70% and the benchmark is 85%. For the category with embryos thawed with ⩾50% of the total intact cells, the competence value is 60% and the benchmark is 85% and for the devitrified embryos, the competence value is 85% and the benchmark is 95%. It should be noted that KPI values do

KPI	Competency	Benchmark
Morphological survival	70%	85%
Cleavage rate	The same as for the comparable population of fresh embryos at the center.	
Embryo development rate	The same as for the comparable population of fresh embryos at the center.	
Implantation rate	No more than 10–30% lower than that for the comparable population of fresh embryos at the center.	

Table 3.
KPIs cryopreserved zygotes.

not prevent the transfer of embryos with suboptimal morphology, as this may be the only opportunity for patients.

2.4.3.2 Development rate indicator after thawing/warming

For the calculation of this key performance indicator, only the embryos with 100% intact morphological structure will be considered after thawing/warming. Post-cryopreservation development includes cleavage and further development at the blastocyst stage, as well as implantation rate, defined as the proportion of ultrasound-confirmed pregnancies with fetal heartbeats relative to the number of embryos transferred.

The competence value for the rate of embryo development after thawing/warming should be at most 10% (relatively) lower than the comparable population of fresh embryos in the laboratory and the benchmark value should be the same as for the comparable population of fresh embryos at the center.

2.4.4 Blastocysts

As the in vitro growth rate is substantially affected by exogenous factors, no key differences were made between the performance indicators of post-freezing/ vitrification blastocysts and blastocyst stages (early, full, expanded blastocyst, hatched). Similarly, there is no recommendation on blastocyst collapse. The decision will be made by each lab accordingly. Regarding the reported results for cryopreserved embryos cryopreserved in the blastocyst stage, they are substantially better after vitrification than after slow freezing.

2.4.4.1 Survival rate

The blastocyst survival rate indicator after cryopreservation is defined as the proportion of surviving blastocysts relative to the total number of thawed/devitrified blastocysts and applies to blastocysts with at least 75% intact morphology.

2.4.4.2 Transfer rate

This KPI has been defined as the proportion of thawed/warmed blastocysts that are of sufficient quality to be transferred. This parameter assumes that the transfer decision is not subject to legislative limitations in terms of the number of embryos transferred per patient and does not take into account the transfer decisions of some suboptimal blastocysts. No matter the type of embryo transfer (single, double, or multiple).

2.4.4.3 Implantation rate

The implant rate indicator was defined as the proportion of ultrasound-confirmed pregnancies with fetal heartbeats relative to the number of blastocysts transferred (**Table 4**).

KPI		Competency	Benchmark
Survival rate	Freezing	70%	85%
	Vitrification	80%	95%
Transfer rate	Freezing	70%	85%
	Vitrification	80%	95%
Implantation rate		⩽10% lower than that for the comparable population of fresh embryos at the center.	The same as for the comparable population of fresh embryos at the center.

Table 4.
KPIs for cryopreserved blastocysts.

2.4.5 Sperm

The performance indicators for sperm are related to:

1. Sperm recovery rate

2. Sperm motility post-wash

The expected proportion of motile spermatozoa in the final washed preparation showed values of 90% for competency and 95% for the benchmark.

Sperm recovery rate, defined as the percentage recovery of progressively motile sperm after washing as compared to pre-washing, can be used as a laboratory KPI, providing useful information for inter-operator comparison and proficiency testing.

2.5 Clinical KPI

Performance indicators (PIs) are a valid method to be sure that the medical facility is of high quality and it operates within acceptable limits. In order to reach these goals in 2019 was published the Maribor consensus [9]. The paper recommends six PIs to be monitored in clinical work in ovarian stimulation for ART: cycle cancelation rate (before oocyte pick-up), rate of cycles with moderate/severe ovarian hyperstimulation syndrome, the proportion of mature oocytes at ICSI, complication rate after OPU, clinical pregnancy rate, and multiple pregnancy rate.

1. Cancelation is an unexpected event that can occur before the oocyte pick-up. The values depend on the population and is ranging from 3% in high responders, 20% in the general population, and up to 40% in poor responders

2. Rate of cycles with moderate/severe ovarian hyperstimulation syndrome: The excessive ovarian response is characterized by the growth of a large number of follicles. Several follicle thresholds have been proposed as critical for predicting the occurrence of OHSS. For example, 14 follicles larger than 11 mm in the general population or > 20 follicles larger than 11 mm for patients with PCOS

(polycystic ovary syndrome) [10]. The value of the rate of cycles with moderate/severe ovarian hyperstimulation syndrome is 6.43% and 10.61% in regular and PCOS groups.

3. The proportion of mature oocytes at ICSI. Oocyte retrieval rate (ORR) or the proportion of oocytes recovered is defined as the number of oocytes retrieved during oocyte pick-up over the number of follicles on the day of trigger (**Table 5**). The proportion of MII (metaphase II) oocytes at ICSI or the rate of mature oocytes was categorized as a reference indicator in Vienna consensus and it is the number of mature oocytes at ICSI over the number of cumulus-oocytes complexes retrieved.

4. The complication rate after oocyte pick-up: Complications of oocyte pick-up include bleeding (severe vaginal, intra-abdominal, or intra-peritoneal bleeding), infections (pelvic or ovarian abscess, pelvic infections), and severe pain or injury of pelvic structures. Vaginal bleeding appears the most common complication, with a reported incidence ranging from 0.01–0.1%. Peritoneal bleeding is a more serious complication of oocyte pick-up and has an incidence of 0.05–0.35%. Pelvic organ (bladder, bowel, and ureters) injury ranges from 0.04–0.77%. Severe pain requiring hospitalization is reported to occur in 0.065to 0.7% of the cases [11, 12].

5. Clinical pregnancy rate: Clinical pregnancy rate (CPR) is a commonly used criterion for measuring the effectiveness of ART, even though is not the final objective of the procedure. However, CPR is associated with clinician skills; therefore, it is relevant to be used as the main PI for ET. Clinical pregnancy is defined as a pregnancy confirmed on ultrasound by visualization of one or more gestational sacs. The benchmark value for CPR is problematic due to a lack of standardization. The Maribor consensus proposed that CPRs competency and benchmark values should be defined at the local level.

6. Multiple pregnancy rate: Multiple pregnancy or gestation is defined as a pregnancy with more than one embryo [13]. Multiple pregnancy is the most frequent and serious iatrogenic complication in ART. The value of it is ranging from 1.1 to 35.7%. lowering the occurrence of multiple pregnancies or deliveries is a desirable goal in ART to increase the safety.

A well-developed system in terms of quality management in the ART clinic must be taken into account the moment when following the monitoring and evaluation of the processes we find that there are problems. That is why an evaluation and correction process must be identified and developed. For a good administration of a scheme for the evaluation and solution of a nonconformity, it is absolutely necessary the root cause analysis (RCA). Such an analysis is the basis of a process that must take place after a problem has arisen.

RI	Benchmark value
Proportion of oocytes recovered	80–95% of follicles measured
Proportion of MII oocytes at ICSI	75–90%

Table 5.
Oocyte retrieval rate and proportion of mature oocytes at ICSI.

DOI: http://dx.doi.org/10.5772/intechopen.106172

In this case, it is necessary to identify the factors that led to the appearance of a nonconformity; therefore, we will classify the factors as follows:

a. No contribution

b. Contributors

c. There is not enough data to establish

In the latter case, the need arises to create or access the necessary data in order to run a new classification. If we identify a number of factors, it is necessary to prioritize them in order to build a risk mold. Following the identification and ranking of contributing factors, an action plan must be developed and implemented. In general, in an ART clinic, the appearance of nonconformities is due to an accumulation of contributing factors and less to a single cause.

Also, the literature recommends that the term "cause" not be used in the reports prepared due to the possible psychological and/or legal impact.

In order for a noncompliance process to be effective, it must be effective and:

1. Leads to the normalization of operations in the shortest time.

2. Leads to a better understanding of the processes, including the performance we want within them.

3. It provides us with both previous and current information about these processes, we must be able to establish at least one key performance indicator, if not more, and be able to make control charts.

4. It offers us the possibility to analyze the processes in depth, using (ideally) additional data that we already have.

5. Leads to minimizing the possibility of similar situations in the future.

Due to technological progress, it has been possible for four decades to get from the first cultures of animal embryos to the culture and transfer of genetically tested human embryos. All these advances require quality control and also quality assurance methods in assisted human reproduction laboratories precisely to ensure repeatable processes. If progress is constant all specialists recommend the introduction of a total quality management system (TQM).

Quality control (QC) in the activities of the bank of reproductive cells and tissues is essential for its smooth running. Quality control must work in parallel with the specific activities of the bank. Recording the temperature of the equipment is an example of a quality control activity. All these control activities have been specially planned to be able to demonstrate and verify if, for example, that equipment produces the same results every time.

In terms of quality assurance (QA), this consists of complex methods of monitoring and evaluating all the processes in a bank. While quality control is concomitant with banking activities, quality assurance is a retrospective process. Also, for good quality management, we have to take into account the qualitative improvements (QI) through which we raise the performance of the activities in the ART clinic.

QI is different from QA and QC and is specifically designed to identify and correct problems or errors in the processes and activities of the ART clinic.

An example of QI is to adapt the laboratory's procedures to new zygote evaluation technologies precisely to improve the criteria for selecting embryos for transfer.

Total quality management (TQM) is a combination of all three of these topics.

This orientation does not change the structure of authority in the organization, nor does it diminish the essential role of top management. The inverted hierarchy emphasizes "service delivery" relationships and the importance of the consumer to the organization, which is why it is the perfect model for healthcare organizations.

An important part of QMS is the environment in the processing space: Laboratory staff must inspect the equipment to ensure that it is in good working order. Instruments used to determine temperature, gas concentration, and relative humidity must be recalibrated at the latest within 1 year.

If the manufacturer recommends another interval, the manufacturer's recommendation will be followed. The maintenance of all equipment must also be considered (according to the manufacturer's instructions and in accordance with the organization's policy).

The recommended monitoring parameters documented measures of continuous evaluation, correction, and monitoring of the activity, as well as, but not limited to:

1. Temperature in incubators (continuous and at three months measurement with separate equipment),

2. Temperature on heated surfaces (daily and at six months measurement with separate equipment),

3. Air temperature in the processing area and/or storage area (continuously and at three months measurement with separate equipment),

4. Temperature in refrigerators (daily and once a month measurement with separate equipment),

5. Temperature in containers of liquid nitrogen (or nitrogen level), (weekly or more often, depending on the evaporation rate of each container);

6. Determination of the level of CO_2 (or mixture, as the case may be) in incubators by direct or indirect measurement—continuous and at three months measurement with separate equipment;

7. Determination of positive pressure (continuous and at 12 months measurement with separate equipment).

2.6 Air quality

The first references to this topic appeared in the 1990s when the first correlations between various toxic agents (bacteria, dust, and VOC = volatile organic components) and embryonic development were reported. Johnson published a study on the influence of VOCs on embryonic culture [14] and Boone published studies on this topic [15]. Other authors published similar findings [16, 17]. Kao published a study that showed improved results based on air quality in the processing area [18]. At present, it is mandatory in most countries to have purified air in the ART laboratory. Most laboratories use HEPA-type ventilation and purification systems (0.3 μm is the average of airborne particles found in measurements). Some of the ART laboratories that process reproductive cells have added ULPA filters, which bring improvements in air quality. It is recommended to have ISO class V regarding the number of airborne particles (grade A). It is also important to monitor the level of VOCs both in the air in the cell processing space and the level inside the incubators [19]. In any case, the HEPA/ULPA filtration system does not exclude the occurrence of VOCs neither in the air in the processing area nor in the incubator environment.

During the measurements carried out in various laboratories, aromatic hydrocarbons like (benzene, toluene, and xylene) were found, probably from the paints used as well as isoflurane due to the fact that the reproductive cell processing space is located in the immediate vicinity of the puncture room. Other VOCs found were propane and hexane, as well as aldehydes, probably from perfume and/or deodorants used by staff [20]. Incubation gas monitoring revealed benzene in CO2 cylinders, which leads to the recommendation to use special filters on the gas transport system [21].

Due to reports of ethylbenzene and benzaldehyde emissions from plastic consumables, special consumables that do not eliminate VOCs are currently being used [22]. Since VOCs are oil-soluble, even the closed culture system (under oil) does not protect embryos from these toxic substances.

Because over time, a number of VOCs from the outside air have been reported, taken over by the HEPA/ULPA ventilation system [23] or the air to be partially recirculated in case the outside air does not correspond to the norms. Fresh air supply of 30% is recommended to use, and also an active charcoal filtration system.

The quality system in an ART clinic is a component part of the total quality management system (TQM). The quality assurance system when performing the tests is formulated in the quality manual and can be developed according to the provisions of SR EN ISO/CEI 17025: 2002.

ISO 17025 is the standard that specifies the requirements for proficiency testing and/or calibration. This standard includes 15 quality management requirements and 10 technical requirements. These requirements show what an ART laboratory needs to do to be accredited.

2.7 Risk analysis

Risk analysis is a process that incorporates three components:

1. Risk evaluation

2. Risk management

3. Risk communication

The person in charge of the reproductive cell and tissue bank has, among other responsibilities, the one related to the implementation of a risk management and prevention policy. According to European Directives and recommendations (European Commission, 2006a, c, 2012; Council of Europe, 2013), work in accordance with a quality management system (QMS) is mandatory. Requirements cover organization, management, personnel, equipment and materials, facilities/premises, documentation, records, and quality assessment. It includes, but is not limited to:

- Providing risk assessment analyses for all activities in the ART clinic.
- Proactive risk assessments and preventive measures must be taken to minimize noncompliance.
- Organize the workspace carefully for the comfort of the operator to provide a safe working environment that minimizes the risk of distraction, fatigue; therefore, the occurrence of an error.
- Informing staff about how viral-positive patients to be treated and awareness of the risks of handling infected biological material.
- Ensuring easy identification of all PTAs (ancillary therapeutic products) to avoid misuse—risk analysis.
- Minimizing any risk of transmitting possible contamination through LN2.

Risk assessment is used to describe the general process or method of identifying hazards and risk factors that have the potential to cause harm (identifying hazards), and analyzing and assessing the risk associated with that hazard (risk analysis and risk assessment).

A danger is anything that can cause harm; these can be physical health hazards, such as chemicals, electricity, working on stairs, an open drawer, or mental health.

The risk is high or low that someone will be injured by these or other hazards, along with an indication of how serious the injury may be.

There are five steps in risk assessment:

1. Hazard identification.
2. Identification of the recipient of the possible injury (staff, patient, embryos, visiting equipment, relatives, etc.)
3. Risk assessment (what is the probability that each identified hazard will cause harm. Also, determine whether to reduce the level of risk. Even after all precautions have been taken, a certain risk usually remains. It must be assessed for each remaining hazard if the risk remains high, medium, or low).
4. Recording all the steps performed.
5. Regular reassessment of all hazards/risks and/or possible new hazards/risks.

For ease of use for biological reproductive material, the Euro-GTP II Guide has been created, which provides structured guidance on how to use the tools and methodologies developed by the EuroGTP II project, namely, the use of a systematic mechanism based on risk analysis from the point of view of the degree of novelty as follows:

- Assessing whether a new or modified process, service, or product has a significant degree of novelty.
- Determining the general risk arising from novelty.

- Determining an appropriate level of preclinical and clinical assessments to address and assess risk.
- Implement the result of risk assessment in routine practice and follow-up the results.

The general process requires to identify specific risks related to potential risk factors and the consequences of the risks. Each of these must be assessed individually to determine the residual risk of implementing the change. Assessment taking into account:

i. The probability of occurrence of the risk.

ii. The severity of the consequences if the risk arises.

iii. The probability that the source of the hazard for the consequences of the risk will be detected before the use of the product/provision of the service.

iv. The instrument does not cover the consequences of risk after embryonic implantation.

v. Any existing evidence that can be used to mitigate the risk.

The instrument shall take into account the number of individual risks assessed to calculate the percentage value of the overall risk.

The result of this risk analysis will be a single global risk score (on a scale of 0 to 100)the final risk score, which can be used to define the extent and/or need for pre-clinical and clinical assessment needed to support the proposal to change or introduce a new type of product or service [24].

3. Conclusion

Due to the fact that infertility is a growing problem in our society, the natality being on a downward trend, medical assisted reproductive technologies have an important role. The success rate depends on numerous factors, patient and non-patient-related. Among the latest, quality management systems with all the components of it play a crucial role in the whole process. The chapter summarizes this part of MART, emphasizing how and why the QMC can and does influence the final result.

Author details

Delia Hutanu[1]* and Ioana Rugescu[2]

1 West University of Timisoara, Biology-Chemistry Department, Timisoara, Romania

2 National Transplant Agency, Bucharest, Romania

*Address all correspondence to: delia.hutanu@e-uvt.ro

References

[1] Alper MM, Brinsden PR, Fischer R, et al. Is your IVF programme good? Human Reproduction. 2002;**17**:8-10

[2] Dale B, Menezo Y, Cohen J, Di Matteo L, Wilding M. Intracellular PH regulation in human ovocyte. Human Reproduction. 1998;**13**:964-970

[3] Heller R, Hindle T. Essential Manager's Manual. New York: DK Publishing; 1998

[4] Available from: https://ec.europa.eu/health/blood-tissues-cells-and-organs/overview/revision-eu-legislation-blood-tissues-and-cells_en

[5] Leape L. L - A systems analysis approach to medical error. JAMA. 1997;**277**:307-311

[6] Mortimer D, Mortimer S. Quality and Risk Management in the IVF Laboratory. UK: Cambridge University Press; 2015

[7] Salinas M, Lopez-Garrigos MG, Lugo J, Sirvent JV, Uris J. Achieving continuous improvement in laboratory organization through performance measurements: A seven-year experience clin. Chemical Lab Medical. 2010;**48**:57-61

[8] The Vienna consensus: Report of an expert meeting on the development of art laboratory performance indicators; ESHRE Special Interest Group of Embryology 1 and Alpha Scientists in Reproductive Medicine

[9] Veljko Vlaisavljevic, Susanna Apter, Antonio Capalbo, Arianna D'Angelo, Luca Gianaroli, Georg Griesinger, Efstratios M Kolibianakis, George Lainas, Tonko Mardesic, Tatjana Motrenko, Sari Pelkonen, Daniela Romualdi, Nathalie Vermeulen, Kelly Tilleman, The Maribor report of an expert meeting on the development of performance indicators for clinical practice in ART, ESHRE Clinic PI Working Group. 2019

[10] Griesinger G, Verweij PJM, Gates D, Devroey P. Prediction of ovarian hyperstimulation syndrome in patients treated with corifollitropin alfa or rFSH in a GnRH antagonist protocol. PloS One. 2016;**11**(3)

[11] Levitt T. Production line approach. Harvard Business Review. 1972:41-52

[12] Özaltın SK, Savan K. Evaluation of complications developing during and after transvaginal ultrasound—guided oocyte retrieval. Ginekologia Polska. 2018;**89**:1-6

[13] Zegers-Hochschild F, Adamson GD, Dyer S, Racowsky C, Mouzon J, Sokol R, et al. The international glossary on infertility and fertility care. Human Reproduction. 2017;**32**(9):1786-1801. DOI: 10.1093/humrep/dex234

[14] Johnson JE, Boone WR, Bernard RS. The effects of volatile compounds (VC) on the outcome of in vitro mouse embryo culture. Fertility and Sterility. 1993;**60**(suppl. 1):S98

[15] Boone WR, Johnson JE, Locke AJ, Crone MM IV, Price TM. Control of air quality in an assisted reproductive technology laboratory. Fertility and Sterility. 1999;**71**:150-154

[16] Cohen J, Alikani M. The time has come to radically rethink assisted reproduction. Reproductive Biomedicine Online. 2013;**27**:323-324

[17] Von Wyl S, Bersinger NA. Air quality in the IVF laboratory: Results and survey.

Journal of Assisted Reproduction and Genetics. 2004;**21**:347-348

[18] Kao YK, Higdon HL III, Graves-Herring JE, Boone WR. Where do mouse embryos thrive best? Comparation of mammalian embryo development under varying laboratory environments. Journal of South Carolina Academy. 2009;**7**(2):29-30

[19] Warrilow KC, Huynh HT, Gwozdziewicz JB, Schillings WA, Peters AYA. Retrospective analysis: The examination of a potential relationship between particulate (P) and volatile organic compound (VOC) levels in a class 100 IVF laboratory cleanroom (CR) and specific parameters of embryogenesis and rates of implantation (IR). Fertility and Sterility. 2001;**76**(suppl. 1):S15-S16

[20] Geisthovel F, Ochsner A, Gilligan AV. Environmental Evaluation of Assisted Reproduction Techniques Laboratories in Germany and the USA. Narasa Publishing Hause; 2001. pp. 184-198

[21] Merton YS, Vermeulen ZL, Otter T, Mullaart E, de Ruigh L, Hasler JF. Carbon activated gas filtration during in vitro culture increased pregnancy rate fallowing transfer of in vitro – Produced bovine embryos. Theriogenology. 2007;**67**:1233-1238

[22] Richardson ME, Trapp AC, Bernard RS. The effect of residual paint fumes on murine embryonic development. Bulletin Academic Science. 1997;**59**:131

[23] Lichtenfels AJFC, Gomes JB, Pieri PC, El Khouri Miraglia SG, Hallak J, Saldiva PHN. Increased levels of air pollution and a decrease in the human and mouse male to female ratio in Sao Paulo, Brasil. Fertility and Sterility. 2007;**87**:230-232

[24] Available from: https://tool.goodtissuepractices.site/

Section 4

Immunology and Infertility, Artificial Intelligence and Ovarian Aging

Chapter 7

Recent Advances in Immunotherapeutic Approaches for Recurrent Reproductive Failure

Samaneh Abdolmohammadi-Vahid, Leili Aghebati-Maleki, Javad Ahmadian-Heris, Shahla Danaii and Mehdi Yousefi

Abstract

Human reproduction is an insufficient process, disturbed by various factors, such as immunologic aberrations of mother. Immunologic abnormalities, including cellular and humoral immunity imbalance, cause dysregulated immune responses against embryo, fetus, and associated components and lack of maternal immunotolerance, which compromise the maintenance of pregnancy. Therefore, evaluation of immunologic parameters, including cellular and humoral immunity assessment (T and B lymphocyte, T helper subtypes, NK cells, cytokines, and autoantibodies), especially in women with a history of pregnancy loss or implantation failure, would help clinicians to manage the disorder and prevent next unfavorable pregnancy outcomes. Moreover, several immunomodulatory approaches have been introduced to modulate the abnormal immunologic responses in patients who experience reproduction failure, especially those diagnosed with immunologic basis. Anticoagulants, corticosteroids, intravenous immunoglobulin, immunosuppressive medications used in inhibition of graft rejection, such as calcineurin inhibitors, recombinant cytokines, and cell therapy approaches, are among these modalities. Here, we discuss the proposed mechanisms of immunologic abnormalities involved in the etiopathogenesis of reproduction disorders, besides the suggested immunologic tests and immunotherapeutic approaches which may be helpful in management of these disorders.

Keywords: reproductive immunology, immunotherapy, recurrent pregnancy loss, repeated implantation failure

1. Introduction

Human reproduction is an incompetent process, as about 70% of conceptions is lost before the first trimester [1]. Approximately, 85% of pregnancy losses are related to failure in implantation or losses prior to clinical diagnosis of pregnancy and only 15% of pregnancy losses are related to clinical miscarriages [2].

Recurrent pregnancy loss (RPL), also known as recurrent miscarriages (RM) and recurrent spontaneous abortion (RSA) or habitual abortion, alongside repeated or recurrent implantation failures (RIF), are among the reproductive disorders, which are included in a broad term called recurrent reproductive failure (RRF) [3]. According to the updated guidelines, including American Society of Reproductive Medicine (ASRM, 2012) and European Society of Human Reproduction and Embryology (ESHRE, 2017) guidelines, RPL is determined as two or more pregnancy losses [4–6]. However, it is determined as three or more consecutive pregnancy losses before the 20th week of gestation, by world health organization (WHO) [7]. As most of the losses happen earlier than clinically recognized or the first missed period, it is difficult to estimate the accurate incidence of RPL. However, it is estimated that RPL accounts for 12–15% of all pregnancies [8]. RPL is divided into two categories, including primary RPL and secondary RPL. Series of pregnancy losses without a previous successful birth is called primary RPL, while a series of pregnancy losses followed by a previous live birth is known as secondary RPL [9].

RIF is also a distressing condition for young couples and an obstacle for human reproduction. Embryo implantation is a critical step in human reproduction. The "window of implantation" is a short and delicately regulated time in which the endometrium is ready for embryo penetration and attachment [10]. A failure in the embryo and the endometrium cross-talk may compromise the embryo attachment and cause implantation failure. In spite of increasing application of assisted reproductive technology (ART) and in vitro fertilization (IVF) still about 10% of couples experience unfavorable outcomes [11]. There are multiple definitions for RIF, based on number of transferred embryos [3–10], unsuccessful IVF cycles (2–6 cycles; the most common, 3 IVF cycles) [12] or both [13]. However, the preimplantation genetic diagnosis (PGD) consortium of ESHRE, defines RIF as >3 failed high quality embryo transfers (ETs) [11, 14].

The exact pathogenesis of RIF and RPL has yet to be understood. However, there are several heterogeneous risk factors, including chromosomal and anatomical abnormalities, infections, endocrine disorders, thrombophilia, and lifestyle [15]. Nevertheless, the etiology of almost 50% of RRFs remains unclear and may be related to maternal immune system abnormalities [16]. Considering the embryo or fetus as a semi-allograft, pregnancy shares similar properties with allogeneic transplantation [17]. In order to survive in a hostile microenvironment, fetus antigens must be recognized and tolerized by maternal immune system. Any abnormalities in the regulatory mechanisms of immune system, which are responsible for establishment of maternal tolerance, may compromise the maintenance of the pregnancy [18]. Here we discuss the different aspects of immune system, which contribute to the pathogenesis of reproductive failure. Immuno-etiology of RRF is summarized in **Figure 1**.

1.1 Cellular immunity

There are solid evidence about the contribution of T cell subsets and their balance in the process of pregnancy, especially the balance between T helper type1 (Th1) and Th2 cells. Th17 and regulatory T (Treg) cells are the other critical population [19]. Embryo implantation requires an aseptic inflammation, created by a shift toward Th1-like cells and cytokines, in the first trimester [3]. Following the implantation, predomination of Th2 responses is required for protection of fetus and balancing the Th1 responses [19]. Th1 associated cytokines, such as interferon-γ (IFNγ) and tumor necrosis factor-α (TNFα), adversely affects the pregnancy, inducing inflammation and thrombotic events in blood vessels of uterus, while Th2 associated cytokines, such as interleukin-4 (IL-4) and IL-10, are known to suppress Th1 immunity and cytokines [16].

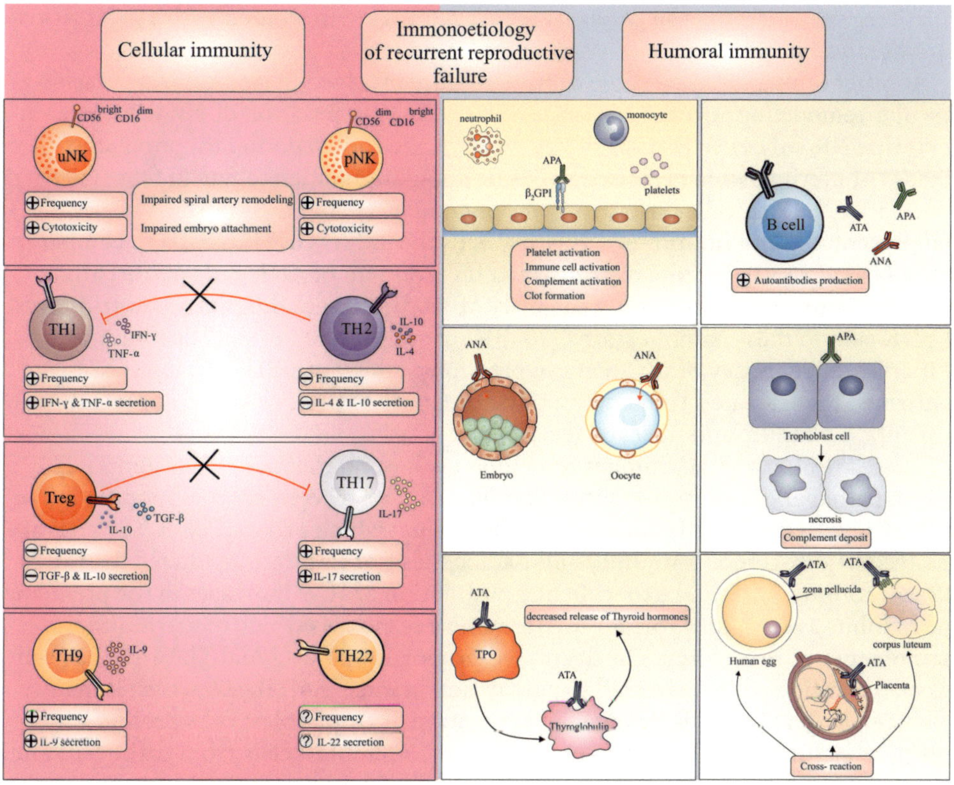

Figure 1.
Immuno-etiology of recurrent reproductive failure. Abnormalities of cellular and humoral immunity are both involved in the pathogenesis of RRF. Cellular immune system abnormalities which are involved in the pathogenesis of RIF and RPL include elevated frequency and cytotoxicity of both uNK and pNK cells, along with upregulation of Th1, Th17, and Th9 cells and associated cytokines. In contrast, immunoregulatory arm is weakened because of reduced frequency and cytokine secretion of Th2 and Treg cells. On the other side, over-production of autoantibodies such as APA, ANA, ACA, and ATA by B lymphocytes in dysregulated humoral immunity, is involved in the pathogenesis of RRF by various mechanisms including cross-reaction with oocyte, placenta, and other vital antigens for human reproduction, inducing thyroid dysfunction, clot formation and necrosis of trophoblast cells. Abbreviation: uNK: uterine natural killer; pNK: peripheral natural killer; TH: T helper; Treg: T regulatory; TNFα: tumor necrosis factor α; IFNγ: interferon γ; IL-4: interleukin-4; IL-10: interleukin-10; IL-17: interleukin-17; TGFβ: Transforming growth factor beta; TPO: thyroid peroxidase; ATA: anti-thyroid antibody; APA: anti-phospholipid antibody; ANA: antinuclear antibody; ACA: anti-cardiolipin antibody; β2GPI: Beta-2-Glycoprotein I.

On the other hand, $CD4^+CD25^+FoxP3^+$ Treg cells play a pivotal role in establishment of maternal immunotolerance toward fetus [20]. Treg cells suppression is mediated through secretion of immunosuppressive cytokines, such as IL-10 and transforming growth factor (TGF-β), or by cell–cell contacts [21]. The frequency of peripheral Treg cells is upregulated in implantation. Following the implantation, Treg cells frequency reaches the highest level in second trimester and decreases after delivery [22]. According to the literature, the frequency of peripheral and uterine Treg cells is downregulated in RPL and RIF women, compared with control group [23–25]. In contrast, Th17 population is upregulated in the decidua and peripheral blood pregnancy complication, besides elevated Th17/Treg ratio [26]. It has been also reported that activation of decidual NK (dNK) is induced by Th17 cells that contribute to vascular dysfunction and embryo resorption [27]. Infertile women exhibited an increased ratio of Th17/$CD4^+$ Treg cell, when compared to normal fertile controls [28]. Therefore,

Th17/Treg cells ratio has the potential to be a biomarker in women with a great risk of reproductive failure.

Another type of immunologic cells, which are involved in trophoblast invasion and vascular remodeling, are natural killer (NK) cells. A population of NK cells, known as uterine NK (uNK) cells ($CD56^{bright}CD16^{dim}$), are the predominant population of mucosa of uterine, which represent 70% of population of leukocyte in feto-maternal interface [29]. UNK cells differ from peripheral NK (pNK) cells ($CD56^{dim}CD16^{bright}$) and present a strong immunomodulatory activity and less cytotoxicity, in comparison with pNK cells [30]. In spite of confirmed involvement of uNK cells in the pathogenesis of reproduction failure, a majority of studies also highlight the contribution of pNK cells in these complications [30, 31]. In addition to the significant impact of increased frequency of uNK cells in pathophysiology of RPL [32], it has been confirmed that elevated frequency and cytotoxicity of pNK cells also contribute to implantation failure and miscarriage [33].

There are only a small number of studies evaluating the role of Th9 and Th22 cells in pathogenesis of reproductive complications. Th9 cells are a subpopulation of Th2 cells, with different functions and phenotype, which produce IL-9. Th9 cells are involved in anti-tumor immunity and pathogenesis of immune-mediated disorders [19]. According to animal experiments, production of IL-9 increases in the pregnancy and exhibits a regulatory role for inflammatory responses which compromise the maintenance of pregnancy. The decreased proportion of decidual Th9 and Treg cell has been confirmed to be related to parturition in mice [34]. IL-22, which is mainly produced by Th22 cells, is involved in promotion of trophoblast cells proliferation, as well as viability. Furthermore, protection of trophoblast cells from pathogens and infiltrated immune cells is mediated by IL-22 [35]. There are limited and conflicting data about the role of Th22 and IL-22 in pregnancy complications. It has been reported that RPL women have a decreased expression of IL-22 receptor, in comparison with control [36]. In the other hand, there are reports about the increased amount of IL-22 of sera in RPL women [37], in contrast, lower gene expression of IL-22 was detected in decidua of these patients [38]. Further studies are required to understand whether IL-22 expression is associated with RPL.

1.2 Humoral immunity

It has been confirmed that some auto-antibodies also contribute to the pathogenesis of RIF and RPL, such as anti-phospholipid antibodies (APAs), anti-nuclear antibodies (ANAs), and anti-thyroid antibodies (ATAs) [39]. Presence of these autoantibodies, regardless of presence of an autoimmune disorder, has been correlated with reproduction failures [40].

Antiphospholipid syndrome (APS), an autoimmune thrombophilia, is associated with the presence of anti-cardiolipin antibodies (ACAs), lupus anticoagulant (LA), and anti-β2-glycoprotein-1 (β2GPI) antibodies. ACAs recognize cardiolipin, a phospholipid of cell membranes, and are the most common antibodies of APS [41]. β2GPI is a cardiolipin-binding factor, which is recognized with anti-β2GPI antibodies, and LA includes various types of autoantibodies [42]. There are accumulated evidence of a direct interaction between serum positivity for APAs and pregnancy complications [42]. The risk of pregnancy wastage increases with higher antibody positivity, as triple positive women experience more pregnancy complications in comparison with double-positive women [41]. Indeed, after recognition of antigens, such as β2GPI, by associated antibody, an intra-placental coagulation-mediated thrombosis may take place, leading in poor pregnancy outcomes [43]. It has been suggested that anti-β2GPI antibodies are capable of recognizing antigenic determinants on trophoblast, stromal decidual, and endometrial endothelial cells [44]. This antibody–antigen reaction would prevent the invasion of trophoblast, inducing apoptosis of trophoblast cells by complement-mediated reactions and recruitment of immune cells, such as neutrophils and monocytes; additionally, a pro-inflammatory microenvironment is created by production of inflammatory products, such as TNF-α, reactive oxygen species (ROS), and chemokines [44, 45]. Lately, there are conflicting data about the contribution of some non-conventional APAs, including antibodies that recognizes prothrombin, phosphatidylethanolamine, and annexin V, in the pathogenesis of obstetric complications [46, 47]; however further investigations are required to confirm the involvement of these APAs in pathogenesis of RIF and RPL.

ANAs, targeting the determinants of cytoplasm and nucleus, are detected in rheumatic and autoimmune diseases, such as systemic lupus erythematosus. In spite of conflicts, it has been reported that increased prevalence of ANA is associated with adverse pregnancy outcomes such as RPL [48] and RIF [49]. A recent meta-analysis confirmed the positive correlation between the presence of ANAs and higher risk for RPL and highlighted the importance of screening test for ANA in women with RPL risk [50]. The exact mechanism of ANAs is not fully understood; however, it is estimated that the presence of ANA adversely affects the quality and development of embryo by inducing the immune complex, which deposits in placental tissue and activates complement cascade [41, 51].

Anti-thyroglobulin (TGAb), anti-thyroid peroxidase (TPOAb), and anti-thyroid stimulating hormone (TSH) receptor (TRAb) antibodies are ATAs found in thyroid autoimmunity (TAI) and recognize antigenic determinants of thyroglobulin, thyroid peroxidase, and TSH receptors (TSHR), respectively [52]. Attachment of these antibodies to associated antigens may disturb the production, secretion, and function of thyroid hormones. Furthermore, ATAs are capable of passing the placental barrier, which enables them to impair the development of the fetus [53]. It has been confirmed that ATAs-positive women, especially positive for TGAbs and TPOAbs, are more prone to pregnancy adverse outcomes. Presence of ATAs increases the risk of miscarriage three times higher, according to the results of a meta-analysis [54]. On the other hand, prevalence of ATAs is also higher in RPL women [41]. Furthermore, ATAs-positive women experience impaired oocyte quality, lower grade A embryos, and implantation rate, in comparison with healthy controls [55]. Sometimes, in spite of overall euthyroidism, ATAs are capable of inducing a slight deficiency in thyroid hormones, which impairs embryo development after implantation [56]. The exact mechanism of ATAs' action in the pathogenesis of obstetric complications has yet to be elucidated. However, there are some suggested mechanisms including dysfunction of thyroid, cross-reaction of ATAs with extra-thymic antigens, such as placenta, zona pellucida, follicular fluid antigens, human chorionic gonadotropin receptors (hCGR), and formation of immune complexes [41, 57, 58]. In addition, the presence of ATAs is a sign of a generalized immune abnormality including abnormal frequency and function of T cell subsets, B lymphocytes, NK cells, and subsequent abnormal cytokines production [59, 60].

Celiac disease is the other disorder that increases the risk of RPL in untreated patients. Celiac is an autoimmune enteropathy of gluten-sensitive susceptible individuals, which involves the mucosa of small intestine. Prevalence of celiac is 1% in general population, while it increases to 2.7% in infertile women. Indeed, celiac women have higher risk for recurrent miscarriage, premature birth, or decreased fetal growth, compared with healthy women [61, 62]. A meta-analysis also indicated a higher risk for celiac in RPL women, when compared to the general population [63]. Anti-transglutaminase and anti-endomysial antibodies are the serum markers of celiac patients, which are recommended to be screened in women with risk of reproductive failure [64]. According to a relevant study, in celiac women, anti-transglutaminase antibody is capable of recognizing antigenic determinants on syncytiotrophoblast, inhibiting the transglutaminase action in the placenta and disturbing the placental function [65]. However, there are studies that do not support the correlation between celiac disease and presence of anti-transglutaminase and anti-endomysial antibodies with adverse pregnancy outcomes, in which screening for these autoantibodies was not recommended in women with RPL history [66–68]. Further investigations are required in order to better understand the correlation between celiac disease and reproductive failures.

1.3 Human leukocyte antigen (HLA) sharing

As suggested by evidence, recurrent miscarriage is associated with elevated rate of HLA sharing. HLA molecules, encoded by a great number of genes on chromosome 6, are known by their broad polymorphism, so the chance of HLA similarity between two individuals is very low. HLA molecules are divided into HLA class I (HLA-A-G antigens) and HLA class II regions (HLA-DR, DQ, and DP antigens) [18]. As suggested by evidence, an increased rate of RPL is associated with higher frequencies of identical HLA-A and HLA-B alleles; however, some studies did not show any relation between HLA sharing and RPL incidence [18]. Increased HLA–sharing with father may suppress the production of blocking antibodies, such as anti-paternal cytotoxic antibodies (APCA), anti-idiotypic antibodies (Ab2), and mixed lymphocyte reaction blocking antibodies (MLR-Bf), which mask the paternal antigens and prohibit their recognition by maternal immune system. Lack of these antibodies compromises the maintenance of pregnancy. Lymphocyte therapy is one of the immunotherapeutic approaches for pregnancy complications, which is able to induce the production of these antibodies [69].

There are increasing evidence about the contribution of immunologic abnormalities in etiopathogenesis of RPL and RIF, including predomination of Th1 and Th17 cells and related cytokines and downregulation of Th2 and Treg cells alongside their cytokines [70], elevated Th1/Th2 and Th17/Treg ratios, increased frequency and function of uNK cells and pNK cells [30], presence of APAs [71] or other autoimmunities like autoimmune thyroiditis [72]. According to the literature, 30.5% of RPL women have increased frequency of NK cells, and 31.6% of them have increased cytotoxicity of NK cells, additionally, 20% of RPL patients and 30% of RIF patients have APAs [73].

Nowadays, there is a strong need for biomarkers and clinical assays for detection of immune abnormalities, besides the helpful immunotherapeutic approaches to improve the immunologic aberration in RIF and RPL patients. This review aims to discuss the immunological approaches in the diagnosis and treatment of pregnancy complications in women with immune-etiology reproductive failures.

2. Immunological tests for RIF and RPL

Analyses of immunologic parameters, addressing immune abnormalities in RIF and RPL women, were not routinely offered by guidelines. In fact, immunological diagnosis tests are generally suggested in the case of "idiopathic" or "unexplained" RIF or RPL, when the other risk factors, including genetic and anatomic complications and infection are excluded. LA, ACA, and anti-β2GPI antibodies screening are more often suggested [74]. On the other hand, it seems that analysis of blood and endometrial immunologic biomarkers prior to immunotherapies would be helpful in selection of a proper candidate, proper therapeutic modality, investigation of altered parameters, and understanding the mechanism of action of therapeutic agent. Here, we summarized the proposed test for evaluation of immunologic imbalances of RIF and RPL women, including cellular and humoral tests [75]. Immunophenotyping and functional assays, besides evaluation of cytokines concentration and autoantibodies titer, are among the proposed immunologic tests.

2.1 Cellular tests

- T, B, and NK immunophenotyping
- Ratio of T CD4/T CD8
- Ratio of Th1/Th2
- TNF-a and IL-10 positive T $CD4^+$
- Regulatory T cells frequency
- NK cells cytotoxicity
- NK cells activator and inhibitory receptors
- Th17/Treg cells
- HLA-typing

2.2 Humoral tests

- ANAs (anti-DNA, anti-histone, anti-Smith (Sm) antibody, anti-ribonucleoprotein, anti-Jo, autoantibodies against topoisomerase (anti-Scl), anti-SSA/Ro, anti-SSB/La antibodies)
- APAs on ≥2 situations with at least 12 weeks intervals and < 5 years prior to clinical manifestations
- Conventional APA (ACA, LA, anti-β2GPI antibodies)
- Non-conventional APA (anti-annexin V antibodies, anti-phosphatidylethalonamine antibodies)
- Anti-transglutaminase and anti-thyroid (TPO and thyroglobulin) antibodies
- Anti-sperm antibodies
- T helper cells cytokines
- APCA

- Anti-HY and anti-HLA antibodies
- Anti-transglutaminase and anti-endomysial antibodies

3. Immunotherapy of RRF

As suggested by evidence, immunologic aberrations play a critical role in pathogenesis of reproductive disorders including RIF and RPL. Obviously, several immunotherapeutic approaches have already been introduced for the management of these complications, such as immunosuppressive and immunomodulatory agents. According to literature, anticoagulants, corticosteroids, and immunosuppressive medications used in inhibition of graft rejection, such as calcineurin inhibitors, recombinant cytokines, and cell therapy approaches are among the immunotherapeutic agents which have been used in animal experiments and clinical trials, in order to modulate the abnormal immune responses and improve the pregnancy consequences. However, the ambiguous evidence provided by this literature need further clarification, as most of these approaches have yet to achieve routine clinical applications, due to concerns about their efficiency and safety. Therefore, further investigations are required to determine the efficacy and safety of novel immunotherapeutic strategies for pregnancy complications. Here, we examine the present immunotherapies, their mechanisms, and related studies, which have been conducted for the management of RIF and RPL patients, especially those with an immunological background. We first

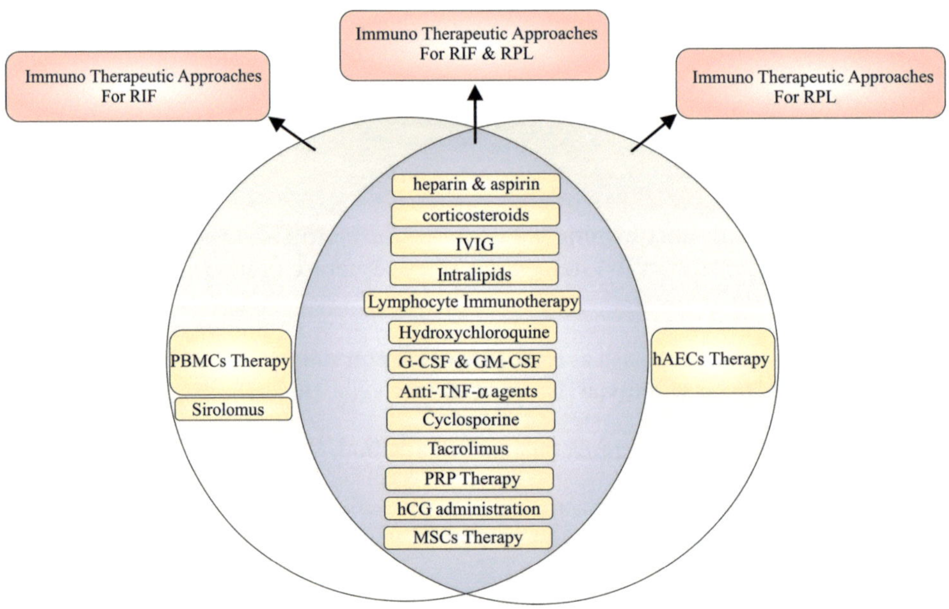

Figure 2.
The classification of immunotherapeutic approaches used for RRF, based on their application for RIF and/or RPL patients. Abbreviation: RPL: recurrent pregnancy failure; RIF: recurrent implantation failure; IVIG: Intravenous immunoglobulin; G-CSF: Granulocyte colony-stimulating factor; GM-CSF: Granulocyte-macrophage colony-stimulating factor; Anti-TNF-α: anti-tumor necrosis factor α; PRP: platelet-rich plasma; hCG: Human chorionic gonadotropin; MSC: mesenchymal stem cells; hAECs: Human amniotic epithelial cells; PBMCs: Peripheral blood mononuclear cells.

describe the proposed mechanisms of action of the immunotherapeutic modalities; afterward, the studies that utilized these agents and related systematic reviews and meta-analyses, for RIF and RPL patients, are described respectively. The classification of these immunotherapeutic approaches, based on their application for RIF and/or RPL patients, is presented in **Figure 2**.

3.1 Immunotherapeutic approaches for RIF and RPL patients

3.1.1 Heparin and aspirin

Heparin is a structural analog of heparan, which is present in reproductive tract and plays a pivotal role in reproduction. Heparin and heparan are capable of binding to growth factors and their receptors, antithrombin, and molecules of extracellular matrix [76]. In addition to anti-thrombotic effect of heparin during implantation, it is able to improve placentation, especially in women with thrombophilia [77]. On the other hand, the proteins involved in the blastocyte invasion and adhesion to endometrium and trophoblastic differentiation are modulated by heparin and it is due to the action of heparin on metalloproteinases, cadherin-E, heparin-binding epidermal growth factor, and free insulin-like growth factor [78]. The anti-inflammatory effect of heparin is also reported, as heparin interferes with the activation of complement [77]. Anti-inflammatory effect of aspirin, a non-steroidal anti-inflammatory drug (NSAIDs), is attributed to the inhibition of prostaglandins synthesis; besides, aspirin is able to induce acetylation of cyclooxygenase-2, which leads to the production of aspirin-triggered lipoxins (ATLs) from arachidonic acid. Aspirin also prohibits platelet generation and exhibits anti-thrombotic effects [79].

According to the ESHRE, ASRM, German/Austrian/Swiss Society of Obstetrics and Gynecology (DGGG/OEGGG/SGGG), and the Royal College of Obstetricians and Gynecologists (RCOG) guidelines, low-dose aspirin and heparin are recommended for treatment of APS [18]. Different studies also reported the positive effect of combination of aspirin and heparin in pregnancy complications, accompanied by APS [80]. Evaluation of effect of heparin therapy around the time of implantation, at/or after egg collection, or at the time of embryo transfer, in subfertile women during assisted reproduction, demonstrated that heparin was able to increase the rate of live birth in comparison with control group [76]. According to the results of Potdar et al. systematic review and meta-analysis, adjunct low molecular weight heparin (LMWH) in women with a history of ≥3 RIF significantly increased the live birth rate in comparison with control group. However, the implantation rate did not show any significant difference [81].

Study by Badawy et al. included 340 women, divided into two groups, one group received LMWH enoxaparin, and the other group received folic acid tablets. The results demonstrated that heparin decreased the incidence of recurrent miscarriages and increased the mean birth weight [82]. A systematic review, investigating the efficacy and safety of aspirin and heparin therapy, in women with at least two unexplained miscarriages, with or without inherited thrombophilia showed no beneficial effect of aspirin and heparin; so, the anticoagulants in women with unexplained RM were not confirmed confirmed in this systematic review [83]. While the cochrane systematic review of Hamulyak et al. confirmed that combination of heparin plus aspirin during pregnancy is capable of improving the live birth rate in RPL women with APS and the efficiency of combination of heparin and aspirin was more than efficiency of aspirin alone [84].

Heparin may be a helpful choice in reproduction complications in the case of known APS or thrombophilia; however, evaluation of the efficacy of heparin in women with reproduction failure has shown almost no improvement of clinical pregnancy or live birth rate in women without known case of thrombophilia. More research is needed about the efficiency of heparin therapy alone or in combination with aspirin in both known and unknown cases of thrombophilia, in order to further evaluate potential benefits of this treatment strategy, and to gain consensus on the ideal treatment.

3.2 Corticosteroids

Along the line of corticosteroids, prednisolone has been widely used in immune-mediated reproductive disorders due to its anti-inflammatory and immunomodulatory effects. The suggested action mechanisms for prednisolone in pregnancy complications include decreasing the Th1/Th2 ratio, secretion of Th1-related cytokine, and downregulation of frequency and cytotoxicity of NK cells [85].

According to the literature, prednisolone may be a helpful choice in improvement of implantation rate of women undergoing IVF procedure, especially the women who are positive for APAs and ANAs [86, 87]. There are evidence about the positive effect of prednisolone, alone or in combination with heparin, on RIF patients through modulation of elevated frequency and function of NK cells [88]. Indeed, expression of glucocorticoid receptors by uNK cells makes these cell to be highly affected by prednisolone [89]. Evaluation of endometrial biopsy of RIF patients indicated that over-activation of immune system in RIF women was modulated after prednisolone administration. The mRNA expression of IL-18/tumor necrosis factor-like weak inducer of apoptosis (TWEAK), which is a reflector of Th1/Th2 ratio, was significantly decreased post-treatment [90]. In addition, a recent study also demonstrated that the dysregulated Th17/Treg axis in RIF patients was modulated by creating a shift toward Treg cell responses after prednisolone administration [91, 92]. On the other hand, there are studies in which prednisolone showed no benefit in the improvement of the outcomes in RIF patients [93]. The results of a recent systematic review about the effect of prednisolone administration in women undergoing IVF or intracytoplasmic sperm injection (ICSI) indicated almost no significant difference in live birth and clinical pregnancy rate of corticoid versus no corticoid or placebo group [94].

Corticosteroid administration for RPL women who have elevated frequency of uNK cells, in cycle days 1–21, was capable of decreasing the frequency of uNK cells [95]. Combination of prednisolone with aspirin and heparin also seemed to be more helpful in pregnancy complications in unexplained recurrent miscarriage, as was confirmed in the study of Gomaa et al. [96]. Evaluation of endometrial samples of RM women showed that the increased percentage of uNK ($CD56^{+}CD16^{-}CD3^{-}$) in RM patients was decreased posttreatment with prednisolone [95]. According to in-vitro experiments, elevation of HLA-G expression post-glucocorticoid therapy may decrease the incidence of RM [97]. Meta-analysis of Don et al. also confirmed that prednisolone may improve pregnancy outcomes in women with idiopathic RM, but its effect was not significant in women undergoing ICSI [98].

There is still a requirement for studies to investigate the efficiency of corticotherapy in RIF and RPL women with immunologic abnormalities; studies which investigate the effect of corticosteroid on improvement of both the immunologic aberrations and pregnancy outcomes. In addition, given the contradictory results about the efficiency of prednisolone and considering the reported adverse effects, such as risk of hypertension and diabetes, further powerful and well-designed placebo-controlled randomized trials with lower doses of prednisolone are required to identify the efficiency of treatment and specific risk factors.

3.3 Intravenous immunoglobulin G (IVIG)

IVIG is an immunomodulatory agent, consisting of natural antibodies and autoantibodies, Fab fragments of IgG, antibodies against antigenic determinants of bacteria, and different cytokines [85, 99]. IVIG is purified from the plasma of 1000 to up to 100,000 healthy donors, and is used for treatment of thrombocytopenia, kawasaki disease, graft versus host disease (GVHD), immune-mediated and pregnancy disorders [100]. There are numerous suggested mechanisms of action, by which IVIG improves the pregnancy outcome, including reducing the number and cytotoxicity of NK cells [101, 102], enhancing the frequency and function of Treg cells [103], inhibiting the production of autoantibodies by B lymphocytes, neutralizing the maternal autoantibodies by its anti-idiotypic antibodies [85, 104], inhibiting the deposition of complement fragment and membrane attack complex (MAC) [105], and upregulation of inhibitory receptors on antigen-presenting cells (APCs) [106]. A reduction in the number of Th1 cells and cytokines secretion and elevation in Th2 responses was also observed after IVIG administration in related studies [107], followed by a reduction in Th1/Th2 ratio [108]. Furthermore, the results of the study of Ahmadi et al. also demonstrated that IVIG is capable of increasing the frequency of Treg cells and mRNA expression of Treg transcription factor, FoxP3, and cytokines such as IL-10 and TGF- β. In addition, the mRNA expression of Th17-associated transcription factor, RORγt was reduced post-treatment [109]. Therefore, the other mechanism of action of IVIG may be attributed to modulation of Th17/Treg axis.

The pregnancy and live birth rates were significantly elevated in RIF patients with an increased level of circulating NK and/or NKT-like cells after IVIG therapy when compared to those not receiving IVIG patients [110]. Additionally, a systematic review and meta-analysis demonstrated that IVIG administration is associated with increased rate of implantation and pregnancy in women undergoing IVF/ICSI cycles, in comparison with placebo group. The results also indicated that IVIG receiving group had a lower rate of miscarriage, therefore the usefulness of IVIG administration was strongly supported in women who had a history of recurrent IVF failure, by this systematic review [111]. A systematic review of our group also confirmed the positive effect of IVIG on RIF patients, especially those with immunologic abnormalities. The results of this systematic review, which included two cohorts, two cross-sectional and one quasi-experimental study, revealed that there is a significant increase in the live birth and pregnancy rate of IVIG group in comparison with control group. However, the miscarriage rate was not significantly affected by IVIG [112].

Numerous studies have assessed the efficiency of IVIG in RPL women with or without known etiologies, including immunologic abnormalities. The group of Yousefi and colleagues evaluated the beneficial effects of IVIG in pregnancy complications, considering the various immunologic abnormalities involved in etiology. For instance, IVIG treatment in RM women with elevated frequency and function of peripheral NK cells resulted in significant decrease in the percentage and cytotoxicity of NK cells and expression of activating receptors. In contrast, expression of inhibitory receptors was significantly elevated, post-treatment. Pregnancy outcome was also improved as a result of IVIG therapy [113]. The other investigation by this group evaluated the effect of IVIG on alteration of Th1 and Th2 responses in RPL women with pre-treatment elevation of

NK cell frequency and cytotoxicity. After IVIG administration, the frequency, mRNA expression level of transcription factor, and secretion of Th1-related cytokine were significantly decreased. In contrast, these parameters for Th2 cells were increased, in comparison with control group. Furthermore, Th1/Th2 ratio was decreased post-treatment. 87.5% of IVIG treated group and 41.6% of untreated groups had live birth [114]. As a new risk factor for recurrent miscarriage, Th17 and Treg cell balance was evaluated in RM patients after IVIG administration. Before and after intravenous administration of 400 mg/kg of IVIG, every 4 weeks through 32 weeks of gestation, the immunologic parameters were evaluated. The results indicated that IVIG therapy is capable of down-regulating Th17 frequency, while Treg frequency is upregulated, in comparison with untreated group. Rate of pregnancy was 86.3% in IVIG treated group and 42% in untreated group [115]. This study confirmed the results of the study of Kim et al. [116]. Exhausted T cells, exhausted Tregs and Treg cell alteration were also evaluated post-IVIG therapy in RM patients. Blood samples were collected twice, prior to treatment at the time of positive pregnancy test and after the latest IVIG administration. The results indicated a significant elevation in frequency of Treg cells and a significant reduction in frequency of exhausted Tregs, in comparison with untreated group; however, the frequency of exhausted T cells was not affected by IVIG. The pregnancy outcome was also significantly higher in IVIG-treated RM patients [117].

There are reports about the lack of beneficial effects of IVIG treatment on the improvement of pregnancy outcomes in obstetric complications, for instance, the study of Christiansen et al. [118] and Stephenson et al. [119], In accordance with these studies, positive effect of IVIG on the improvement of live birth was not confirmed in systematic review of Wang et al. [120]. However, a recent systematic review and meta-analysis by Parhizkar et al. assessed the results of IVIG therapy on RPL women with immunologic abnormalities in five studies (two cohorts and three quasi experimental studies). The results revealed that IVIG therapy significantly increased the live birth rate, when compared with untreated group and emphasized the efficiency of IVIG for RPL patients, especially those with immunologic aberrations [121].

As reported by several studies, IVIG may be used in combination with other therapeutic approaches, such as prednisolone and TNF-α inhibitor, in order to improve the pregnancy consequences. The combination of TNF-α inhibitor and IVIG showed promising results in improvement of implantation, clinical pregnancy, and live birth rate in women with elevated Th1/Th2 cytokine ratio, who undergo IVF cycles [122]. Furthermore, combination of IVIG with prednisolone also was helpful as indicated by the study of Nyborg et al. [123].

Keeping in view of all the above studies, there are controversies about the efficiency of IVIG in the improvement of pregnancy outcomes alongside immunologic abnormalities in RM and RIF women. Small sample size, lack of randomization, using the less potent IVIG like Gamimune, which was not able to effectively suppress elevated NK cells [75], and lack of evaluation of immune abnormalities prior to treatment, are among the reasons for the heterogeneities of studies. It is inferred that final conclusion about the efficiency of IVIG in improvement of pregnancy outcomes requires more well-designed and powered prospective and randomized controlled trials with appropriate sample size and protocols.

3.4 Intralipids

Intralipids are 20% parenteral sterile fat emulsion, with main components of polyunsaturated fatty acids (PUFAs), especially linoleic acid, in addition to soybean oil, egg phospholipids, glycerin, and water [124]. According to the literature, intravenous administration of intralipids is capable of suppressing the proliferation of immune cells, by altering the composition of cell membrane phospholipids, which subsequently modulates the fluidity and receptors of membrane [124]. Reducing the cytotoxicity of NK cells and inhibition of Th1 responses are attributed to fatty acids and soybean oil of intralipids, respectively [125]. Intralipids also diminish the signals, which are required for T and B lymphocyte activation, by inhibition of IL-2 production and downregulating pro-inflammatory mediators such as IL-1β and TNF-α [15, 126]. However, intralipids are often known to influence the NK cell expansion and function [127].

There are studies that reported the effect of intralipids on NK cell function in women with reproductive disorders [128, 129], and its ability to improve clinical pregnancy and live birth rate in RIF patients [126]. Results of a similar study demonstrated that abnormal NK cell function in patients who received intralipids was modulated to the normal range, after the first or second infusions [129]. According to a systematic review, a significant elevation in clinical pregnancy and live birth rate was observed after intravenous intralipid in RIF women [130]. There are several studies that indicated no beneficial effect of intralipid administration for RIF patients including the study of Shreeve et al. [124] and Check et al. [131].

Intralipids were also capable of elevating the live birth rate in RM patients, according to the meta-analysis of Placais et al., in which live birth was observed in 70% of pregnancies of women with elevated pNK cells, who received intralipids, when compared to untreated group [132]. The other recent systematic review and meta-analysis showed the efficiency of intralipids administration on live birth rate in unexplained infertility and RM patients with known immunological risk factors, but still not as a routine intervention for reproductive disorders [133]. On the contrary, there are studies that do not confirm the beneficial effect of intralipid supplementation in RSA women, even with elevated NK cells such as the study of Dakhly et al. [134].

There is heterogeneity across the studies, which evaluate the efficiency of intralipids in reproductive failures. Moreover, there are limited data about the exact mechanism of action of intralipids for decreasing the elevated number and cytotoxicity of NK and about the safety of intralipids administration during pregnancy. Large-scaled and well-designed research are required for safe conclusions on the efficiency of intralipid therapy in reproductive disorders.

3.5 Lymphocyte immunotherapy (LIT)

LIT or peripheral blood mononuclear cell (PBMCs) therapy includes paternal lymphocyte immunization (PLI), third-party lymphocyte immunization, or insemination of patients' own lymphocytes, in which the lymphocytes are gathered and administrated to the prospective mother [69].

The proposed mechanisms by which LIT improves pregnancy outcomes include stimulation of the maternal immune system in order to produce antibodies, such as APCA, and Ab2, including anti-T cells receptor (TCR) idiotypic antibodies, MLR-Bf, and progesterone-induced blocking factor (PIBF), which avoid recognition of paternal HLA antigens by maternal immune system, especially T and NK cells, by blocking these antigens [135, 136]. Furthermore, it is reported that LIT is capable of reducing the activity of NK cells, downregulating the expression of maternal IL-2 receptors [137], creating a shift toward Th1 responses, improving the Th1/Th2 equilibrium and increasing Treg responses over Th17 responses [138, 139]. Considering the amount and dose of lymphocytes (100–500 × 10^6 cells) [140], route (Intradermal, intravenous and fewer subcutaneous, intracutaneous and intramuscular routes) [141] and time (before pregnancy, during pregnancy, before and during pregnancy: the most helpful) of administration [69], there are multiple protocols for LIT [85].

3.5.1 Intradermal LIT

There are evidence that confirms the positive effect of LIT in improvement of pregnancy outcome in women with immunologic abnormalities by inducing maternal tolerance toward fetus and decreasing the risk of pregnancy wastage; however, most of these studies emphasize the beneficial effect of LIT, especially intradermal LIT, on RPL patients more than RIF women [142, 143]. The recent systematic review of Cavalcante and colleagues indicated that the use of LIT would be a beneficial treatment in RM patients; however, it was not recommended for RIF patients [144]. Gao et al. investigated the immunologic parameters of pre- and post-intradermal paternal lymphocyte immunization in women with unexplained RSA. Before LIT, RSA patients showed an increased rate of lymphocyte counts, CD4/CD8 cell ratios, and frequency of NK cells, in comparison with control group. LIT was capable of reducing all the mentioned parameters in RSA women, except T cell frequency, which was increased post-treatment. Considering the abnormal activation of immune system in RSA patients, lymphocyte immunotherapy was helpful in modulation of these abnormalities [145]. In addition, it has been confirmed that intradermal paternal or third-party lymphocyte immunization increased the $CD4^{+}CD25^{bright}$ T cells frequency in RSA women while decreasing the percentage of $CD4^{+}CD25^{dim}$ cells. This study suggested that $CD4^{+}CD25^{+}$ regulatory T cells serve as a biomarker for monitoring the efficiency of LIT in RSA patients [146]. LIT was also capable of elevating the pregnancy outcome in RSA patients. Abortion rate was significantly decreased after LIT in RSA women, in comparison with patients who received routine treatment. Furthermore, LIT significantly increased the pregnancy success rate [147]. On the contrary, there are studies that reported no beneficial effect of LIT for the improvement of pregnancy outcomes in RM patients [134]. However, the efficiency and safety of LIT for RM patients were confirmed in the systematic review and meta-analysis of Cavalcante et al. [139].

3.5.2 Intrauterine LIT

Intrauterine administration of each patient's own PBMCs, mostly used for RIF women, is suggested to improve the immunologic balance of endometrium which is required for successful implantation and pregnancy, in addition to enhancing the endometrial receptivity [148]. Indeed, PBMCs improve the invasion of trophoblast and implantation by increasing the expression level of matrix metalloproteinase-2 (MMP-2) and MMP-9 and decreasing the expression of tissue inhibitors of metalloproteinase [149]. PBMCs also create a shift toward Th2 prominent responses by induction of progesterone from luteal cells [150]. Peripheral blood of each patient is collected 3–5 days before the embryo transfer, subsequently, PBMCs are isolated and infused into the uterine cavity via an intrauterine insemination catheter [151]. It has been observed that co-culture of PBMCs with human chorionic gonadotropin (HCG), corticotropin-releasing hormone (CRH), and human menopausal gonadotropin (HMG), prior to infusion, may be a useful approach in improving the rate of implantation, as the secretion of essential cytokines and mediators for implantation would be increased [152, 153].

There are solid evidence of the positive effect of intrauterine implementation of PBMCs, leading to favorable outcomes in RIF patients [154], including the study of Yoshioka and colleagues [155]. The results of our previous study also confirmed the efficiency of intrauterine administration of autologous hCG-activated PBMCs in improving the live birth rate and decreasing the miscarriage rate of RIF patients with a history of at least three IVF/ET failures [156]. The systematic review of Wu et al., demonstrated that PBMC therapy improved clinical pregnancy implantation and live birth rate of RIF patients, in comparison with placebo or no treatment group [149]. The next systematic review and meta-analysis indicated that clinical pregnancy and live birth, irrespective of embryo stage and cycle type, were increased after PBMC therapy [150]. The most recent systematic review belongs to our group, in which we investigated the effect of intrauterine PBMC-therapy before IVF in women with at least three IVF/ET failures. The results demonstrated that PBMC therapy in RIF women is associated with significantly higher implantation, pregnancy, and live birth rate and reduced miscarriage rate, in comparison with non-treated group [157].

Further RCTs are still required with a larger population and high-quality study design and less heterogeneous study populations, for recommending PBMC administration as a helpful immunologic approach in treatment protocol of RIF patients.

3.6 Hydroxychloroquine

Hydroxychloroquine, known as an anti-malaria drug, has been considered an immunomodulatory drug in inflammatory and autoimmune disorders such as systemic lupus erythematosus and rheumatoid arthritis [158]. The proposed mechanisms of action of hydroxychloroquine from the immunologic point of view, include downregulation of prostaglandins and inflammatory cytokines such as TNF-α and IFN-γ, reducing the antigen presentation and chemotaxis of immune cells, blocking the receptor signaling of B and T lymphocytes [159], restoring the Th1/Th2 balance and creating a shift toward Th2 responses [160], promotion of Treg cells, inhibition of phospholipase activity and lysosomal acidification and prevention of platelet aggregation and matrix metalloproteinases action [161]. In recent years, hydroxychloroquine has gained attention for its immunomodulatory properties in improvement of reproductive disorders. The efficiency of hydroxychloroquine in reducing the titer of autoantibodies in APS has been reported, therefore it serves an anti-thrombotic effect [158]. In addition, binding of anti-β2GPI antibodies to phospholipid bilayers in trophoblasts is decreased by hydroxychloroquine [160]. In other words, hydroxychloroquine saves the fusion and differentiation of trophoblast, which were compromised because of APAs [162].

In the study of Ghasemnejad-berenji et al., the effect of 400 mg/per day of oral hydroxychloroquine was investigated on immunologic parameters of RIF women with increased TNF-α/IL-10 ratio. Post-treatment with hydroxychloroquine, the serum level of TNF-α was significantly downregulated, while the serum level of IL-10 was increased. Moreover, the expression of Th1 cells transcription factor, T-bet, and Th2 transcription factor, GATA-3, were significantly decreased and increased, respectively, in comparison with pre-treatment [163]. A clinical trial that evaluated the effect of hydroxychloroquine on Th17/Treg axis in RIF women, reported that hydroxychloroquine was able to downregulate the function and cytokines of Th17 cells, while Treg cells function and cytokines were significantly upregulated post-treatment. The expression level of Th17 and Treg cells associated transcription factors was significantly decreased and increased, respectively. However, no significant difference in pregnancy outcomes was observed post-treatment with hydroxychloroquine [161].

The effectiveness of hydroxychloroquine was also evaluated in RPL patients, but the studies are limited. Hydroxychloroquine administration for autoimmune-related RPL women who did not gain benefit of the low-dose aspirin and LMWH in previous pregnancies, indicated that hydroxychloroquine was able to significantly increase the live birth rate, gestational age at delivery and the mean birth weight, in comparison to placebo group [164]. There are some ongoing clinical trials assessing the impact of hydroxychloroquine on RPL or RM women [165–167]. Nevertheless, the results of a systematic review by Yang et al. suggested that combination of hydroxychloroquine with current treatment regimens used in the prevention of RM in APS patients, including low-dose aspirin and heparin, has been shown to have beneficial effects. However, this study also suggested further large-scale and well-designed RCTs to confirm these findings [168].

3.7 Granulocyte colony-stimulating factor (G-CSF)

G-CSF is a cytokine, produced by various types of cells, such as monocytes and macrophages, endothelial, decidual, and bone marrow cells, which act as a stimulator of neutrophils differentiation, proliferation, and function [169]. According to experimental studies, G-CSF positively affects trophoblast growth and placenta metabolism and supports the embryo [170]. It is also reported that G-CSF promotes Th2-type responses, and cytokines decreases the cytotoxicity of NK cells and enhances the function of Treg cells [15]. Moreover, G-CSF is involved in endometrial vascular remodeling which is essential for implantation [171].

According to the literature, G-CSF is capable of enhancing the thickness of endometrium and improves the quality of embryo [172]. As shown in an endometrial ex vivo model, the endometrial genes which are involved in fetus adhesion, cell migration, and remodeling of endometrial vascular are regulated by recombinant human G-CSF [173]. Subcutaneous injection of G-CSF prior to embryo transfer in RIF women, resulted in increased clinical pregnancy and implantation rates when compared to control group [174]. Study by Xu et al. showed positive effect of intrauterine administration of G-CSF for thickening of thin endometrium and significantly increasing the embryo implantation and clinical pregnancy rates [175]. Systematic review and meta-analysis of Jiang et al. indicated that G-CSF administration was capable of enhancing the implantation and clinical pregnancy rate by both the intrauterine and subcutaneous routes, however, subcutaneous injection was more efficient [176]. Almost the same beneficial effect was reported in Li. et al. meta-analysis, about the effect of transvaginal perfusion of G-CSF [177].

G-CSF treatment was also capable of elevating the Foxp3 expressing cells, indicating Treg cells, in the decidua of RPL women. Expression of G-CSF and vascular endothelial growth factor (VEGF) in trophoblast was also upregulated as a result of G-CSF treatment. These findings showed the efficiency of G-CSF therapy for RPL women, probably by modulating the immune responses by induction and recruitment of Treg cell in decidua of RPL women [178]. Subcutaneous G-CSF administration for primary RM patients showed that 82.8% of women who received G-CSF, had live birth, while the rate of live birth was 48.5% in placebo group [179]. However, a RCT by Eapen et al. indicated no improvement in pregnancy outcome after administration of recombinant human G-CSF in the first trimester of pregnancy for RPL patients

[180]. Lack of beneficial effect after intrauterine G-CSF injection was also confirmed in another RCT including RM women [181].

Considering the heterogeneities in studies, besides inexpensive cost of G-CSF and no report of the newborn's abnormalities or malformations and minor maternal side effect [75], G-CSF has the potential to be a promising approach in management of reproductive disorders. Nevertheless, administration of G-CSF for improvement of pregnancy outcome and immunologic aberrations in RIF and RPL women, requires further high-quality researches.

3.8 Granulocyte-macrophage colony-stimulating factor (GM-CSF)

GM-CSF is a cytokine, produced by T lymphocytes, macrophages, endothelial cells, and fibroblasts, which stimulates the differentiation, survival, and activation of granulocytes and macrophages [182]. GM-CSF is also produced by epithelial cells of uterine glands or lumen during the pregnancy, furthermore, placental trophoblasts express GM-CSF receptor [75]. GM-CSF production increases significantly during embryo implantation and pregnancy, especially in the first trimester; however, the elevated production of GM-CSF in normal pregnancy, is not observed in reproductive disorders [15]. It is estimated that GM-CSF is essential for normal development of blastocyst, through inhibition of apoptosis and stimulation of glucose uptake by blastocyst [183]. The addition of GM-CSF to the embryo culture medium, enhanced the survival of transferred embryo, implantation rate in addition to live birth rate [184]. The same improvement in the implantation and progressive clinical pregnancy rate was obtained in the study of Tevkin et al. [185]. Study by Akgul et al. indicated that GM-CSF activity was decreased in decidua of RPL patients, while moderate and severe GM-CSF activity was observed in fertile women. In addition, GM-CSF rate and distribution were different in various compartments of decidua [186].

Considering the positive effects of GM-CSF on human reproduction, it may be effective in women with reproductive disorders; however, there are limited studies evaluating the effect of GM-CSF in RIF and RM patients, which highlights the importance of further large-scale studies.

3.9 Anti-tumor necrosis factor-α (anti-TNF-α) for RIF patients

Anti-TNF-α medications target TNF-α cytokine and are utilized for the treatment of autoimmune disorders like rheumatoid arthritis [187]. These medications, including adalimumab (humira-fully human recombinant immunoglobulin G1 monoclonal antibody) and etanercept (dimeric Fc fusion protein), reduce inflammation, thus they are suggested to be useful in improving the pregnancy outcome in reproductive disorders [188]. Elevated level of TNF-α is responsible for higher Th1 type responses, increasing the rate of prostaglandin E2, uterine muscle contraction, and activation of coagulation cascade, which leads to thrombosis of placental vascular and adverse pregnancy outcome [189]. In fact, TNF-α is involved in thrombosis-mediated fetal loss by increasing the expression of fibrinogen-like protein 2 (FGL2), a fibrinogen-related prothrombinase, which induces the synthesis of thrombin, deposition of fibrin and activation of C5 component of complement and neutrophils [75].

The study of Santiago et al., which used etanercept for endometrial preparation at the time of embryo transfer in women suffering from RIF, indicated 75.9% of embryo implantation and 62.7% of ongoing pregnancy/live birth rate, post-treatment [190]. The effect of Adalimumab on pregnancy complications is often investigated in combination with other therapeutic approaches such as IVIG. For instance, the study of Winger et al. investigated the efficiency of adalimumab alone or in combination with IVIG in RIF patients, who had an increased Th1/Th2 ratio. The implantation rate for adalimumab receiving group was 31% (4/13), while it was 59% (50/85) in combination with adalimumab and IVIG. The clinical pregnancy and live birth rates were also higher in combination treatment group [122]. Another investigation by this author, evaluated the effect of preconception Adalimumab and IVIG in group I with severe TNF-α/IL-10 cytokine elevation, before the conception and treatment (>39.0) and group II with a moderate TNF-α/IL-10 ratio (>30.6 and ≤ 39.0). The implantation, clinical pregnancy, delivery, and live birth rate was higher in group II when compared to group I; however, the difference was not significant. The TNF-α/IL-10 ratio was also significantly decreased post-treatment. This study supported the beneficial effect of modulating the elevated inflammatory cytokines in improving the success rate of IVF cycles with immunomodulatory approaches, such as anti-TNF-α and IVIG [191].

It has been proved that the frequency of TNF-α producing Th1 cells, and TNF-α/IL-10 ratio is significantly higher in RPL patients [192]. Increased serum concentration of TNF-α in immune-dependent RM patients was decreased after treatment with etanercept [193]. In the study of Fu et al. etanercept was able to downregulate the levels of TNF-α and NK cell activity and increased the rate of live birth, in refractory RSA patients with immunologic abnormalities [194]. Moreover, etanercept was able to significantly downregulate the activity of NK cells, however, no significant difference was observed in Treg cells level. Therefore, beneficial effect of etanercept in RM patients was attributed to the immunomodulatory effect of etanercept [195]. Combination of TNF inhibitors and IVIG for the treatment of RSA women was investigated in study of Winger et al. Study population was divided into three groups, receiving anticoagulant (group I), anticoagulant and IVIG (group II) and anticoagulant, IVIG and etanercept or adalimumab (group III). The live birth rate was 19%, 54%, and 71% for groups I, II, and III, respectively. Moreover, a significant increase was observed in the pregnancy outcome of group III, in comparison with group I [196].

3.10 Cyclosporine

Cyclosporine, an immunosuppressive agent, is widely utilized in order to prevent graft rejection post-transplantation and in treatment of autoimmune disorders [197]. Cyclosporine impairs both humoral and cellular immunity and prevents IL-2, TNF-α, and IFN-γ expression and T cell proliferation, by inhibiting calcium-dependent signaling pathways [198]. According to the literature, cyclosporine upregulates IL-4 secretion and creates a shift in favor of Th2-type responses in addition to suppression of Th1 lymphocytes and associated cytokines [199]. Furthermore, NK cells, macrophages, and dendritic cells' function is also impaired by cyclosporine [85]. Cyclosporine is capable of improving the trophoblast invasion by regulation of MMP9 and MMP2, in first trimester [200]. Indeed, animal investigations proved the positive effect of cyclosporine on trophoblast cells and its ability in inducing maternal immunotolerance by downregulation of co-stimulatory molecules, upregulation of inhibitory mediators, and modulation of Th1/Th2 and Th17/Treg equilibrium [201, 202].

There are limited studies that explore the efficiency of cyclosporine in improvement of outcomes of RIF patients. In a recent retrospective cohort study by Cheng et al., the beneficial effect of cyclosporine after embryo transfer on pregnancy

DOI: http://dx.doi.org/10.5772/intechopen.108869

outcome was investigated among RIF patients. Implantation, clinical pregnancy, and live birth rate of subjects were significantly improved post-cyclosporine application, while there was no elevation in the risk of obstetric and pediatric complications after this treatment protocol [17]. It is inferred that the beneficial effect of cyclosporine in improvement of pregnancy outcomes is associated with immunomodulatory effect of this agent, which hampers maternal immune system's attack on the embryo. Cyclosporin effect was also explored on women with a history of unexplained transfer failure in frozen-thawed embryo transfer (FET) cycles in the study of Qu et al. However, the results of this study showed no significant differences between cyclosporine-treated group and control group in implantation, clinical pregnancy, and take-home baby rate [203].

Refractory immune RSA patients who were positive for APS were treated with cyclosporine after unsuccessful treatments with aspirin, prednisone, heparin, LIT, and IVIG. Cyclosporine was capable of reducing the titer of autoantibodies besides 76.92% successful pregnancy was achieved [204]. In the study of Ling et al. the effect, safety, and mechanism of low-dose cyclosporine in RSA patients were assessed. At the time of positive pregnancy test, 100 mg/day oral cyclosporine was started for treatment group for 30 days, control group received progesterone. Immunologic parameters were evaluated pre- and post-treatment. CD3 level of maternal blood was upregulated while CD8 level was downregulated after treatment. Moreover, the live birth rate was significantly higher in cyclosporine group. No side effects and adverse pregnancy outcomes were reported [205]. In the study of Azizi et al., 76 RPL women were recruited (38 in cyclosporine group, 38 in control group) and alteration of immunologic parameters besides pregnancy outcome were assessed pre- and post-treatment. According to the results, the frequency of Th1 cells, Th1/Th2 ratio, expression of T-bet, Th1-related transcription factor, and secretion of IFN-γ and TNF-α were significantly downregulated after cyclosporine administration, when compared to pre-treatment. Control group exhibited no significant differences. Moreover, cyclosporine significantly upregulated the frequency of Th2 cells, expression of GATA-3, and secretion of IL-10. A significant elevation in the rate of successful childbirth was observed in cyclosporine group [206]. Another study evaluated the effect of cyclosporine on Th17/Treg axis in peripheral blood of RSA patients. The study group included 30 women with normal early pregnancy, 25 RSA women, 27 pregnant women with RSA history receiving progesterone, and 24 pregnant women with RSA history receiving cyclosporine. Cyclosporine significantly increased the frequency of Treg cells, production of IL-10 and TGF-β, and decreased Th17 cells, by upregulation of co-inhibitory molecules expression [207]. A recent RCT by Zhao et al. Investigated the effectiveness of intrauterine perfusion of cyclosporine in RSA women with endometrial alloimmune dysfunction. Live birth rate of cyclosporine group was significantly higher than control group, while the frequency of $CD56^+$ cell and $CD57^+$ cell at the luteal phase of the second menstrual cycle was lower [208]. A recent meta-analysis, in which effects of oral immunosuppressants were assessed on pregnancy outcome of RM patients, indicated that cyclosporine or prednisolone was able to significantly enhance the rate of live birth (OR = 3.6, 95% CI: 2.1–6.15, $p < 0.00001$) and ongoing pregnancy (OR = 8.82, 95% CI: 2.91–26.75, $p = 0.0001$) in idiopathic RM patients. Rate of miscarriage was decreased post-treatment. However, the study reported significant heterogeneity and a moderate-to-severe risk of bias [209].

There is still a lack of high-quality evidence about cyclosporine efficiency for RSA and RIF patients. Due to limited evidence, cyclosporine is not recommended for these patients and cyclosporine application must be limited to clinical trials.

3.11 Sirolimus

Sirolimus, also known as rapamycin, is an immunomodulator agent approved by FDA for prevention of solid organ transplant rejection, furthermore, anti-tumor effect of sirolimus has been also documented. The immunosuppressive effect of sirolimus is mediated by its inhibitory action on mammalian target of rapamycin (mTOR) kinase pathway, blocking the downstream of co-stimulatory signals [210]. The proposed mechanisms of action of sirolimus for modulation of immune system include expansion of Treg cells and prevention of the differentiation of Th17 cells, inhibition of B and T lymphocytes proliferation by prevention of IL-2 and IL-4 production, and attenuation of inflammatory responses [211, 212].

According to a report from the national transplantation pregnancy registry (NTPR), more than 14,000 female transplant recipients worldwide, had a history of successful pregnancies, therefore, it is concluded that sirolimus is not a contraindication for pregnancy [213]. In addition, animal studies also confirmed the positive effect of sirolimus on gestation. An animal study on murine model of RIF demonstrated that Sirolimus was able to promote the expansion of Treg cells in the depletion of regulatory T cell (DEREG) mice and improved the implantation rate [214]. A phase II randomized clinical trial by Ahmadi et al. evaluated the immunomodulatory effect of Sirolimus on immunologic abnormalities in RIF women with a history of at least 3 implantation failures. Patients with increased Th17/Treg ratio, who received Sirolimus showed an expansion of Treg cells, besides a reduction in frequency of Th17 cells and Th17/Treg ratio. Subsequently, an elevated rate of clinical pregnancy and live birth was observed in treated group, compared with non-treated control group [215].

There is no study assessing the efficiency of sirolimus in improvement of pregnancy outcomes in RPL women and by today, sirolimus has been used in animal model of RIF and for improvement of pregnancy consequences of RIF women in Ahamdi et al. study. Nevertheless, there are limited evidence about the efficiency of sirolimus in reproductive failure. Considering the immunomodulatory effect of sirolimus, it has the potential to provide a promising option to ameliorate reproductive disorders on immunologic basis.

3.12 Tacrolimus

Tacrolimus (FK506), is an immunosuppressive agent, approved for inhibition of allograft transplant rejection, by diminishing the recipient's immune systems' alloreactivity toward graft [216]. It has been also documented that Tacrolimus is also efficient in management of GVHD and autoimmune disorders, such as rheumatoid arthritis and degenerative inflammatory brain diseases [15]. Binding of Tacrolimus to FK506 binding protein (immunophilin FKBP12), and subsequent creation of a complex with calcineurin, prevents the production of IFN-γ, IL-2, TNFα, IL-1β, and IL-6 and activation and proliferation of T lymphocyte [85].

It is postulated that tacrolimus may be a plausible choice in management of reproductive disorders, such as RIF and RPL, especially in patients with an elevated level of Th1 cells, as it was investigated in the study of Nakagawa et al. In this prospective cohort study, RIF patients with elevated Th1 ($CD4^+$/IFN-γ^+)/Th2 ($CD4^+$/IL-4^+) ratio, received tacrolimus 2 days before embryo transfer, continued until a positive pregnancy test. The results indicated that RIF women who received tacrolimus had a significantly higher rate of clinical pregnancy and live birth rate, compared to control group, while the miscarriage rate was significantly decreased post-treatment [217].

The other prospective cohort study by this group included larger population of RIF patients, who had elevated Th1/Th2 ($CD4^{+}IFN\text{-}\gamma^{+}/CD4^{+}IL\text{-}4^{+}$) cells ratios (≥10.3) and were treated with tacrolimus. Dose of tacrolimus was adjusted based on the initial Th1/Th2 ratio. Th1 cells level were divided as low, medium, and high. Clinical pregnancy rates of low, middle, and high Th1 level groups were not statistically different. Successful ongoing pregnancy rate was statistically elevated in the low Th1 group when compared with the high Th1 group. However, the rate of live births was not significantly different between groups [218]. In Bahrami-Asl and colleagues' study, 10 RIF women with increased Th1/Th2 ratio were evaluated after tacrolimus treatment for expression of p53, leukemia inhibitory factor (LIF), IL-4, IL-10, IL-17, and IFN-γ in the endometrium. LIF, IL-10, and IL-17 expression were upregulated and IL-4, IFN-γ expression, and IFN-γ/IL-10 ratio were downregulated post-treatment. Moreover, rate of implantation, clinical pregnancy, and live birth were 40, 50, and 35% respectively, in RIF women without a history of previous successful pregnancy [219]. Considering the results of these studies, Th1/Th2 ratio may be a biomarker for predicting ART outcomes in RIF patients and selection of suitable candidates for tacrolimus administration. Of note, due to presence of a congenital heart abnormality in one of the babies in study of Nakagawa, careful considerations must be taken in administration of tacrolimus.

There are limited studies evaluating the effectiveness of tacrolimus for RPL and RSA patients. A case report study utilized tacrolimus for an RM patient with a history of 11 consecutive miscarriages in spite of receiving different treatments including low-dose aspirin, LMWH, prednisolone, and IVIG. After 12th conception, the patient showed an elevated rate of Th1/Th2 ratio, so she received tacrolimus (1 mg/d). In spite of this treatment, the patient miscarried. However, 13th conception of this patient was successful by receiving 2 mg/d of tacrolimus. The authors suggested the efficiency of immunosuppressive treatment with tacrolimus for RM patients with increased Th1/Th2 ratio [220].

There are studies that investigated the effectiveness of tacrolimus on both RIF and RPL patients. A study including 58 subjects, who were divided into two groups: (I) 31 subjects in RIF-alone group; and (II) 27 subjects in RIF-plus-RPL group was done by Hisano et al., in order to investigate the effect of tacrolimus on these patients. Frequency of Th1 was decreased after treatment in both groups, however, the reduction in Th1 frequency was delayed in Group II [221]. One hundred nine RIF or RPL women with increased peripheral Th1/Th2 ($CD4^{+}IFN\text{-}\gamma^{+}/CD4^{+}IL\text{-}4^{+}$) cell ratio received tacrolimus. One hundred thirteen babies, including 4 twins, were born. Obstetric complications including hypertension and one congenital abnormality were reported [222].

Further, well-designed and ideally randomized double-blind controlled studies are required to confirm the efficiency of tacrolimus in pregnancy complications with immunologic aberrations.

3.13 Platelet-rich plasma (PRP)

Recently, there is accumulating interest in the efficiency of intrauterine infusion of PRP in improving the pregnancy outcome in RIF patients. PRP is an autologous blood product, containing concentrated platelets in a small volume of plasma [223]. PRP may be able to promote endometrial receptivity through the various growth factors, cell adhesion molecules, and cytokines, stored in platelets' granules, including fibroblast growth factor (FGF), epidermal growth factor (EGF), platelet-derived growth factor (PDGF), VEGF, transforming growth factor (TGF), insulin-like growth factor I, II (IGF-I, II), connective tissue growth factor (CTGF) and IL-8 [151, 224]. Intrauterine administration of PRP induces the activation of platelets and release of above mentioned mediators in the uterus space, leading to cellular proliferation and differentiation, endometrial cell migration, and neu-angiogenesis alongside alteration of local immunologic responses [151]. In fact, platelets are capable of regulating immune responses. The TGFβ content of platelets mediates the immunosuppressive effect on T cells, furthermore, platelets can suppress the $CD8^+$ T cell's function [225].

There are limited studies investigating PRP therapy for reproductive disorders. Study by Nazeri et al. indicated that intrauterine infusion of 0.5 ml of PRP, 48 hours before ET, was effective in improvement of pregnancy outcomes in RIF patients [226]. Another study revealed that endometrial thickness, implantation rate, and per-cycle clinical pregnancy rate were higher in PRP administration [227]. The same positive effect of increasing the thickness of endometrium by PRP in RIF subjects was reported in the study of Mouanness et al. [228] and Coksuer et al. [229]. To our knowledge, there is only one study investigating the effectiveness of autologous PRP for improvement of pregnancy outcomes in RPL patients. Sixty-three RPL patients with a history of at least two previous pregnancy losses were divided into PRP receiving group and control group. The rate of clinical pregnancy and live birth was higher in patients who received intrauterine PRP. This study confirmed the efficiency of PRP administration in RPL women for the first time [230].

However, there is a lack of studies that investigate the effect of PRP on alteration of immunologic parameters in RIF and RPL women. Additionally, larger RCTs are still required to prove the efficiency of intrauterine PRP administration for reproductive failures.

3.14 Human chorionic gonadotropin (hCG)

HCG is an embryo-derived glycoprotein, which is involved in the process of implantation and regulation of endometrium receptivity. Prior to implantation, production of hCG is started by the blastocyst; after the implantation, the syncytiotrophoblast is responsible for hCG synthesis; furthermore, hCG is secreted by endometrium in the secretory phase [231]. Endometrial decidualization, receptivity, and immune system are regulated by hCG, through expressed hCG receptors on endothelium, in a paracrine manner. Additionally, the cytotrophoblast synthesizes a hyperglycosylated form of hCG, which plays a role in embryo implantation and trophoblast invasion [232].

The results of intrauterine infusion of hCG at the time of embryo transfer in RIF women, in an RCT, demonstrated increased implantation, pregnancy, clinical pregnancy, ongoing pregnancy, and live delivery rate in treated women [233]. Significantly higher implantation, clinical pregnancy, and ongoing pregnancy rate were observed in intrauterine administration of recombinant hCG (rhCG), prior to embryo transfer [234]. However, the positive effects of hCG were not confirmed in the study of Kathleen et al., in which no improvement in pregnancy outcome was achieved post-infusion of hCG [235]. Giuliani et al. investigated the effect of a single intrauterine hCG infusion at the time of embryo transfer on the distribution of NK cells in the uterine, in fertile oocyte donors. Stromal $CD56^+CD16^+$NK cells were evaluated in endometrial biopsies. Intrauterine hCG infusion was capable of enhancing the percentage of stromal $CD16^+$ cells; however, no statistical differences were observed in $CD56^+$ staining in hCG receiving group, compared with control group [232]. The systematic review and meta-analysis of Gao et al. confirmed the efficiency of intrauterine injection of hCG in improvement of live birth, clinical pregnancy and ongoing pregnancy and implantation rate after IVF cycles. This study also emphasized that different effects of hCG on IVT-ET outcomes are related to different timing and dosages of hCG injection [236]. Further studies, including multicenter, randomized controlled trials, are suggested in order to confirm the conclusion of these meta-analysis, because of the great heterogeneity among the studies.

Swart et al. found that hCG supplementation during the mid-secretory phase for RPL women was able to significantly reduce the miscarriage rate [237]. The immunomodulatory effect of hCG was assessed in a cohort study, in which intrauterine infusion of hCG was administrated for infertile women with a decreased rate of FoxP3$^+$ Treg cells in mid-luteal phase. As a result, frequency of Treg cells and the clinical pregnancy rate were significantly elevated post-treatment [238]. The results of a cochrane database systematic review, assessing the efficacy of hCG in preventing further miscarriage in RM women indicated that hCG significantly decreased the miscarriage rate, but in the case of excluding two studies with lower methodological quality, no significant difference was observed. This study suggested well-designed RCTs of sufficient power and methodological quality to determine efficiency of hCG in RM patients [239].

It is concluded that there is a requirement for further studies including multicenter, randomized controlled trials, and preferential studies that consider immunologic aberration, in order to assess the efficiency of hCG administration for reproductive failures.

3.15 Mesenchymal stem cells (MSCs)

MSCs are stromal cells, derived from adipose tissue, umbilical cord blood, Wharton's jellies, endometrium, and amniotic fluid, which exhibit the ability of self-renewal, multilineage differentiation, secretion of multiple factors, and regulation of immune responses [240]. Considering these potentials, MSCs may be a promising approach for immunotherapy. According to the literature, the efficiency of MSCs, derived from different sources, has been evaluated in pregnancy-associated disorders, especially RPL, in animal models. According to animal studies, the action mechanisms of MSCs in improvement of pregnancy outcome in abortion-prone mice includes downregulation of Th1 cytokines, upregulation of Th2 cytokines, induction of switch of M1 macrophages to anti-inflammatory M2 type, reducing of lymphocytes proliferation, increasing the secretion of anti-inflammatory cytokines, such as IL-10 and TGF-β, which are mediated by mediators produced by MSCs or by cell–cell interaction [241].

Most of the animal studies were conducted on abortion-prone mice and RSA mouse models, however, only Tersoglio et al. study investigated the effect of MSCs on thin endometrium with repeated implantation failure. Endometrial changes were evaluated before and after administration of endometrial mesenchymal stem cells in 29 RIF patients with thin endometrium, hypo-responsive/unresponsive to estrogens. Endometrial thickness was increased significantly and immunologic parameters including T and B lymphocytes and NK cells were normalized post-treatment, resulting in an improvement in pregnancy outcomes [242].

Wharton jelly of human umbilical cord was utilized for isolation of MSCs for treatment of spontaneous-abortion rat model. Intravenous injection of bromocriptine was used for induction of abortion model, inducing degeneration of decidual cells. Transplantation of MSCs prevented the damage caused by injection and restored the changes in expression and secretion of IL-10, IFN-γ, and IL-17, with IL-10 increasing and IFN-γ, IL-17 decreasing [243]. A recent study by Zhang et al. investigated the effect of umbilical MSCs on the expansion of Treg cells. Co-culture of MSCs with decidual Treg cells showed that MSCs are capable of promoting the expansion and suppressive function of decidual Treg cells besides elevating the IL-10 and TGF-β production, in vitro. Additionally, in vivo experiments, including transfer of bone marrow-derived MSCs to LPS-induced abortion model and spontaneous abortion model promoted the decidual Treg cell, meanwhile, the rate of absorption was decreased in both models [244]. The same immunoregulatory effect was confirmed for adipose-derived MSCs in abortion-prone mice, including reduction of IL-2 and IFN-γ and up-regulation of IL-4 and IL-10 production, reduction of IL-12, IL-2, and IFN-γ and upregulation of IL-4, IL-6, IL-10, and GM-CSF gene expression besides significant decrease in abortion rate [245]. Modulation of uNK cells and promotion of secretion of tolerogenic cytokines rather than inflammatory cytokines [246], switching off the decidual macrophages to an M2 phenotype and prevention of CD4+ T cells proliferation [247], decreasing the rate of Th1 cells while upregulating the Th2 responses and downregulation of lymphocytes proliferation against paternal antigens [246, 248] are among the immunoregulatory mechanism of MSCs, on animal models of abortion or RPL.

It seems that MSCs derived from adipose, bone marrow, Wharton jelly, and other resources are helpful in improvement of pregnancy consequences and modulation of abnormal immune systems in animal models. It is estimated that MSCs could be efficiently used in the immunotherapy of patients with reproductive failures, however further well-designed RCTs are required to confirm these findings.

3.16 Human amniotic epithelial cells (hAECs)

hAECs are derived from the closest layer of the term placenta to the fetus and have a high potential for proliferation and multilineage differentiation capacity. hAECs have gained considerable attention in recent years because of their stem cell characteristics, which differentiate into various cell lineages [249]. hAECs are also able to produce prostaglandin E2 and TGF-β and possess immunomodulatory effects on the proliferation and function of immune cells. Activity of NK cells, switch of M1 type macrophages to M2 type cells, apoptosis induction in T and B lymphocytes, and prevention of NK cells and macrophage migration, are mediated by the cytokines secreted from hAECs [250]. Immunomodulatory potential and low immunogenicity due to reduced expression of major histocompatibility complex (MHC) type I, make hAECs a promising approach for clinical applications [250].

To our knowledge, there is only one study that investigates the effects of hAEC on the immune cells of unexplained RSA patients, in vitro. Co-culture of naive $CD4^+$ T cells of URSA patients with hAECs indicated that proliferation of naive $CD4^+$ T cells and secretion of Th1 and Th17 cytokines were inhibited by hAECs, while secretion of Th2 cytokines and differentiation of Tregs alongside production of Treg associated cytokines were increased. Considering the immunosuppressive ability of hAECs, the authors suggested that these cells may be a promising choice in treatment of RSA patients [251].

4. Future prospective

In recent years, considerable progress has been made in the management of reproductive failures, including immunotherapeutic approaches. However, there is a paucity of clinical data and well-designed qualified studies in this field, especially studies in which candidates for immunotherapy are selected based on evaluation of immunologic aberration. In addition, there is an urgent need for experiments that evaluate the pre- and post-treatment alteration of immunologic parameters, in addition to pregnancy outcome, to further determine the mechanism of action of the immunologic treatment in obstetric complications. Moreover, a "benefit to risk" evaluation of these therapeutic agents is required in order to determine the probable risk of pregnancy adverse outcome or fetus malformation. Further research is also required to update the knowledge about the newly introduced immunotherapeutic agents such as calcineurin inhibitors. There is also a need for studies which determine the immunological status of uterine, rather than peripheral blood, as immune status of peripheral blood does not always reflect the uterine immune status.

Among immunomodulator and immunosuppressive therapies which have already been introduced to clinical practice for the management of reproductive complications, including RIF and RPL, some still need further investigations. Immunosuppressive medications, such as cyclosporine, sirolimus, and tacrolimus seem to be beneficial, however, future studies are required to determine the appropriate candidates besides side effects.

Nowadays, therapeutic modalities with minimal side effects and ethical issues, besides high efficiency have gained a great deal of attention. In recent years, there has been increasing attention on the role of endometrial microbiota in reproductive disorders. Administration of probiotic formulation that includes species of lactobacillus or bifidobacterium, as most commonly used probiotic strains, or other probiotic strains, by different routes has been investigated in literatures. Probiotics consist of bacteria or non-pathogenic yeast, which colonize the gastrointestinal tract and exhibit health benefits when applied to the body [252]. It has been suggested that probiotics are capable of modulating the abnormalities of immune system in animal models, including upregulation of suppressive immune cells and mediators and downregulation of pro-inflammatory microenvironment [253]. The data on probiotics efficiency and mechanisms in pregnancy complications and its immunomodulatory effect, are limited and conflicting due to the heterogeneity of the studies [254]. Therefore, well-designed high-quality randomized controlled trials are required to comprehend the effectiveness of probiotics in reproductive complications, considering the probable immunomodulatory effect of probiotics.

Stem cells are the other promising approaches, which have gained attention in recent years based on their wide sources, easy sampling, low immunogenicity, and minimum ethical issues, which make stem cells an attractive therapeutic modality. There is increasing evidence indicating the exciting results of MSC therapy in autoimmune diseases, cancers, GVHD and etc. Nevertheless, a small number of studies have been conducted investigating the effectiveness of MSC-based therapy in RIF and RPL women [255]. Considering the immunomodulatory action of MSCs, it can be a promising approach in reproductive disorders with immunologic basis. In addition, extracellular vesicles derived from MSCs have also provided a novel insight into cell-free therapies for treatment of various diseases, as a safer and more suitable treatment for clinical applications. Therefore, MSC-derived extracellular vesicles may serve as an attractive modality, with similar therapeutic and immunomodulatory effects with MSCs, in the field of reproduction disorders.

The proposed action mechanism of immunotherapeutic approaches in improvement of pregnancy consequences in RRF patients is summarized in **Figure 3**.

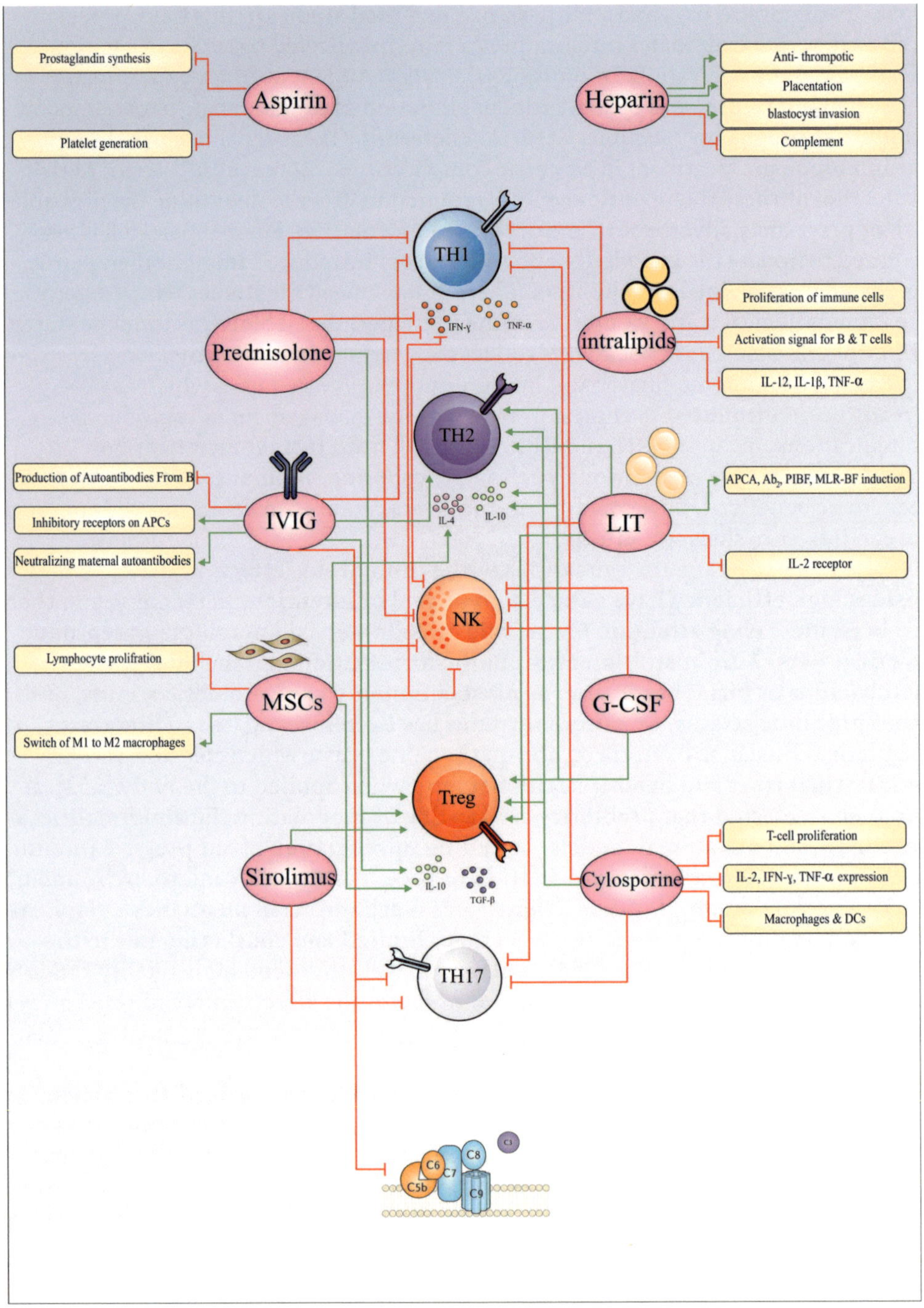

Figure 3.

The proposed action mechanism of immunotherapeutic approaches in improvement of pregnancy consequences in RRF patients. The common immune cells which are affected by immunotherapeutic modalities include Th1 and Th17 cells, which are downregulated by these approaches, in contrast, NK cell and Th2 and Treg cells frequency and/or cytokine secretion are upregulated by these immunologic methods. Abbreviation: NK: natural killer; Th1: T helper 1; Th2: T helper 2; Th17: T helper 17; Treg: T regulatory; TNFα: tumor necrosis factor α; IFNγ: interferon γ; IL-4: interleukin-4; IL-10: interleukin-10; IL-17: interleukin-17; TGFβ: Transforming growth factor beta; IVIG: Intravenous immunoglobulin; G-CSF: Granulocyte colony stimulating factor; MSC: mesenchymal stem cells; LIT: lymphocyte immunotherapy.

5. Conclusion

RRF is a frustrating condition for both couples and clinicians in the field of reproductive treatment and a significant concern for women who have already undergone ART treatments without favorable outcomes. Here, we discussed the immunologic aspects of reproductive failure, proposed mechanisms, and immunologic tests, besides the immunotherapeutic modalities. Given the limited number and quality of available research and heterogeneity of studies (sample size, patients' selection, dose, route, duration, etc.) which investigate the mechanism of immunologic imbalances in pathogenesis of RRF, further investigations are required to update the current knowledge about the immunoetiology of RRF. Additionally, considering the novelty of immunotherapy in the field of reproductive disorders, more experiments are required to determine the effectiveness of mentioned approaches in improvement of pregnancy consequences, besides their mechanisms and side effects. Nevertheless, the involvement of immunologic aberrations in pathogenesis of RRF (excluding other etiologies) and beneficial effects of immunotherapeutic approaches in the treatment of patients who are selected based on their immunologic basis, are indisputable. Therefore, selection of immunotherapeutic approach, based on the immunologic origin of complication, or personalized medicine in other word, is maybe the best solution for the dilemma.

Further advancement of the immunologic diagnostic test, is also helpful to assess the underlying immunoetiology of subject, prior to treatment. Nevertheless, considering the novel promising approaches, such as calcineurin inhibitors, MSCs therapy and related extracellular vesicles, and probiotics, already available therapeutic modalities, such as PBMC therapy and TNF-α inhibitors, immunologic-based RRF diagnosis and treatment have the potential to be the next great forthcoming development in the field of human reproduction.

Author details

Samaneh Abdolmohammadi-Vahid[1], Leili Aghebati-Maleki[2,3], Javad Ahmadian-Heris[4], Shahla Danaii[5] and Mehdi Yousefi[3,6*]

1 Department of Immunology, School of Medicine, Shahid Beheshti University of Medical Sciences, Tehran, Iran

2 Immunology Research Center, Tabriz University of Medical Sciences, Tabriz, Iran

3 Department of Immunology, Faculty of Medicine, Tabriz University of Medical Sciences, Tabriz, Iran

4 Department of Allergy and Clinical Immunology, Pediatric Hospital, Tabriz University of Medical Sciences, Tabriz, Iran

5 Gynecology Department, Eastern Azerbaijan ACECR ART center, Eastern Azerbaijan branch of ACECR, Tabriz, Iran

6 Stem Cell Research Center, Tabriz University of Medical Science, Tabriz, Iran

*Address all correspondence to: yousefime@tbzmed.ac.ir

References

[1] Macklon NS, Geraedts JP, Fauser BC. Conception to ongoing pregnancy: The 'black box' of early pregnancy loss. Human Reproduction Update. 2002;**8**(4):333-343

[2] Robillard P-Y, Hulsey TC, Dekker GA, Chaouat G. Preeclampsia and human reproduction: An essay of a long term reflection. Journal of Reproductive Immunology. 2003;**59**(2):93-100

[3] Makrigiannakis A, Petsas G, Toth B, Relakis K, Jeschke U. Recent advances in understanding immunology of reproductive failure. Journal of Reproductive Immunology. 2011;**90**(1):96-104

[4] No RG-tG. The Investigation and Treatment of Couples with Recurrent First-trimester and Second-trimester Miscarriage. London, UK: RCOG; 2011

[5] Medicine PCotASfR. Evaluation and treatment of recurrent pregnancy loss: A committee opinion. Fertility and Sterility. 2012;**98**(5):1103-1111

[6] RPL EGGo, Bender Atik R, Christiansen OB, Elson J, Kolte AM, Lewis S, et al. ESHRE guideline: Recurrent pregnancy loss. Human Reproduction Open. 2018;**2018**(2):hoy004

[7] Dbstet A. WHO: Recommended definitions, terminology and format for statistical tables related to the perinatal period and use of a new certificate for cause of perinatal deaths. Acta Obstetricia et Gynecologica Scandinavica. 1977;**56**(3):247-253

[8] Divya P, Gupta S. Current update on recurrent pregnancy loss. Journal of Basic and Clinical Reproductive Sciences. 2019;**8**(1):1-6

[9] Medicine PCotASfR. Definitions of infertility and recurrent pregnancy loss: A committee opinion. Fertility and Sterility. 2013;**99**(1):63

[10] Sebastian-Leon P, Garrido N, Remohí J, Pellicer A, Diaz-Gimeno P. Asynchronous and pathological windows of implantation: Two causes of recurrent implantation failure. Human Reproduction. 2018;**33**(4):626-635

[11] Padvi NV, Singh PP, Nadkarni PK, Nadkarni AA. Knowing a cross-talk between embryo and endometrium can help to achieve successful pregnancy outcome in recurrent implantation failure. International Journal of Reproduction, Contraception, Obstetrics and Gynecology. 2017;**6**(2):739-743

[12] Tan BK, Vandekerckhove P, Kennedy R, Keay SD. Investigation and current management of recurrent IVF treatment failure in the UK. BJOG: An International Journal of Obstetrics & Gynaecology. 2005;**112**(6):773-780

[13] Cimadomo D, Craciunas L, Vermeulen N, Vomstein K, Toth B. Definition, diagnostic and therapeutic options in recurrent implantation failure: An international survey of clinicians and embryologists. Human Reproduction. 2021;**36**(2):305-317

[14] Coughlan C, Ledger W, Wang Q, Liu F, Demirol A, Gurgan T, et al. Recurrent implantation failure: Definition and management. Reproductive Biomedicine Online. 2014;**28**(1):14-38

[15] Parhizkar F, Motavalli-Khiavi R, Aghebati-Maleki L, Parhizkar Z, Pourakbari R, Kafil HS, et al. The impact of new immunological therapeutic

strategies on recurrent miscarriage and recurrent implantation failure. Immunology Letters. 2021;**236**:20-30

[16] Kwak-Kim J, Chung-Bang H, Ng S, Ntrivalas E, Mangubat C, Beaman K, et al. Increased T helper 1 cytokine responses by circulating T cells are present in women with recurrent pregnancy losses and in infertile women with multiple implantation failures after IVF. Human Reproduction. 2003;**18**(4):767-773

[17] Cheng W, Wu Y, Wu H, Zou Q, Meng Q, Wang F, et al. Improved pregnancy outcomes of cyclosporine A on patients with unexplained repeated implantation failure in IVF/ICSI cycles: A retrospective cohort study. American Journal of Reproductive Immunology. 2022;**87**(4):e13525

[18] Vomstein K, Feil K, Strobel L, Aulitzky A, Hofer-Tollinger S, Kuon R-J, et al. Immunological risk factors in recurrent pregnancy loss: Guidelines versus current state of the art. Journal of Clinical Medicine. 2021;**10**(4):869

[19] Wang W, Sung N, Gilman-Sachs A, Kwak-Kim J. T helper (Th) cell profiles in pregnancy and recurrent pregnancy losses: Th1/Th2/Th9/Th17/Th22/Tfh cells. Frontiers in Immunology. 2020;**11**:2025

[20] Yang F, Zheng Q, Jin L. Dynamic function and composition changes of immune cells during normal and pathological pregnancy at the maternal-fetal interface. Frontiers in Immunology. 2019;**10**:2317

[21] Huber S, Schramm C, Lehr HA, Mann A, Schmitt S, Becker C, et al. Cutting edge: TGF-β signaling is required for the in vivo expansion and immunosuppressive capacity of regulatory CD4+ CD25+ T cells. The Journal of Immunology. 2004;**173**(11):6526-6531

[22] Sasaki Y, Sakai M, Miyazaki S, Higuma S, Shiozaki A, Saito S. Decidual and peripheral blood CD4+ CD25+ regulatory T cells in early pregnancy subjects and spontaneous abortion cases. MHR: Basic Science of Reproductive Medicine. 2004;**10**(5):347-353

[23] Ghaebi M, Abdolmohammadi-Vahid S, Ahmadi M, Eghbal-Fard S, Dolati S, Nouri M, et al. T cell subsets in peripheral blood of women with recurrent implantation failure. Journal of Reproductive Immunology. 2019;**131**:21-29

[24] Abdolmohammadi Vahid S, Ghaebi M, Ahmadi M, Nouri M, Danaei S, Aghebati-Maleki L, et al. Altered T-cell subpopulations in recurrent pregnancy loss patients with cellular immune abnormalities. Journal of Cellular Physiology. 2019;**234**(4):4924-4933

[25] Keller CC, Eikmans M, van der Hoorn M-LP, Lashley LE. Recurrent miscarriages and the association with regulatory T cells; A systematic review. Journal of Reproductive Immunology. 2020;**139**:103105

[26] Wang W-J, Hao C-F, Yin G-J, Bao S-H, Qiu L-H, Lin Q-D. Increased prevalence of T helper 17 (Th17) cells in peripheral blood and decidua in unexplained recurrent spontaneous abortion patients. Journal of Reproductive Immunology. 2010;**84**(2):164-170

[27] Travis OK, White D, Pierce WA, Ge Y, Stubbs CY, Spradley FT, et al. Chronic infusion of interleukin-17 promotes hypertension, activation of cytolytic natural killer cells, and vascular dysfunction in pregnant rats. Physiological Reports. 2019;7(7):e14038

[28] Lee S, Kim J, Hur S, Kim C, Na B, Lee M, et al. An imbalance in interleukin-17-producing T and Foxp3+ regulatory T cells in women with idiopathic recurrent pregnancy loss. Human Reproduction. 2011;**26**(11):2964-2971

[29] Moffett A, Shreeve N. First do no harm: uterine natural killer (NK) cells in assisted reproduction. Human Reproduction. 2015;**30**(7):1519-1525

[30] Seshadri S, Sunkara SK. Natural killer cells in female infertility and recurrent miscarriage: A systematic review and meta-analysis. Human reproduction Update. 2014;**20**(3):429-438

[31] Karami N, Boroujerdnia MG, Nikbakht R, Khodadadi A. Enhancement of peripheral blood CD56dim cell and NK cell cytotoxicity in women with recurrent spontaneous abortion or in vitro fertilization failure. Journal of Reproductive Immunology. 2012;**95**(1-2):87-92

[32] Matsubayashi H, Shida M, Kondo A, Suzuki T, Sugi T, Izumi SI, et al. Preconception peripheral natural killer cell activity as a predictor of pregnancy outcome in patients with unexplained infertility. American Journal of Reproductive Immunology. 2005;**53**(3):126-131

[33] Emmer PM, Nelen WL, Steegers EA, Hendriks JC, Veerhoek M, Joosten I. Peripheral natural killer cytotoxicity and CD56posCD16pos cells increase during early pregnancy in women with a history of recurrent spontaneous abortion. Human Reproduction. 2000;**15**(5):1163-1169

[34] Gomez-Lopez N, Olson DM, Robertson SA. Interleukin-6 controls uterine Th9 cells and CD8+ T regulatory cells to accelerate parturition in mice. Immunology and Cell Biology. 2016;**94**(1):79-89

[35] Dambaeva S, Schneiderman S, Jaiswal MK, Agrawal V, Katara GK, Gilman-Sachs A, et al. Interleukin 22 prevents lipopolysaccharide-induced preterm labor in mice. Biology of Reproduction. 2018;**98**(3):299-308

[36] Wang Y, Xu B, Li M-Q, Li D-J, Jin L-P. IL-22 secreted by decidual stromal cells and NK cells promotes the survival of human trophoblasts. International Journal of Clinical and Experimental Pathology. 2013;**6**(9):1781

[37] Roomandeh N, Saremi A, Arasteh J, Pak F, Mirmohammadkhani M, Kokhaei P, et al. Comparing serum levels of Th17 and treg cytokines in women with unexplained recurrent spontaneous abortion and fertile women. Iranian Journal of Immunology. 2018;**15**(1):59-67

[38] Perfetto COH, Fan X, Dahl S, Krieg S, Westphal LM, Lathi RB, et al. Expression of interleukin-22 in decidua of patients with early pregnancy and unexplained recurrent pregnancy loss. Journal of Assisted Reproduction and Genetics. 2015;**32**(6):977-984

[39] Bashiri A, Halper KI, Orvieto R. Recurrent Implantation Failure-update overview on etiology, diagnosis, treatment and future directions. Reproductive Biology and Endocrinology. 2018;**16**(1):1-18

[40] Carp HJ, Selmi C, Shoenfeld Y. The autoimmune bases of infertility and pregnancy loss. Journal of Autoimmunity. 2012;**38**(2-3):J266-JJ74

[41] D'Ippolito S, Ticconi C, Tersigni C, Garofalo S, Martino C, Lanzone A, et al. The pathogenic role of autoantibodies in recurrent pregnancy loss. American Journal of Reproductive Immunology. 2020;**83**(1):e13200

[42] Schreiber K, Sciascia S, De Groot PG, Devreese K, Jacobsen S, Ruiz-Irastorza G, et al. Antiphospholipid syndrome. Nature reviews Disease Primers. 2018;**4**(1):1-20

[43] Saccone G, Berghella V, Maruotti GM, Ghi T, Rizzo G, Simonazzi G, et al. Antiphospholipid antibody profile based obstetric outcomes of primary antiphospholipid syndrome: The pregnants study. American Journal of Obstetrics and Gynecology. 2017;**216**(5):-525 e1.e12

[44] Di Simone N, Raschi E, Testoni C, Castellani R, D'Asta M, Shi T, et al. Pathogenic role of anti-β2-glycoprotein I antibodies in antiphospholipid associated fetal loss: Characterisation of β2-glycoprotein I binding to trophoblast cells and functional effects of anti-β2-glycoprotein I antibodies in vitro. Annals of the Rheumatic Diseases. 2005;**64**(3):462-467

[45] Girardi G, Berman J, Redecha P, Spruce L, Thurman JM, Kraus D, et al. Complement C5a receptors and neutrophils mediate fetal injury in the antiphospholipid syndrome. The Journal of Clinical Investigation. 2003;**112**(11):1644-1654

[46] Mekinian A, Bourrienne M-C, Carbillon L, Benbara A, Noémie A, Chollet-Martin S, et al., editors. Non-conventional antiphospholipid antibodies in patients with clinical obstetrical APS: Prevalence and treatment efficacy in pregnancies. In: Seminars in Arthritis and Rheumatism. United Kingdom: W.B. Saunders Ltd., Elsevier; 1 Oct 2016;**46**(2):232-237)

[47] Shi H, Zheng H, Yin Y-F, Hu Q-Y, Teng J-L, Sun Y, et al. Antiphosphatidylserine/prothrombin antibodies (aPS/PT) as potential diagnostic markers and risk predictors of venous thrombosis and obstetric complications in antiphospholipid syndrome. Clinical Chemistry and Laboratory Medicine (CCLM). 2018;**56**(4):614-624

[48] Sakthiswary R, Rajalingam S, Norazman M, Hussein H. Antinuclear antibodies predict a higher number of pregnancy loss in unexplained recurrent pregnancy loss. La Clinica Terapeutica. 2015;**166**(2):e98-e101

[49] Kikuchi K, Shibahara H, Hirano Y, Kohno T, Hirashima C, Suzuki T, et al. Antinuclear antibody reduces the pregnancy rate in the first IVF-ET treatment cycle but not the cumulative pregnancy rate without specific medication. American Journal of Reproductive Immunology. 2003;**50**(4):363-367

[50] Chen S, Yang G, Wu P, Sun Y, Dai F, He Y, et al. Antinuclear antibodies positivity is a risk factor of recurrent pregnancy loss: A meta-analysis. In: Seminars in Arthritis and Rheumatism: WB Saunders. 1 Aug 2020;**50**(4):534-543

[51] Ying Y, Zhong YP, Zhou CQ, Xu YW, Ding CH, Wang Q, et al. A further exploration of the impact of antinuclear antibodies on in vitro fertilization–embryo transfer outcome. American Journal of Reproductive Immunology. 2013;**70**(3):221-229

[52] Maghsoudi R, Mirhosseini M. Spontaneous abortion and anti-thyroid antibodies in mother's serum. Life Science Journal. 2014;**11**(SPEC):41-44

[53] Fröhlich E, Wahl R. Thyroid autoimmunity: Role of anti-thyroid antibodies in thyroid and extra-thyroidal diseases. Frontiers in Immunology. 2017;**8**:521

[54] Thangaratinam S, Tan A, Knox E, Kilby MD, Franklyn J, Coomarasamy A.

Association between thyroid autoantibodies and miscarriage and preterm birth: Meta-analysis of evidence. BMJ. 9 May 2011;**342**:d2616

[55] Monteleone P, Parrini D, Faviana P, Carletti E, Casarosa E, Uccelli A, et al. Female infertility related to thyroid autoimmunity: The ovarian follicle hypothesis. American Journal of Reproductive Immunology. 2011;**66**(2):108-114

[56] Łukaszuk K, Kunicki M, Kulwikowska P, Liss J, Pastuszek E, Jaszczołt M, et al. The impact of the presence of antithyroid antibodies on pregnancy outcome following intracytoplasmatic sperm injection-ICSI and embryo transfer in women with normal thyreotropine levels. Journal of Endocrinological Investigation. 2015;**38**(12):1335-1343

[57] Rahnama R, Mahmoudi A-R, Kazemnejad S, Salehi M, Ghahiri A, Soltanghoraee H, et al. Thyroid peroxidase in human endometrium and placenta: A potential target for anti-TPO antibodies. Clinical and Experimental Medicine. 2021;**21**(1):79-88

[58] Kelkar RL, Meherji PK, Kadam SS, Gupta SK, Nandedkar TD. Circulating auto-antibodies against the zona pellucida and thyroid microsomal antigen in women with premature ovarian failure. Journal of Reproductive Immunology. 2005;**66**(1):53-67

[59] Twig G, Shina A, Amital H, Shoenfeld Y. Pathogenesis of infertility and recurrent pregnancy loss in thyroid autoimmunity. Journal of Autoimmunity. 2012;**38**(2-3):J275-JJ81

[60] Vissenberg R, Manders V, Mastenbroek S, Fliers E, Afink G, Ris-Stalpers C, et al. Pathophysiological aspects of thyroid hormone disorders/thyroid peroxidase autoantibodies and reproduction. Human Reproduction Update. 2015;**21**(3):378-387

[61] Hajder E, Hajder M, Brkic M, Hajder E. Immune mechanisms in recurrent pregnancy loss (RPL) and recurrent implantation failure (RIF). HealthMED. 2016;**10**(4):179

[62] Khashan A, Henriksen T, Mortensen P, McNamee R, McCarthy F, Pedersen M, et al. The impact of maternal celiac disease on birthweight and preterm birth: A Danish population-based cohort study. Human Reproduction. 2010;**25**(2):528-534

[63] Tersigni C, Castellani R, De Waure C, Fattorossi A, De Spirito M, Gasbarrini A, et al. Celiac disease and reproductive disorders: Meta-analysis of epidemiologic associations and potential pathogenic mechanisms. Human Reproduction Update. 2014;**20**(4):582-593

[64] Butler M, Kenny L, McCarthy F. Coeliac disease and pregnancy outcomes. Obstetric Medicine. 2011;**4**(3):95-98

[65] Anjum N, Baker PN, Robinson NJ, Aplin JD. Maternal celiac disease autoantibodies bind directly to syncytiotrophoblast and inhibit placental tissue transglutaminase activity. Reproductive Biology and Endocrinology. 2009;**7**(1):1-7

[66] Sharshiner R, Romero ST, Bardsley TR, Branch DW, Silver RM. Celiac disease serum markers and recurrent pregnancy loss. Journal of Reproductive Immunology. 2013;**100**(2):104-108

[67] Kutteh MA, Abiad M, Norman GL, Kutteh WH. Comparison of celiac disease markers in women with early recurrent pregnancy loss and normal controls. American Journal of Reproductive Immunology. 2019;**82**(1):e13127

[68] Sarikaya E, Tokmak A, Aksoy RT, Pekcan MK, Alisik M, Alkan A. The association between serological markers of celiac disease and idiopathic recurrent pregnancy loss. Fetal and Pediatric Pathology. 2017;**36**(5):373-379

[69] Pandey MK, Thakur S, Agrawal S. Lymphocyte immunotherapy and its probable mechanism in the maintenance of pregnancy in women with recurrent spontaneous abortion. Archives of Gynecology and Obstetrics. 2004;**269**(3):161-172

[70] Leber A, Teles A, Zenclussen AC. Regulatory T cells and their role in pregnancy. American Journal of Reproductive Immunology. 2010;**63**(6):445-459

[71] Buckingham K, Chamley L. A critical assessment of the role of antiphospholipid antibodies in infertility. Journal of Reproductive Immunology. 2009;**80**(1-2, 132):-45

[72] Kim NY, Cho HJ, Kim HY, Yang KM, Ahn HK, Thornton S, et al. Thyroid autoimmunity and its association with cellular and humoral immunity in women with reproductive failures. American Journal of Reproductive Immunology. 2011;**65**(1):78-87

[73] Saab W, Seshadri S, Huang C, Alsubki L, Sung N, Kwak-Kim J. A systemic review of intravenous immunoglobulin G treatment in women with recurrent implantation failures and recurrent pregnancy losses. American Journal of Reproductive Immunology. 2021;**85**(4):e13395

[74] Dimakou DB, Tamblyn J, Justin C, Coomarasamy A, Richter A. Diagnosis and management of idiopathic recurrent pregnancy loss (RPL): Current immune testing and immunomodulatory treatment practice in the United Kingdom. Journal of Reproductive Immunology. 1 Sep 2022;**153**:103662

[75] Mekinian A, Cohen J, Alijotas-Reig J, Carbillon L, Nicaise-Roland P, Kayem G, et al. Unexplained recurrent miscarriage and recurrent implantation failure: Is there a place for immunomodulation? American Journal of Reproductive Immunology. 2016;**76**(1):8-28

[76] Akhtar MA, Sur SD, Raine-Fenning N, Jayaprakasan K, Thornton JG, Quenby S. Heparin for assisted reproduction. Cochrane Database of Systematic Reviews. 2013;**8**:CD009452

[77] Quaranta M, Erez O, Mastrolia SA, Koifman A, Leron E, Eshkoli T, et al. The physiologic and therapeutic role of heparin in implantation and placentation. PeerJ. 2015;**3**:e691

[78] Berker B, Taşkın S, Kahraman K, Taşkın EA, Atabekoğlu C, Sönmezer M. The role of low-molecular-weight heparin in recurrent implantation failure: A prospective, quasi-randomized, controlled study. Fertility and Sterility. 2011;**95**(8):2499-2502

[79] Cadavid AP. Aspirin: The mechanism of action revisited in the context of pregnancy complications. Frontiers in Immunology. 2017;**8**:261

[80] Alijotas-Reig J, Esteve-Valverde E, Ferrer-Oliveras R, Sáez-Comet L, Lefkou E, Mekinian A, et al. Comparative study of obstetric antiphospholipid syndrome (OAPS) and non-criteria obstetric APS (NC-OAPS): Report of 1640 cases from the EUROAPS registry. Rheumatology. 2020;**59**(6):1306-1314

[81] Potdar N, Gelbaya TA, Konje JC, Nardo LG. Adjunct low-molecular-weight heparin to improve live birth rate after recurrent implantation

failure: A systematic review and meta-analysis. Human Reproduction Update. 2013;**19**(6):674-684

[82] Badawy A, Khiary M, Sherif L, Hassan M, Ragab A, Abdelall I. Low-molecular weight heparin in patients with recurrent early miscarriages of unknown aetiology. Journal of Obstetrics and Gynaecology. 2008;**28**(3):280-284

[83] de Jong PG, Kaandorp S, Di Nisio M, Goddijn M, Middeldorp S. Aspirin and/or heparin for women with unexplained recurrent miscarriage with or without inherited thrombophilia. Cochrane Database of Systematic Reviews. 2014;7:CD004734

[84] Hamulyák EN, Scheres LJ, Marijnen MC, Goddijn M, Middeldorp S. Aspirin or heparin or both for improving pregnancy outcomes in women with persistent antiphospholipid antibodies and recurrent pregnancy loss. Cochrane Database of Systematic Reviews. 2020;**5**:CD012852

[85] Abdolmohammadi-Vahid S, Danaii S, Hamdi K, Jadidi-Niaragh F, Ahmadi M, Yousefi M. Novel immunotherapeutic approaches for treatment of infertility. Biomedicine & Pharmacotherapy. 2016;**84**:1449-1459

[86] Taniguchi F. Results of prednisolone given to improve the outcome of in vitro fertilization-embryo transfer in women with antinuclear antibodies. The Journal of Reproductive Medicine. 2005;**50**(6):383-388

[87] Ando T, Suganuma N, Furuhashi M, Asada Y, Kondo I, Tomoda Y. Successful glucocorticoid treatment for patients with abnormal autoimmunity on in vitro fertilization and embryo transfer. Journal of Assisted Reproduction and Genetics. 1996;**13**(10):776-781

[88] Fawzy M, El-Refaeey A-AA. Does combined prednisolone and low molecular weight heparin have a role in unexplained implantation failure? Archives of Gynecology and Obstetrics. 2014;**289**(3):677-680

[89] Tang A-W, Alfirevic Z, Turner MA, Drury JA, Small R, Quenby S. A feasibility trial of screening women with idiopathic recurrent miscarriage for high uterine natural killer cell density and randomizing to prednisolone or placebo when pregnant. Human Reproduction. 2013;**28**(7):1743-1752

[90] Lédée N, Prat-Ellenberg L, Petitbarat M, Chevrier L, Simon C, El Irani E, et al. Impact of prednisone in patients with repeated embryo implantation failures: Beneficial or deleterious? Journal of Reproductive Immunology. 2018;**127**:11-15

[91] Huang Q, Wu H, Li M, Yang Y, Fu X. Prednisone improves pregnancy outcome in repeated implantation failure by enhance regulatory T cells bias. Journal of Reproductive Immunology. 2021;**143**:103245

[92] Tang A-W, Alfirevic Z, Turner MA, Drury J, Quenby S. Prednisolone Trial: Study protocol for a randomised controlled trial of prednisolone for women with idiopathic recurrent miscarriage and raised levels of uterine natural killer (uNK) cells in the endometrium. Trials. 2009;**10**(1):1-7

[93] Cooper S, Laird SM, Mariee N, Li TC, Metwally M. The effect of prednisolone on endometrial uterine NK cell concentrations and pregnancy outcome in women with reproductive failure. A retrospective cohort study. Journal of reproductive immunology. 2019;**131**:1-6

[94] Boomsma CM, Kamath MS, Keay SD, Macklon NS. Peri-implantation

glucocorticoid administration for assisted reproductive technology cycles. Cochrane Database of Systematic Reviews. 2022;**6**:CD005996

[95] Quenby S, Kalumbi C, Bates M, Farquharson R, Vince G. Prednisolone reduces preconceptual endometrial natural killer cells in women with recurrent miscarriage. Fertility and Sterility. 2005;**84**(4):980-984

[96] Gomaa MF, Elkholy AG, El-Said MM, Abdel-Salam NE. Combined oral prednisolone and heparin versus heparin: The effect on peripheral NK cells and clinical outcome in patients with unexplained recurrent miscarriage. A double-blind placebo randomized controlled trial. Archives of Gynecology and Obstetrics. 2014;**290**(4):757-762

[97] Akhter A, Faridi R, Das V, Pandey A, Naik S, Agrawal S. In vitro up-regulation of HLA-G using dexamethasone and hydrocortisone in first-trimester trophoblast cells of women experiencing recurrent miscarriage. Tissue Antigens. 2012;**80**(2):126-135

[98] Dan S, Wei W, Yichao S, Hongbo C, Shenmin Y, Jiaxiong W, et al. Effect of prednisolone administration on patients with unexplained recurrent miscarriage and in routine intracytoplasmic sperm injection: A meta-analysis. American Journal of Reproductive Immunology. 2015;**74**(1):89-97

[99] Sokos DR, Berger M, Lazarus HM. Intravenous immunoglobulin: Appropriate indications and uses in hematopoietic stem cell transplantation. Biology of Blood and Marrow Transplantation. 2002;**8**(3):117-130

[100] Branch DW, Porter TF, Paidas MJ, Belfort MA, Gonik B. Obstetric uses of intravenous immunoglobulin: Successes, failures, and promises. Journal of Allergy and Clinical Immunology. 2001;**108**(4):S133-S1S8

[101] Morikawa M, Yamada H, Kato EH, Shimada S, Kishida T, Yamada T, et al. Massive intravenous immunoglobulin treatment in women with four or more recurrent spontaneous abortions of unexplained etiology: Down-regulation of NK cell activity and subsets. American Journal of Reproductive Immunology. 2001;**46**(6):399-404

[102] Shimada S, Takeda M, Nishihira J, Kaneuchi M, Sakuragi N, Minakami H, et al. A high dose of intravenous immunoglobulin increases CD94 expression on natural killer cells in women with recurrent spontaneous abortion. American Journal of Reproductive Immunology. 2009;**62**(5):301-307

[103] Caspi RR. Expanding tregs with IVIg. Blood. 2008;**111**(2):481-482

[104] Carp HJ, Sapir T, Shoenfeld Y. Intravenous immunoglobulin and recurrent pregnancy loss. Clinical Reviews in Allergy & Immunology. 2005;**29**(3):327-332

[105] Sewell W, Jolles S. Immunomodulatory action of intravenous immunoglobulin, Immunology. 2002;**107**(4):387

[106] Omwandho CO, Gruessner SE, Roberts TK, Tinneberg HR. Intravenous immunoglobulin (IVIG): Modes of action in the clinical management of recurrent pregnancy loss (RPL) and selected autoimmune disorders. Clinical Chemistry and Laboratory Medicine (CCLM). 2004;**42**(4):359-370

[107] Graphou O, Chioti A, Pantazi A, Tsekoura C, Kontopoulou V, Georgiadou E, et al. Effect of intravenous immunoglobulin treatment on the Th1/Th2 balance in women with recurrent

spontaneous abortions. American Journal of Reproductive Immunology. 2003;**49**(1):21-29

[108] Yamada H, Morikawa M, Furuta I, Kato EH, Shimada S, Iwabuchi K, et al. Intravenous immunoglobulin treatment in women with recurrent abortions: Increased cytokine levels and reduced Th1/Th2 lymphocyte ratio in peripheral blood. American Journal of Reproductive Immunology. 2003;**49**(2):84-89

[109] Ahmadi M, Abdolmohammadi-Vahid S, Ghaebi M, Aghebati-Maleki L, Dolati S, Farzadi L, et al. Regulatory T cells improve pregnancy rate in RIF patients after additional IVIG treatment. Systems Biology in Reproductive Medicine. 2017;**63**(6):350-359

[110] Ramos-Medina R, García-Segovia A, Gil J, Carbone J, Aguaron de la Cruz A, Seyfferth A, et al. Experience in IVI g therapy for selected women with recurrent reproductive failure and NK cell expansion. American Journal of Reproductive Immunology. 2014;**71**(5):458-466

[111] Li J, Chen Y, Liu C, Hu Y, Li L. Intravenous immunoglobulin treatment for repeated IVF/ICSI failure and unexplained infertility: A systematic review and a meta-analysis. American Journal of Reproductive Immunology. 2013;**70**(6):434-447

[112] Abdolmohammadi-Vahid S, Pashazadeh F, Pourmoghaddam Z, Aghebati-Maleki L, Abdollahi-Fard S, Yousefi M. The effectiveness of IVIG therapy in pregnancy and live birth rate of women with recurrent implantation failure (RIF): A systematic review and meta-analysis. Journal of Reproductive Immunology. 2019;**134**:28-33

[113] Ahmadi M, Ghaebi M, Abdolmohammadi-Vahid S, Abbaspour-Aghdam S, Hamdi K, Abdollahi-Fard S, et al. NK cell frequency and cytotoxicity in correlation to pregnancy outcome and response to IVIG therapy among women with recurrent pregnancy loss. Journal of Cellular Physiology. 2019;**234**(6):9428-9437

[114] Ahmadi M, Abdolmohammadi-Vahid S, Ghaebi M, Aghebati-Maleki L, Afkham A, Danaii S, et al. Effect of Intravenous immunoglobulin on Th1 and Th2 lymphocytes and improvement of pregnancy outcome in recurrent pregnancy loss (RPL). Biomedicine & Pharmacotherapy. 2017;**92**:1095-1102

[115] Ahmadi M, Nouri M, Babaloo Z, Farzadi L, Ghasemzadeh A, Hamdi K, et al. Intravenous immunoglobulin (IVIG) treatment modulates peripheral blood Th17 and regulatory T cells in recurrent miscarriage patients: Non randomized, open-label clinical trial. Immunology Letters. 2017;**192**:12-19

[116] Kim DJ, Lee SK, Kim JY, Na BJ, Hur SE, Lee M, et al. Intravenous immunoglobulin G modulates peripheral blood T h17 and F oxp3+ regulatory T cells in pregnant women with recurrent pregnancy loss. American Journal of Reproductive Immunology. 2014;**71**(5):441-450

[117] Jafarzadeh S, Ahmadi M, Dolati S, Aghebati-Maleki L, Eghbal-Fard S, Kamrani A, et al. Intravenous immunoglobulin G treatment increases live birth rate in women with recurrent miscarriage and modulates regulatory and exhausted regulatory T cells frequency and function. Journal of Cellular Biochemistry. 2019;**120**(4):5424-5434

[118] Christiansen OB, Larsen E, Egerup P, Lunoee L, Egestad L, Nielsen H. Intravenous immunoglobulin treatment for secondary recurrent

miscarriage: A randomised, double-blind, placebo-controlled trial. BJOG: An International Journal of Obstetrics & Gynaecology. 2015;**122**(4):500-508

[119] Stephenson MD, Kutteh WH, Purkiss S, Librach C, Schultz P, Houlihan E, et al. Intravenous immunoglobulin and idiopathic secondary recurrent miscarriage: A multicentered randomized placebo-controlled trial. Human Reproduction. 2010;**25**(9):2203-2209

[120] Wong LF, Porter TF, Scott JR. Immunotherapy for recurrent miscarriage. Cochrane Database of Systematic Reviews. 2014;**10**:CD000112

[121] Parhizkar F, Parhizkar Z, Mojahedi M, Chakari-Khiavi A, Salehnia F, Chakari-Khiavi F, et al. The impact of IVIG therapy on live birth rates in women with RPL: A systematic review and meta-analysis. Gene Reports. 2022;**10**:101490

[122] Winger EE, Reed JL, Ashoush S, Ahuja S, El-Toukhy T, Taranissi M. Treatment with adalimumab (Humira®) and intravenous immunoglobulin improves pregnancy rates in women undergoing IVF. American Journal of Reproductive Immunology. 2009;**61**(2):113-120

[123] Nyborg KM, Kolte AM, Larsen EC, Christiansen OB. Immunomodulatory treatment with intravenous immunoglobulin and prednisone in patients with recurrent miscarriage and implantation failure after in vitro fertilization/intracytoplasmic sperm injection. Fertility and Sterility. 2014;**102**(6):1650-1655 e1

[124] Shreeve N, Sadek K. Intralipid therapy for recurrent implantation failure: New hope or false dawn? Journal of Reproductive Immunology. 2012;**93**(1):38-40

[125] Granato D, Blum S, Rössle C, Le Boucher J, Malnoë A, Dutot G. Effects of parenteral lipid emulsions with different fatty acid composition on immune cell functions in vitro. Journal of Parenteral and Enteral Nutrition. 2000;**24**(2):113-118

[126] Singh N, Davis AA, Kumar S, Kriplani A. The effect of administration of intravenous intralipid on pregnancy outcomes in women with implantation failure after IVF/ICSI with non-donor oocytes: A randomised controlled trial. European Journal of Obstetrics & Gynecology and Reproductive Biology. 2019;**240**:45-51

[127] Coulam CB. Intralipid treatment for women with reproductive failures. American Journal of Reproductive Immunology. 2021;**85**(4):e13290

[128] Roussev RG, Ng SC, Coulam CB. Natural killer cell functional activity suppression by intravenous immunoglobulin, intralipid and soluble human leukocyte antigen-G. American Journal of Reproductive Immunology. 2007;**57**(4):262-269

[129] Roussev RG, Acacio B, Ng SC, Coulam CB. Duration of intralipid's suppressive effect on NK cell's functional activity. American Journal of Reproductive Immunology. 2008;**60**(3):258-263

[130] Zhou P, Wu H, Lin X, Wang S, Zhang S. The effect of intralipid on pregnancy outcomes in women with previous implantation failure in in vitro fertilization/intracytoplasmic sperm injection cycles: A systematic review and meta-analysis. European Journal of Obstetrics & Gynecology and Reproductive Biology. 2020;**252**:187-192

[131] Check J, Check D. Intravenous intralipid therapy is not beneficial in

having a live delivery in women aged 40-42 years with a previous history of miscarriage or failure to conceive despite embryo transfer undergoing in vitro fertilization-embryo transfer. Clinical and Experimental Obstetrics & Gynecology. 2016;**43**(1):14-15

[132] Plaçais L, Kolanska K, Kraiem YB, Cohen J, Suner L, Bornes M, et al. Intralipid therapy for unexplained recurrent miscarriage and implantation failure: Case-series and literature review. European Journal of Obstetrics & Gynecology and Reproductive Biology. 2020;**252**:100-104

[133] Kumar P, Marron K, Harrity C. Intralipid therapy and adverse reproductive outcome: Is there any evidence? Reproduction and Fertility. 2021;**2**(3):173-186

[134] Dakhly DM, Bayoumi YA, Sharkawy M, Allah SHG, Hassan MA, Gouda HM, et al. Intralipid supplementation in women with recurrent spontaneous abortion and elevated levels of natural killer cells. International Journal of Gynecology & Obstetrics. 2016;**135**(3):324-327

[135] Pandey MK, Saxena V, Agrawal S. Characterization of mixed lymphocyte reaction blocking antibodies (MLR-Bf) in human pregnancy. BMC Pregnancy and Childbirth. 2003;**3**(1):1-7

[136] Check JH, Arwitz M, Gross J, Peymer M, Szekeres-Bartho J. Lymphocyte immunotherapy (LI) increases serum levels of progesterone induced blocking factor (PIBF). American Journal of Reproductive Immunology. 1997;**37**(1):17-20

[137] Kilpatrick DC. Soluble interleukin-2 receptors in recurrent miscarriage and the effect of leukocyte immunotherapy. Immunology Letters. 1992;**34**(3):201-206

[138] Wu L, Luo L-H, Zhang Y-X, Li Q, Xu B, Zhou G-X, et al. Alteration of Th17 and Treg cells in patients with unexplained recurrent spontaneous abortion before and after lymphocyte immunization therapy. Reproductive Biology and Endocrinology. 2014;**12**(1):1-9

[139] Cavalcante MB, Sarno M, Araujo Júnior E, Da Silva CF, Barini R. Lymphocyte immunotherapy in the treatment of recurrent miscarriage: Systematic review and meta-analysis. Archives of Gynecology and Obstetrics. 2017;**295**(2):511-518

[140] Smith JB, Cowchock FS, Lata JA, Hankinson BT. The number of cells used for immunotherapy of repeated spontaneous abortion influences pregnancy outcome. Journal of Reproductive Immunology. 1992;**22**(3):217-224

[141] Illeni MT, Marelli G, Parazzini F, Acaia B, Bocciolone L, Bontempelli M, et al. Immunology: Immunotherapy and recurrent abortion: A randomized clinical trial. Human Reproduction. 1994;**9**(7):1247-1249

[142] Günther V, Alkatout I, Meyerholz L, Maass N, Görg S, von Otte S, et al. Live birth rates after active immunization with partner lymphocytes. Biomedicine. 2021;**9**(10):1350

[143] Liu M, Zhen X, Song H, Chen J, Sun X, Li X, et al. Low-dose lymphocyte immunotherapy rebalances the peripheral blood Th1/Th2/Treg paradigm in patients with unexplained recurrent miscarriage. Reproductive Biology and Endocrinology. 2017;**15**(1):1-7

[144] Cavalcante MB, Sarno M, Barini R. Lymphocyte immunotherapy in recurrent miscarriage and recurrent

implantation failure. American Journal of Reproductive Immunology. 2021;**85**(4):e13408

[145] Gao L, Zhang J, Chen H, Zhang S, Chen L, Tan J, et al. Characteristics of immune cell changes before and after immunotherapy and their clinical significance in patients with unexplained recurrent spontaneous abortion. Genetics and Molecular Research. 2014;**13**(1):1169-1178

[146] Yang H, Qiu L, Di W, Zhao A, Chen G, Hu K, et al. Proportional change of CD4+ CD25+ regulatory T cells after lymphocyte therapy in unexplained recurrent spontaneous abortion patients. Fertility and Sterility. 2009;**92**(1):301-305

[147] Chen J-L, Yang J-M, Huang Y-Z, Li Y. Clinical observation of lymphocyte active immunotherapy in 380 patients with unexplained recurrent spontaneous abortion. International Immunopharmacology. 2016;**40**:347-350

[148] Fujiwara H. Immune cells contribute to systemic cross-talk between the embryo and mother during early pregnancy in cooperation with the endocrine system. Reproductive Medicine and Biology. 2006;**5**(1):19-29

[149] Wu Y, Li L, Liu L, Yang X, Yan P, Yang K, et al. Autologous peripheral blood mononuclear cells intrauterine instillation to improve pregnancy outcomes after recurrent implantation failure: A systematic review and meta-analysis. Archives of Gynecology and Obstetrics. 2019;**300**(5):1445-1459

[150] Maleki-Hajiagha A, Razavi M, Rezaeinejad M, Rouholamin S, Almasi-Hashiani A, Pirjani R, et al. Intrauterine administration of autologous peripheral blood mononuclear cells in patients with recurrent implantation failure: A systematic review and meta-analysis. Journal of Reproductive Immunology. 2019;**131**:50-56

[151] Turocy J, Williams Z. Novel therapeutic options for treatment of recurrent implantation failure. Fertility and Sterility. 2021;**116**(6):1449-1454

[152] Li S, Wang J, Cheng Y, Zhou D, Yin T, Xu W, et al. Intrauterine administration of hCG-activated autologous human peripheral blood mononuclear cells (PBMC) promotes live birth rates in frozen/thawed embryo transfer cycles of patients with repeated implantation failure. Journal of Reproductive Immunology. 2017;**119**:15-22

[153] Makrigiannakis A, Vrekoussis T, Makrygiannakis F, Ruso H, Kalantaridou SN, Gurgan T. Intrauterine CRH-treated PBMC in repeated implantation failure. European Journal of Clinical Investigation. 2019;**49**(5):e13084

[154] Yu N, Zhang B, Xu M, Wang S, Liu R, Wu J, et al. Intrauterine administration of autologous peripheral blood mononuclear cells (PBMC s) activated by HCG improves the implantation and pregnancy rates in patients with repeated implantation failure: A prospective randomized study. American Journal of Reproductive Immunology. 2016;**76**(3):212-216

[155] Yoshioka S, Fujiwara H, Nakayama T, Kosaka K, Mori T, Fujii S. Intrauterine administration of autologous peripheral blood mononuclear cells promotes implantation rates in patients with repeated failure of IVF–embryo transfer. Human Reproduction. 2006;**21**(12):3290-3294

[156] Pourmoghadam Z, Soltani-Zangbar MS, Sheikhansari G, Azizi R, Eghbal-Fard S, Mohammadi H, et al.

Intrauterine administration of autologous hCG-activated peripheral blood mononuclear cells improves pregnancy outcomes in patients with recurrent implantation failure; A double-blind, randomized control trial study. Journal of Reproductive Immunology. 2020;**142**:103182

[157] Pourmoghadam Z, Abdo-lmohammadi-Vahid S, Pashazadeh F, A nsari F, Yousefi M. Efficacy of intrauterine administration of autologous peripheral blood mononuclear cells on the pregnancy outcomes in patients with recurrent implantation failure: A systematic review and meta-analysis. Journal of Reproductive Immunology. 2020;**137**:103077

[158] Mekinian A, Costedoat-Chalumeau N, Masseau A, Tincani A, De Caroli S, Alijotas-Reig J, et al. Obstetrical APS: Is there a place for hydroxychloroquine to improve the pregnancy outcome? Autoimmunity Reviews. 2015;**14**(1):23-29

[159] Kaplan YC, Ozsarfati J, Nickel C, Koren G. Reproductive outcomes following hydroxychloroquine use for autoimmune diseases: A systematic review and meta-analysis. British Journal of Clinical Pharmacology. 2016;**81**(5):835-848

[160] de Moreuil C, Alavi Z, Pasquier E. Hydroxychloroquine may be beneficial in preeclampsia and recurrent miscarriage. British Journal of Clinical Pharmacology. 2020;**86**(1):39-49

[161] Sadeghpour S, Ghasemnejad Berenji M, Nazarian H, Ghasemnejad T, Nematollahi MH, Abroon S, et al. Effects of treatment with hydroxychloroquine on the modulation of Th17/Treg ratio and pregnancy outcomes in women with recurrent implantation failure: Clinical trial. Immunopharmacology and Immunotoxicology. 2020;**42**(6):632-642

[162] Marchetti T, Ruffatti A, Wuillemin C, De Moerloose P, Cohen M. Hydroxychloroquine restores trophoblast fusion affected by antiphospholipid antibodies. Journal of Thrombosis and Haemostasis. 2014;**12**(6):910-920

[163] Ghasemnejad-Berenji H, Novin MG, Hajshafiha M, Nazarian H, Hashemi S, Ilkhanizadeh B, et al. Immunomodulatory effects of hydroxychloroquine on Th1/Th2 balance in women with repeated implantation failure. Biomedicine & Pharmacotherapy. 2018;**107**:1277-1285

[164] Elsenity M, Abdelrazeq M, Fayed S, Elsokkary M, Ghaleb M. Hydroxychloroquine therapy in women with autoimmune recurrent pregnancy loss, refractory to low dose aspirin and heparin: A randomized controlled trial. Вопросы гинекологии. 2022;**21**(1):19-28

[165] Pasquier E, de Saint-Martin L, Marhic G, Chauleur C, Bohec C, Bretelle F, et al. Hydroxychloroquine for prevention of recurrent miscarriage: Study protocol for a multicentre randomised placebo-controlled trial BBQ study. BMJ Open. 2019;**9**(3):e025649

[166] Yang S, Ni R, Lu Y, Wang S, Xie F, Zhang C, et al. A three-arm, multicenter, open-label randomized controlled trial of hydroxychloroquine and low-dose prednisone to treat recurrent pregnancy loss in women with undifferentiated connective tissue diseases: Protocol for the Immunosuppressant regimens for LIving FEtuses (ILIFE) trial. Trials. 2020;**21**(1):1-9

[167] Schreiber K, Breen K, Cohen H, Jacobsen S, Middeldorp S, Pavord S, et al., editors. Hydroxychloroquine to improve pregnancy outcome in women with antiphospholipid antibodies (HYPATIA) protocol: A multinational randomized controlled trial of

hydroxychloroquine versus placebo in addition to standard treatment in pregnant women with antiphospholipid syndrome or antibodies. In: Seminars in Thrombosis and Hemostasis; United States. Thieme Medical Publishers Inc. Sep 2017;**43**(06):562-571

[168] Yang Z, Shen X, Zhou C, Wang M, Liu Y, Zhou L. Prevention of recurrent miscarriage in women with antiphospholipid syndrome: A systematic review and network meta-analysis. Lupus. 2021;**30**(1):70-79

[169] Demetri GD, Griffin JD. Granulocyte Colony-stimulating Factor and its Receptor. Blood. 1991;**78**(11):2791-2808

[170] Würfel W. Treatment with granulocyte colony-stimulating factor in patients with repetitive implantation failures and/or recurrent spontaneous abortions. Journal of Reproductive Immunology. 2015;**108**:123-135

[171] Eftekhar M, Naghshineh E, Khani P. Role of granulocyte colony-stimulating factor in human reproduction. Journal of Research in Medical Sciences: The Official Journal of Isfahan University of Medical Sciences. 2018;**23**:7

[172] Lédée N, Lombroso R, Lombardelli L, Selva J, Dubanchet S, Chaouat G, et al. Cytokines and chemokines in follicular fluids and potential of the corresponding embryo: The role of granulocyte colony-stimulating factor. Human Reproduction. 2008;**23**(9):2001-2009

[173] Kalem Z, Namli Kalem M, Bakirarar B, Kent E, Makrigiannakis A, Gurgan T. Intrauterine G-CSF administration in recurrent implantation failure (RIF): An Rct. Scientific Reports. 2020;**10**(1):1-7

[174] Aleyasin A, Abediasl Z, Nazari A, Sheikh M. Granulocyte colony-stimulating factor in repeated IVF failure, a randomized trial. Reproduction. 2016;**151**(6):637-642

[175] Xu B, Zhang Q, Hao J, Xu D, Li Y. Two protocols to treat thin endometrium with granulocyte colony-stimulating factor during frozen embryo transfer cycles. Reproductive Biomedicine Online. 2015;**30**(4):349-358

[176] Jiang Y, Zhao Q, Zhang Y, Zhou L, Lin J, Chen Y, et al. Treatment of G-CSF in unexplained, repeated implantation failure: A systematic review and meta-analysis. Journal of Gynecology Obstetrics and Human Reproduction. 2020;**49**(10):101866

[177] Li J, Mo S, Chen Y. The effect of G-CSF on infertile women undergoing IVF treatment: A meta-analysis. Systems Biology in Reproductive Medicine. 2017;**63**(4):239-247

[178] Scarpellini F, Klinger FG, Rossi G, Sbracia M. Immunohistochemical study on the expression of G-CSF, G-CSFR, VEGF, VEGFR-1, Foxp3 in first trimester trophoblast of recurrent pregnancy loss in pregnancies treated with G-CSF and controls. International Journal of Molecular Sciences. 2019;**21**(1):285

[179] Scarpellini F, Sbracia M. Use of granulocyte colony-stimulating factor for the treatment of unexplained recurrent miscarriage: A randomised controlled trial. Human Reproduction. 2009;**24**(11):2703-2708

[180] Eapen A, Joing M, Kwon P, Tong J, Maneta E, De Santo C, et al. Recombinant human granulocyte–colony stimulating factor in women with unexplained recurrent pregnancy losses: A randomized clinical trial. Human Reproduction. 2019;**34**(3):424-432

[181] Zafardoust S, Akhondi MM, Sadeghi MR, Mohammadzadeh A, Karimi A, Jouhari S, et al. Efficacy of intrauterine injection of granulocyte colony stimulating factor (G-CSF) on treatment of unexplained recurrent miscarriage: A pilot RCT study. Journal of Reproduction & Infertility. 2017;**18**(4):379

[182] Egea L, Hirata Y, Kagnoff MF. GM-CSF: A role in immune and inflammatory reactions in the intestine. Expert Review of Gastroenterology & Hepatology. 2010;**4**(6):723-731

[183] Behr B, Mooney S, Wen Y, Polan ML, Wang H. Preliminary experience with low concentration of granulocyte-macrophage colony-stimulating factor: A potential regulator in preimplantation mouse embryo development and apoptosis. Journal of Assisted Reproduction and Genetics. 2005;**22**(1):25-32

[184] Ziebe S, Loft A, Povlsen BB, Erb K, Agerholm I, Aasted M, et al. A randomized clinical trial to evaluate the effect of granulocyte-macrophage colony-stimulating factor (GM-CSF) in embryo culture medium for in vitro fertilization. Fertility and Sterility. 2013;**99**(6):1600-1609 e2

[185] Tevkin S, Lokshin V, Shishimorova M, Polumiskov V. The frequency of clinical pregnancy and implantation rate after cultivation of embryos in a medium with granulocyte macrophage colony-stimulating factor (GM-CSF) in patients with preceding failed attempts of ART. Gynecological Endocrinology. 2014;**30**(sup1):9-12

[186] Akgül ÖK, Kasımoğulları EV, Güraslan H, Akgül C. The role of granulocyte-macrophage colony stimulating factor in recurrent pregnancy losses. Bagcılar Medical Bulletin= Bağcılar Tıp Bülteni. 2019;**4**(3):61

[187] Chambers CD, Johnson DL. Emerging data on the use of anti-tumor necrosis factor-alpha medications in pregnancy. Birth Defects Research Part A: Clinical and Molecular Teratology. 2012;**94**(8):607-611

[188] Alijotas-Reig J, Esteve-Valverde E, Ferrer-Oliveras R, Llurba E, Gris JM. Tumor necrosis factor-alpha and pregnancy: focus on biologics. An updated and comprehensive review. Clinical Reviews in Allergy & Immunology. 2017;**53**(1):40-53

[189] Zhang C, Deng X, Zhang X, Pan Z, Zhao W, Zhang Y, et al. Association between serum TNF-α levels and recurrent spontaneous miscarriage: A meta-analysis. American Journal of Reproductive Immunology. 2016;**75**(2):86-93

[190] Santiago KY, Porchia LM, López-Bayghen E. Endometrial preparation with etanercept increased embryo implantation and live birth rates in women suffering from recurrent implantation failure during IVF. Reproductive Biology. 2021;**21**(1):100480

[191] Winger EE, Reed JL, Ashoush S, El-Toukhy T, Ahuja S, Taranissi M. Degree of TNF-α/IL-10 cytokine elevation correlates with IVF success rates in women undergoing treatment with adalimumab (Humira) and IVIG. American Journal of Reproductive Immunology. 2011;**65**(6):610-618

[192] Lee SK, Na BJ, Kim JY, Hur SE, Lee M, Gilman-Sachs A, et al. Determination of clinical cellular immune markers in women with recurrent pregnancy loss. American Journal of Reproductive Immunology. 2013;**70**(5):398-411

[193] Ohams MJ, Jerzak M, Górski A. Effects of sildenafil citrate and

etanercept treatment on TNF-α levels in peripheral blood of women with recurrent miscarriage. Ginekologia Polska. 2015;**86**(7):520-524

[194] Fu J, Li L, Qi L, Zhao L. A randomized controlled trial of etanercept in the treatment of refractory recurrent spontaneous abortion with innate immune disorders. Taiwanese Journal of Obstetrics and Gynecology. 2019;**58**(5):621-625

[195] Jerzak M, Ohams M, Górski A, Baranowski W. Etanercept immunotherapy in women with a history of recurrent reproductive failure. Ginekologia polska. 2012;**83**(4):260-264

[196] Winger EE, Reed JL. Treatment with tumor necrosis factor inhibitors and intravenous immunoglobulin improves live birth rates in women with recurrent spontaneous abortion. American Journal of Reproductive Immunology. 2008;**60**(1):8-16

[197] Borel JF. History of the discovery of cyclosporin and of its early pharmacological development. Wiener Klinische Wochenschrift. 2002;**114**:433-437

[198] Germano V, Ferlito C, Podestà E, Salemi S, Migliore A, D'Amelio R, et al. Cyclosporine A in the long-term management of systemic lupus erythematosus. Journal of Biological Regulators and Homeostatic Agents. 2011;**25**(3):397-403

[199] Piao H-L, Wang S-C, Tao Y, Zhu R, Sun C, Fu Q, et al. Cyclosporine A enhances Th2 bias at the maternal-fetal interface in early human pregnancy with aid of the interaction between maternal and fetal cells. 2012

[200] Zhou W-H, Du M-R, Dong L, Zhu X-Y, Yang J-Y, He Y-Y, et al. Cyclosporin A increases expression of matrix metalloproteinase 9 and 2 and invasiveness in vitro of the first-trimester human trophoblast cells via the mitogen-activated protein kinase pathway. Human Reproduction. 2007;**22**(10):2743-2750

[201] Huang Y-H, Ma Y-L, Ma L, Mao J-L, Zhang Y, Du M-R, et al. Cyclosporine A improves adhesion and invasion of mouse preimplantation embryos via upregulating integrin β3 and matrix metalloproteinase-9. International Journal of Clinical and Experimental Pathology. 2014;7(4):1379

[202] Zhou W-H, Dong L, Du M-R, Zhu X-Y, Li D-J. Cyclosporin A improves murine pregnancy outcome in abortion-prone matings: Involvement of CD80/86 and CD28/CTLA-4. Reproduction. 2008;**135**(3):385

[203] Qu D, Tian X, Ding L, Li Y, Zhou W. Impacts of Cyclosporin A on clinical pregnancy outcomes of patients with a history of unexplained transfer failure: A retrospective cohort study. Reproductive Biology and Endocrinology. 2021;**19**(1):1-8

[204] Fu J. Analysis of the use of cyclosporin A to treat refractory immune recurrent spontaneous abortion. Clinical and Experimental Obstetrics & Gynecology. 2015;**42**(6):739-742

[205] Ling Y, Huang Y, Chen C, Mao J, Zhang H. Low dose Cyclosporin A treatment increases live birth rate of unexplained recurrent abortion-initial cohort study. Clinical and Experimental Obstetrics & Gynecology. 2017;**44**(2):230-235

[206] Azizi R, Ahmadi M, Danaii S, Abdollahi-Fard S, Mosapour P, Eghbal-Fard S, et al. Cyclosporine A improves pregnancy outcomes in

women with recurrent pregnancy loss and elevated Th1/Th2 ratio. Journal of Cellular Physiology. 2019;**234**(10):19039-19047

[207] Wang S, Li M, Sun F, Chen C, Ye J, Li D, et al. Th17/Treg-cell balance in the peripheral blood of pregnant females with a history of recurrent spontaneous abortion receiving progesterone or cyclosporine A. Experimental and Therapeutic Medicine. 2021;**21**(1):1

[208] Zhao L, Qi L, Fu J, Bi S, Li L, Fu Y. Efficacy of intrauterine perfusion of cyclosporin A for intractable recurrent spontaneous abortion patients with endometrial alloimmune disorders: A randomized controlled trial. Frontiers in Physiology. 2021;**12**:737878

[209] Ma N, Qin R, Qin W, Liao M, Zhao Y, Hang F, et al. Oral immunosuppressants improve pregnancy outcomes in women with idiopathic recurrent miscarriage: A meta-analysis. Journal of Clinical Pharmacy and Therapeutics. 2022;**47**(7):870-878

[210] Law BK. Rapamycin: An anti-cancer immunosuppressant? Critical Reviews in Oncology/Hematology. 2005;**56**(1):47-60

[211] Mehrabi A, Fonouni H, Kashfi A, Schmied B, Morath C, Sadeghi M, et al. The role and value of sirolimus administration in kidney and liver transplantation. Clinical Transplantation. 2006;**20**:30-43

[212] Kopf H, Gonzalo M, Howard OZ, Chen X. Rapamycin inhibits differentiation of Th17 cells and promotes generation of FoxP3+ T regulatory cells. International Immunopharmacology. 2007;7(13):1819-1824

[213] Coscia LA, Constantinescu S, Moritz MJ, Frank AM, Ramirez CB, Maley WR, et al. Report from the National transplantation pregnancy registry (NTPR): Outcomes of pregnancy after transplantation. Clinical Transplants. 2010:65-85

[214] Royster GD, Harris JC, Nelson A, Castro Y, Weitzel RP, Tisdale J, et al. Rapamycin corrects T regulatory cell depletion and improves embryo implantation and live birth rates in a murine model. Reproductive Sciences. 2019;**26**(12):1545-1556

[215] Ahmadi M, Abdolmohamadi-Vahid S, Ghaebi M, Dolati S, Abbaspour-Aghdam S, Danaii S, et al. Sirolimus as a new drug to treat RIF patients with elevated Th17/Treg ratio: A double-blind, phase II randomized clinical trial. International Immunopharmacology. 2019;**74**:105730

[216] Rath T. Tacrolimus in transplant rejection. Expert Opinion on Pharmacotherapy. 2013;**14**(1):115-122

[217] Nakagawa K, Kwak-Kim J, Ota K, Kuroda K, Hisano M, Sugiyama R, et al. Immunosuppression with tacrolimus improved reproductive outcome of women with repeated implantation failure and elevated peripheral blood TH1/TH2 cell ratios. American Journal of Reproductive immunology. 2015;**73**(4):353-361

[218] Nakagawa K, Kwak-Kim J, Kuroda K, Sugiyama R, Yamaguchi K. Immunosuppressive treatment using tacrolimus promotes pregnancy outcome in infertile women with repeated implantation failures. American Journal of Reproductive Immunology. 2017;**78**(3):e12682

[219] Bahrami-Asl Z, Farzadi L, Fattahi A, Yousefi M, Quinonero A, Hakimi P, et al. Tacrolimus improves the implantation rate in patients with elevated Th1/2 helper cell ratio and

repeated implantation failure (RIF). Geburtshilfe und Frauenheilkunde. 2020;**80**(08):851-862

[220] Nakagawa K, Kuroda K, Sugiyama R, Yamaguchi K. After 12 consecutive miscarriages, a patient received immunosuppressive treatment and delivered an intact baby. Reproductive Medicine and Biology. 2017;**16**(3):297-301

[221] Hisano M, Nakagawa K, Kwak-Kim J, Sugiyama R, Sago H, Yamaguchi K. Changes in the T-helper 1 and 2 cell populations during pregnancy in tacrolimus-treated women with repeated implantation failure and recurrent pregnancy loss. Human Fertility. 2021:1-8

[222] Nakagawa K, Kwak-Kim J, Hisano M, Kasahara Y, Kuroda K, Sugiyama R, et al. Obstetric and perinatal outcome of the women with repeated implantation failures or recurrent pregnancy losses who received pre-and post-conception tacrolimus treatment. American Journal of Reproductive Immunology. 2019;**82**(2):e13142

[223] Eppley BL, Woodell JE, Higgins J. Platelet quantification and growth factor analysis from platelet-rich plasma: Implications for wound healing. Plastic and reconstructive surgery. 2004;**114**(6):1502-1508

[224] Garcia-Velasco JA, Acevedo B, Alvarez C, Alvarez M, Bellver J, Fontes J, et al. Strategies to manage refractory endometrium: State of the art in 2016. Reproductive BioMedicine Online. 2016;**32**(5):474-489

[225] Luzo AC, Fávaro WJ, Seabra AB, Durán N. What is the potential use of platelet-rich-plasma (PRP) in cancer treatment? A mini review. Heliyon. 2020;**6**(3):e03660

[226] Nazari L, Salehpour S, Hoseini S, Zadehmodarres S, Ajori L. Effects of autologous platelet-rich plasma on implantation and pregnancy in repeated implantation failure: A pilot study. International Journal of Reproductive Biomedicine. 2016;**14**(10):625

[227] Eftekhar M, Neghab N, Naghshineh E, Khani P. Can autologous platelet rich plasma expand endometrial thickness and improve pregnancy rate during frozen-thawed embryo transfer cycle? A randomized clinical trial. Taiwanese Journal of Obstetrics and Gynecology. 2018;**57**(6):810-813

[228] Mouanness M, Ali-Bynom S, Jackman J, Seckin S, Merhi Z. Use of intra-uterine injection of platelet-rich plasma (PRP) for endometrial receptivity and thickness: A Literature review of the mechanisms of action. Reproductive Sciences. 2021;**28**(6):1659-1670

[229] Coksuer H, Akdemir Y, Ulas BM. Improved in vitro fertilization success and pregnancy outcome with autologous platelet-rich plasma treatment in unexplained infertility patients that had repeated implantation failure history. Gynecological Endocrinology. 2019;**35**(9):815-818

[230] Nazari L, Salehpour S, Hosseini S, Hashemi T, Borumandnia N, Azizi E. Effect of autologous platelet-rich plasma for treatment of recurrent pregnancy loss: A randomized controlled trial. Obstetrics & Gynecology Science. 2022;**65**(3):266-272

[231] Xie H, Zeng H, He D, Liu N. Effect of intrauterine perfusion of human chorionic gonadotropin before embryo transfer after two or more implantation failures: A systematic review and meta-analysis. European Journal of Obstetrics

& Gynecology and Reproductive Biology. 2019;**243**:133-138

[232] Giuliani E, Olson M, Strug M, Young J, Shavell V, Dodds W, et al. Intrauterine hCG infusion affects the distribution of natural killer cells in the endometrium of fertile oocyte donors. Fertility and Sterility. 2015;**104**(3):e149-ee50

[233] Aaleyasin A, Aghahosseini M, Rashidi M, Safdarian L, Sarvi F, Najmi Z, et al. In vitro fertilization outcome following embryo transfer with or without preinstillation of human chorionic gonadotropin into the uterine cavity: A randomized controlled trial. Gynecologic and Obstetric Investigation. 2015;**79**(3):201-205

[234] Zarei A, Parsanezhad ME, Younesi M, Alborzi S, Zolghadri J, Samsami A, et al. Intrauterine administration of recombinant human chorionic gonadotropin before embryo transfer on outcome of in vitro fertilization/intracytoplasmic sperm injection: A randomized clinical trial. Iranian Journal of Reproductive Medicine. 2014;**12**(1):1

[235] Hong KH, Forman EJ, Werner MD, Upham KM, Gumeny CL, Winslow AD, et al. Endometrial infusion of human chorionic gonadotropin at the time of blastocyst embryo transfer does not impact clinical outcomes: A randomized, double-blind, placebo-controlled trial. Fertility and Sterility. 2014;**102**(6):1591-1595 e2

[236] Gao M, Jiang X, Li B, Li L, Duan M, Zhang X, et al. Intrauterine injection of human chorionic gonadotropin before embryo transfer can improve in vitro fertilization-embryo transfer outcomes: A meta-analysis of randomized controlled trials. Fertility and Sterility. 2019;**112**(1):89-97 e1

[237] Swart L, Holoch K, Amalfitano K, Forstein D, Lessey B. 212: Luteal phase hCG improves outcomes but not pregnancy rates in unexplained recurrent pregnancy loss. American Journal of Obstetrics & Gynecology. 2012;**206**(1):S106

[238] Cai S, Lin R, Liu S, Wang X, Wei H, Huang C, et al. Intrauterine infusion of human chorionic gonadotropin improves the endometrial FoxP3+ Tregs level and pregnancy outcomes in patients with lower endometrial FoxP3+ Tregs. Journal of Reproductive Immunology. 2022;**153**:103678

[239] Morley LC, Simpson N, Tang T. Human chorionic gonadotrophin (hCG) for preventing miscarriage. Cochrane Database of Systematic Reviews. 2013;**1**:CD008611

[240] Alhadlaq A, Mao JJ. Mesenchymal stem cells: isolation and therapeutics. Stem Cells and Development. 2004;**13**(4):436-448

[241] Pourakbari R, Ahmadi H, Yousefi M, Aghebati-Maleki L. Cell therapy in female infertility-related diseases: Emphasis on recurrent miscarriage and repeated implantation failure. Life Sciences. 2020;**258**:118181

[242] Tersoglio AE, Tersoglio S, Salatino DR, Castro M, Gonzalez A, Hinojosa M, et al. Regenerative therapy by endometrial mesenchymal stem cells in thin endometrium with repeated implantation failure. A novel strategy. JBRA Assisted Reproduction. 2020;**24**(2):118

[243] Chen X, Yang X, Wu R, Chen W, Xie H, Qian X, et al. Therapeutic effects of Wharton jelly-derived mesenchymal stem cells on rat abortion models. Journal of Obstetrics and Gynaecology Research. 2016;**42**(8):972-982

[244] Zhang D, Lin Y, Li Y, Zhao D, Du M. Mesenchymal stem cells enhance Treg immunosuppressive function at the fetal-maternal interface. Journal of Reproductive Immunology. 2021;**148**:103366

[245] Farrokhi AS, Zarnani A-H, Moazzeni SM. Mesenchymal stem cells therapy protects fetuses from resorption and induces Th2 type cytokines profile in abortion prone mouse model. Transplant Immunology. 2018;**47**:26-31

[246] Rezaei Kahmini F, Shahgaldi S, Moazzeni SM. Mesenchymal stem cells alter the frequency and cytokine profile of natural killer cells in abortion-prone mice. Journal of Cellular Physiology. 2020;**235**(10):7214-7223

[247] Li Y, Zhang D, Xu L, Dong L, Zheng J, Lin Y, et al. Cell–cell contact with proinflammatory macrophages enhances the immunotherapeutic effect of mesenchymal stem cells in two abortion models. Cellular & Molecular Immunology. 2019;**16**(12):908-920

[248] Sadighi-Moghaddam B, Salek Farrokhi A, Namdar Ahmadabad H, Barati M, Moazzeni SM. Mesenchymal stem cell therapy prevents abortion in CBA/J× DBA/2 mating. Reproductive Sciences. 2018;**25**(8):1261-1269

[249] Insausti CL, Blanquer M, García-Hernández AM, Castellanos G, Moraleda JM. Amniotic membrane-derived stem cells: Immunomodulatory properties and potential clinical application. Stem Cells and Cloning: Advances and Applications. 2014;**7**:53

[250] Miki T. Stem cell characteristics and the therapeutic potential of amniotic epithelial cells. American Journal of Reproductive Immunology. 2018;**80**(4):e13003

[251] Motedayyen H, Zarnani A-H, Tajik N, Ghotloo S, Rezaei A. Immunomodulatory effects of human amniotic epithelial cells on naive CD4+ T cells from women with unexplained recurrent spontaneous abortion. Placenta. 2018;**71**:31-40

[252] Dugoua J-J, Machado M, Zhu X, Chen X, Koren G, Einarson TR. Probiotic safety in pregnancy: A systematic review and meta-analysis of randomized controlled trials of *Lactobacillus*, *Bifidobacterium*, and *Saccharomyces* spp. Journal of Obstetrics and Gynaecology Canada. 2009;**31**(6):542-552

[253] Tao Y, Huang F, Zhang Z, Tao X, Wu Q, Qiu L, et al. Probiotic Enterococcus faecalis Symbioflor 1 ameliorates pathobiont-induced miscarriage through bacterial antagonism and Th1-Th2 modulation in pregnant mice. Applied Microbiology and Biotechnology. 2020;**104**(12):5493-5504

[254] Corbett G, Crosby D, McAuliffe F. Probiotic therapy in couples with infertility: A systematic review. European Journal of Obstetrics & Gynecology and Reproductive Biology. 2021;**256**:95-100

[255] Li Y-H, Zhang D, Du M-R. Advances and challenges of mesenchymal stem cells for pregnancy-related diseases. Cellular & Molecular Immunology. 2021;**18**(8):2075-2077

Chapter 8

Artificial Intelligence for Ovarian Stimulation

Jean-Claude Emperaire and J. Charles Eldridge

Abstract

Ovarian stimulation, the basis of treatment strategies for infertility, from anovulation to in vitro fertilization, is a highly efficient therapeutic procedure. The stimulation should ensure a complete development of the follicle(s) along with maturation of the oocyte(s), all without risking hyperstimulation and multiple pregnancies. For these reasons, a stimulation protocol should be personalized, and its evolution must be continually scrutinized using measures of both blood hormone levels and ovarian responses by ultrasound. Essentially all of the stimulation algorithms proposed to date focus only on determination of the starting dose of gonadotropin. But ovarian stimulation should be continually monitored until the final decision is made to trigger or to abort the cycle. This decision can be achieved through use of an experience-based computer software system that monitors menstrual cycles through a beginning pregnancy. This software (*StimXpert®*) should work effectively with a classical stimulation as well as a controlled hyperstimulation for IVF. It may also be modified from experience-based to evidence-based programming through progressive learning.

Keywords: ovarian stimulation, ovulation stimulation, medical software, infertility

1. Introduction

Ovarian stimulation is an essential component of nearly all contemporary approaches for management of a couples' infertility: for mono-follicular stimulation in cases of anovulation, for mono- or bi-follicular stimulation in idiopathic infertility, for assisted procreation to prepare for intra-uterine insemination (IUI), and also for controlled hyperstimulation for in vitro fertilization (IVF).

A successful stimulation requires achievement of both fertilization and then nidation without complications. Each stimulation must be uniquely customized for each patient. A critical factor for success depends on estimation or anticipation of the ovarian response, which in turn relies on the choice of gonadotropin preparation plus an understanding of the patient's own ovarian sensitivity. All of this comes together when deciding on the starting dose, to be administered over 5–7 days. Choices for subsequent stimulation are typically a bit less challenging, as they are likely to be smaller adjustments in light of previous responses. Nonetheless, monitoring of responses may reveal unpleasant surprises, so careful attention is necessary until the process ends with a decision to trigger ovulation or to cancel the cycle.

 IntechOpen

2. Can computer applications facilitate ovarian stimulation decisions?

Numerous variables must be taken into account when stimulating ovulation. For the starting dose, one must consider patient age, weight, body mass index (BMI), antral follicle count (AFC), plus serum levels of follicle stimulating hormone (FSH) and anti-mullerian hormone (AMH). During stimulation, the ovarian response must be monitored by hormone levels of estradiol (E), luteinizing hormone (LH), progesterone (P), and also by sonographic parameters such as the number and size of growing follicles. Because these parameters, while diverse, are interacting with each other, it becomes conceivable that algorithms might be developed to integrate the entire treatment cycle, for each stimulation protocol.

Curiously, few experience-based proposals have appeared for programs of this sort, despite the fact that ovarian stimulation protocols have been in use for more than 50 years. For this reason alone, a software system should originate with a large clinical practice group having sufficient experience with various stimulation protocols used over a long time. The resulting algorithms should then be validated by peers. Finally, the software needs to be inherently self-evaluating, so that responses can be compared with stored information from previous trials to develop an optimal evidence-based stimulation tool.

The system proposed here represents an initial step derived from the author's personal experience of more than 40,000 ovarian stimulation cycles conducted over 50 years of clinical infertility practice and, in particular, the most recent 1200 stimulation cycles that resulted in a beginning pregnancy [1].

3. Characteristics of the stimXpert system

Ideally, a protocol for ovarian stimulation must compute not only the starting gonadotropin dose, as several existing systems do, but also cover the entire treatment sequence up to the ovulation triggering step, or cycle cancelation, if necessary. It should be designed to optimize the number of mature follicles in concert with the specific stimulation goal and should avoid complications such as the ovarian hyperstimulation syndrome (OHS) or a multiple pregnancies.

StimXpert is a software system designed to initiate and guide all therapeutic decisions for ovarian stimulation using the gonadotropins FSH, LH, and hCG. Because evidence-based algorithms for ovarian stimulation have not existed, this experience-based application was developed to fill the need. The present configuration includes 10 specific protocols: four for mono-follicular anovulatory stimulation (step-up low dose, step-up chronic low dose, step-down and sequential), two for ovulatory patients preparing for intrauterine insemination (mono- or bi-follicular), and four utilized for controlled hyperstimulation (long agonist, short agonist, fixed antagonist, flexible antagonist). For each protocol, the starting dose is dictated by the patient's weight and her level of plasma AMH [1, 2].

Initial Monitoring Control: define the FSH dose and the number of stimulation days. After the first 5–7 days, adjust the dose in accordance with the ovarian response, based on serum hormone levels (LH, estradiol, progesterone) and on sonographic observation (number and diameter of the largest growing follicles).

Additional Monitoring Controls: in patients who continue stimulation after the first control.

Triggering Criteria: computed within the security limits to avoid both hyperstimulation and multiple pregnancies.

Reasons for Aborting the Stimulation Cycle:

- Identified risk for multiple pregnancy in a mono-follicular stimulation
- Need to add LH when sonography and hormonal levels are dissociated
- Abnormal pre-ovulatory increase of plasma progesterone (> 1.5 ng/ml)
- Identified risk for ovarian hyperstimulation, e.g., estradiol rises above 500 pg./ml in a classic stimulation, or above 2500 pg./ml and/or with more than 15 follicles observed during a controlled hyperstimulation for IVF, or when
- Fewer than four follicles are observed during a controlled hyperstimulation for IVF

Of course, all of the signals from the software application may be modified or overruled by the clinician's judgment, in line with his/her own experience and/or knowledge of the situation with each particular patient.

4. Parameters for each protocol

While most of the parameters are basically common to all stimulation protocols, the software needs to include specific aspects of each protocol. To illustrate this importance, two examples are presented here of the application's success:

4.1 Mono-follicular stimulation in a case of anovulation

- ***Stimulation Protocol***: the usual experience with an anovulatory patient producing estrogen favors the low-dose step-up protocol. The rationale is to increase the gonadotropin dose, by 50% of the starting dose, at 7-day intervals until a minimal response of the most sensitive follicle is observed. The same dose is then continued until the follicle attains the pre-ovulatory stage ready for ovulation trigger. The StimXpert application will propose alternative protocols to consider: the standard step-up, chronic low-dose step-up, step-down, or sequential protocols.
- ***Nature of the Gonadotropin:*** with exception of a few rare instances, all commercial FSH preparations are equally efficacious for mono-follicular stimulation. None seems at present to be superior, whether extracted or recombinant, or whether the preparation includes LH. The software includes characteristics of each brand without favoring any. However, one exception of note is that in cases of hypogonadotropic hypogonadism, where LH must be included, recombinant LH is not among the available choices. The software instead offers gonadotropin preparations that already contain FSH and LH, thereby avoiding two separate hormone injections for a better patient's compliance.

- ***Starting Dose:*** mono-follicular cycles do not have a consensus starting dose of gonadotropin, and referencing an AMH level is of little help in making this decision. A very low level is expected in hypogonadotropic hypogonadism [3], while a high level does not establish a need to start with the lowest possible dose [4–6]. StimXpert will suggest two starting levels of 50 and 75 IU to be decided according to the patient's age and BMI.

- ***Monitoring:*** hormonal measures and a sonogram should be done after the starting dose is continued for 7 days. If no significant ovarian response is detected, the software will recommend increasing the dose by 50% for 7 more days, with identical increases initiated each 7 days until a 10 mm follicle appears. At that point, the dosing will be maintained until optimum maturity is reached, a follicle at least 16 mm in diameter with a suitable serum estradiol level. If an adequate response does not appear after three 7-day steps of increased dosing, the program will cancel the stimulation protocol. A new stimulation series should begin with a number of FSH units just over the last used dose in the previous protocol.

- ***Triggering ovulation:*** this should be done when a single 16-mm follicle is reached, and with no other follicles of 12-mm diameter or larger being detected, so that multiple ovulations and pregnancies will be avoided. Serum estradiol should not exceed 500 pg./ml. Note that numerous responsive small follicles may contribute to the estradiol pool, but the risk for ovarian hyperstimulation (OHS) must also be taken into account: the program will cancel the process if maximum limits of follicular size or hormone levels are exceeded. Alternatively, the program may allow for triggering to proceed by using a GnRH agonist, which decreases but does not obviate risk for multiple pregnancies or OHS.

- ***At each step of the StimXpert protocol, the clinician can still decide to override the software decisions.*** **Figure 1** illustrates an example algorithm for mono-follicular stimulation.

4.2 Multi-follicular stimulation for in vitro fertilization (IVF)

This type of stimulation aims to recruit 8–15 follicles to full maturation. Large numbers may actually be less necessary at present, with so-called "friendly stimulations" being recommended. To be sure, high numbers are inadvisable when risks of OHS are present, even when embryo freezing for later transfer is considered.

- ***Stimulation Protocol***: StimXpert offers a choice of the two main types of controlled follicular hyperstimulation, using GnRH analogs. There appears to be no recognized difference among analog products; the choice of the GnRH preparation or its mode of administration (daily or long-acting) does not influence the program algorithm.

- ***Agonist Stimulation Protocols***: the "long protocol," where ovarian stimulation is preceded by agonist-driven ovarian desensitization, continues to be the gold standard approach. The "short protocol," where GnRH agonist and gonadotropin are administered together, yields somewhat poorer results, and thus is relegated to special situations, such as the case of a low responder.

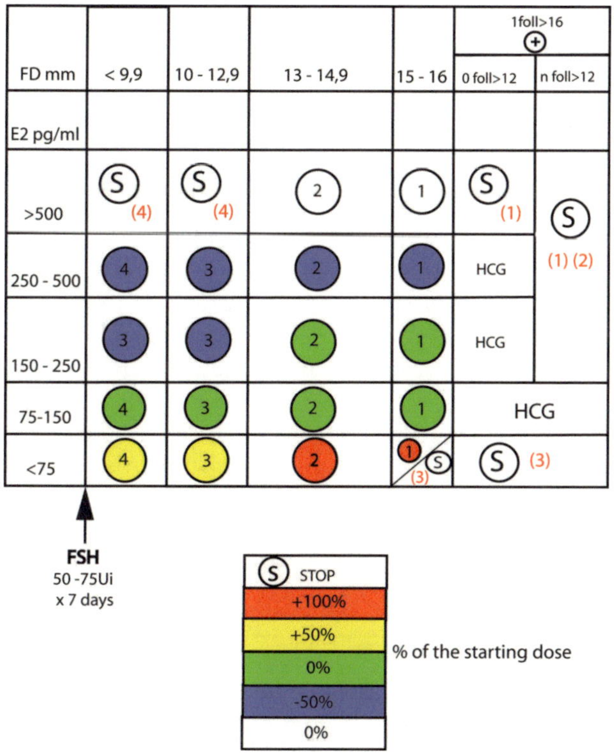

Figure 1.
Standard step-up protocol for a mono-follicular stimulation: example of an algorithm showing the possible scenarios after the administration of 50–75 UI FSH for 5 days (StimXpert).

- ***Antagonist Stimulation Protocols***: a progressive shift to this approach has occurred, with the need for more "friendly stimulations." It results in pregnancy rates comparable to the long agonist protocol and appears to include a lower risk for ovarian hyperstimulation. GnRH antagonist may be introduced along with gonadotropins, on a fixed stimulation day (fixed antagonist), or at a later time when ovarian response meets specified sonographic and/or hormonal levels (flexible antagonist). *All four protocols (long/short agonist, fixed/flexible antagonist) are available with StimXpert*

- ***Nature of the Gonadotropin***: All FSH gonadotropins are suitable for multi-follicular stimulations. Although the isoforms of each hormone differ from each other, research has never established one to be superior. Thus, StimXPert offers a choice from among all products, and clinicians may choose their favorite without affecting the algorithm.

- **Starting Dose:** Most controversies appear in choices at this step, and multiple algorithms have emerged in relation to the patient characteristics: age, weight, BMI, antral follicular count (AFC), and blood levels of FSH or AMH [7, 8]. This program offers a starting dose based on only two of these parameters, namely weight and AMH level. There is no concrete evidence that BMI has a significant predictive effect over weight, while age, FSH, and AFC appear to be consistently related to AMH level. Note that the recommended starting dose for follitropin delta is based on these same two variables [9].

- ***Monitoring:*** Initial monitoring should occur after 5 days of FSH injections (or 4 days for the short agonist protocol). The StimXpert software will, as usual, adapt the continued dosing and monitoring schedules according to ovarian responses. One exception, when using follitropin alpha: the starting dose level continues unchanged during the entire stimulation period [9]. In case of a poor ovarian response, e.g., when fewer than five developing follicles are detected, the program will recommend cancelation of the cycle. This decision may be overcome by the physician, who remains free to override any programmed recommendations. The software remains ready to recalculate after modifications by the clinician.

- ***Ovulation Triggering***: Ovulation is triggered using hCG when 5–15 follicles are present, and estradiol level is less than 2500 pg./ml. StimXpert will recommend cancelation at higher sonographic and hormonal levels, in order to avoid risk of OHS. If the antagonist protocol is being used, the program will propose to trigger using a GnRH agonist, even though the risk of OHS is not completely absent.

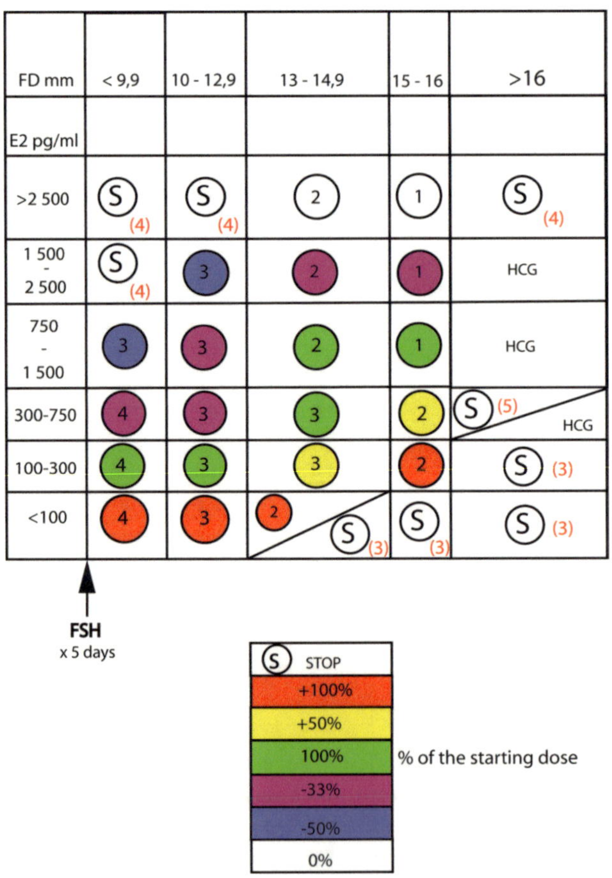

Figure 2.
Long agonist multifollicular stimulation protocol with a target of 6–14 follicles: example of an algorithm showing the possible scenarios after 5 days of FSH (StimXpert).

Again, the clinician can override these recommendations and trigger with hCG, to enable freezing of embryos for later transfer as well as to avoid a secondary OHS. The software also will recommend cancelation of the cycle in a case of poor ovarian response, for example, with fewer than five mature follicles, and this too may be overridden.

Figure 2 illustrates an example of the algorithm used by the software for the agonist long protocol.

5. Software for whom?

The StimXpert program does not pretend to cover the whole field of ovarian stimulation possibilities, as different decisions might attain similar results otherwise. It does, however, establish how using programmed recommendations can enable a stimulation cycle to result in a successful beginning pregnancy without numerous complications. This system is not intended for clinicians with established experience in ovarian stimulations, although its utilization within a team of clinicians may help to harmonize varied practices of each member. In particular, it should limit the more predictable complications associated with human factors, working toward creation of a "hyperstimulation-free" clinic.

More directly, StimXpert is recommended for:

- Medical students and trainees learning the principles of ovarian stimulation.
- Gynecologist and endocrinologist practitioners assuming direct care of their infertility patients, but who have had apprehensions about the undertaking.
- Any practitioner who feels inexperienced in ovarian stimulation protocols, thus seeking some assistance in the decision-making process.
- Clinicians in developing countries where infertility therapy remains scarce.

6. What about other algorithm-based systems?

Only one computer decision support system encompasses the whole stimulation cycle with day-to-day decisions, but exclusively for IVF controlled hyperstimulation [10]. The few other algorithm-based treatments ever published take into account only one of two specific steps of the stimulation cycle and quite exclusively for IVF purposes: the starting dose [7–11] or the criteria for ovulation triggering [12, 13]. To date, StimXpert represents the only stimulation software available assuming both 1 – the entire treatment cycle, and 2 – all validated protocols, from mono-follicular classic stimulation to multi-follicular controlled hyperstimulation.

7. Conclusion

The StimXpert software aims to facilitate the acquisition of technical principles of ovarian stimulation and to optimize the chances of pregnancy together with diminishing risks for complications such as multiple pregnancies and OHS. As designed, the program may be modified, completed, and turned into an evidence-based stimulation software protocol, or it can alternatively be converted into a self-learning system by integrating increasing numbers of cycles leading to safe beginning pregnancies.

Author details

Jean-Claude Emperaire[1*] and J. Charles Eldridge[2]

1 Clinique Bordeaux Nord, Bordeaux, France

2 Wake Forest University School of Medicine, Winston-Salem, NC, USA

*Address all correspondence to: dr.jc.emperaire@gmail.com

References

[1] Emperaire JC. Ovulation Stimulation with Gonadotropins. London: Springer Verlag; 2015

[2] Emperaire JC. Stimulation ovulatoire: développement d'un logiciel d'initiation et d'aide à la décision. Med Reprod Gyn Endocrinol. 2017;**19**:206-213

[3] Bry-Gauillard H, Larrat-Ledoux F, Levaillant JF. Anti-Mullerian hormone and ovarian morphology in women with isolated hypogonadotropic hypogonadism/Kallmann syndrome: Effects of recombinant human FSH. Clinics in Endocrinology and Metabolism. 2017;**102**:1102-1111

[4] Fischer D, Reisenbüchler C, Rösner S. Avoiding OHSS: Controlled ovarian low-dose stimulation in women with PCOS. Gebursthilfe Frauenheilkunde. 2016;**76**:718-726

[5] Mumford SL, Legros RS, Diamond MP. Baseline AMH levels associated with ovulation following ovulation induction in women with polycystic ovary syndrome. The Journal of Clinical Endocrinology and Metabolism. 2016;**101**:3288-3296

[6] Kamel A, Ramadan W, Hussein AF. Can AMH levels predict the need for increased medication during IVF/ ICSI in PCOS women? The Journal of Maternal-Fetal & Neonatal Medicine. 2017;**12**:1-10

[7] Papaleo E, Zaffagnini S, Munaretto M, et al. Clinical application of a normogram based on age, serum FSH and AMH to select the FSH starting dose in IVF/ ICSI cycles: A retrospective two-centers study. European Journal of Obstetrics, Gynecology, and Reproductive Biology. 2016;**207**:94-99

[8] Yovitch JL, Alsbjerq B, Coceicao JL. PIVET rFSH dosing algorithms for controlled hyper- stimulation enables optimized pregnancy rates and avoidance of ovarian hyperstimulation syndrome. Dru Des Devel Ther. 2016;**10**:256-273

[9] Andersen AN, Nelson SM, Fauser BCJM, et al. Individual versus conventional ovarian stimulation for *in vitro* fertilization: A multicenter, randomized, controlled, assessor-blind phase 3 non-inferiority trial. Fertility and Sterility. 2017;**107**:387-396

[10] Letterie G, Mac DA. Artificial intelligence in in vitro fertilization: A computer decision support system for day to day management of ovarian stimulation during in vitro fertilization. Fertility and Sterility. 2020;**114**:1026-1031

[11] Bachmann A, Kissler S, Laubert I, et al. An eight centre, retrospective, clinical practice data analysis on algorithm-based treatment with follitropin delta. Reproductive BioMedical Online. 2022;**44**:853-857

[12] Hariton E, Chi EA, Chi G. et al, A machine learning algorithm can optimize the day of trigger to improve in vitro fertilization outcomes. Fertility and Sterility. 2021;**116**:1227-1235

[13] Fanton M, Nutting V, Solano F. et al, An interpretable machine learning model for predicting the optimal day of trigger during ovarian stimulation. Fertility and Sterility. 2022;**118**(1):101-108

Chapter 9

Perspective Chapter: Ovarian Reproductive Aging and Rejuvenation Strategies

Antonio Díez-Juan and Iavor K. Vladimirov

Abstract

The ovarian milieu, which includes increased vasculature, different growth factors, necessary hormone synthesis, and appropriate granulosa cell function, is essential for oocyte maturation. Keeping the microenvironment in a state of equilibrium is crucial for healthy ovarian function. However, as people age, their tissues rebuild less effectively, leading to an imbalance in the microenvironment's homeostasis and ovarian fibrosis, which finally causes ovarian function to deteriorate. As a result, full restoration of ovarian microenvironment health is required to enhance ovarian function. The precise identification of the molecular pathways involved in ovarian aging can help to devise therapy techniques that can decrease ovarian decay and boost the amount and quality of oocytes available for IVF. Antioxidants, melatonin, growth hormones, and mitochondrial and cell therapy are among the available treatments. All of these treatments must be considered in light of every couple's history and current biological parameters, and a personalized (patient-tailored) therapy program must be developed. In this chapter, we aim to give an overview on the identified mechanism involved in female reproductive aging and potential therapeutic approaches to amend reproductive efficiency.

Keywords: ovary, aging, human reproduction, therapy, infertility

1. Introduction

Aging in humans is an incredibly complex process characterized by time-dependent functional decline, resulting in a decrease in the quality of life [1]. There is a relationship between the longevity of a species and its reproductive capacity. The parameters that determine reproductive efficiency are (i) gestation length, (ii) litter size, (iii) time to reach adulthood, (iv) litter intervals, and (v) duration of fertility for the duration of the overall lifespan. We as humans are the longest-lived land mammal, at the top of the long-living mammals and far from other primates. Although our reproductive efficiency is low, our social structure and creative thinking create a formidable life-history combination that most likely played a significant role in the successful colonization of hunter-gatherers around the world.

IntechOpen

Social behavior is evolving, and reproductive efficiency in humans is decreasing, the average age of motherhood has been increasing since 1980, reducing the reproductive time, litter size, and intervals. The risk of childlessness increases with age, with reproductive aging being the most obvious factor.

Reproductive aging is a process involving a variety of intrinsic and extrinsic factors that affect the entire organism. Specifically, the reproductive organs and germ cell quality [2]. Reproductive aging causes infertility, increased miscarriages, and birth defects because gamete quality declines more rapidly in women than in men [3]. Menopause is the final menstrual cycle in women and other primates, which can be ovulatory or not. Fertility usually ends before menopause [4].

For decades, researchers have studied reproductive aging in humans and laboratory animals at the physiological, hormonal, cellular, and molecular levels.

2. Reproductive system aging

Aging is characterized by the progressive decline of multiple organ functions and the onset of degenerative diseases [5]. One aspect of aging is the decline in reproductive function. The reproductive system is a network of organs that generate gametes together with sex hormones. It fosters the birth of healthy offspring and coordinates physiological functions by sustaining endocrine homeostasis. When a female partner is over the age of 35, the risk of infertility tends to increase [6]. Furthermore, aging-related menopause in women is accompanied by an endocrine disorder as well as an increased risk of several major health complications, which include osteoporosis, cardiovascular disease, recurrent depression, and others [7]. Male fertility declines with age as well, but it happens more gradually and is associated with endocrine equilibrium disorders like late-onset hypogonadism (LOH). LOH symptoms include libido loss, sexual dysfunction, and declines in bone and muscle mass density. Moreover, benign prostatic hypertrophy (BPH) as well as prostate cancer (PCa), are common age-related diseases that impact the male reproductive system and impair the elderly's quality of life [8].

Reproductive aging leads to a variety of age-related disorders in both men and women since reproductive health is so tightly connected to overall health.

3. Female reproductive aging

Age-related infertility is a multifactorial process and understanding factors affecting follicle/oocyte aging requires the comparison of the theories on aging mechanisms based on studies on tissues and organs other than the ovary [9].

Female fecundity capacity peaks in their 20s, declines in their late 30s in defiance of regular menstrual cycles, and ends in menopause at the average age of 50–51 years [10]. Data from in vitro fertilization (IVF) shows that the mother's age is an important factor that leads to impressive differences in clinical results [11]. While the fraction of first births in women over the age of 30 increased sixfold between 1970 and 2002. According to an American study of over 120.000 assisted reproduction technologies (ART), the successful delivery rate per embryo transfer reduced from 43.2% in women 35 years old to 15.1% in women 41–42 years old and 5.9% in women over 42 years old [12].

Changes in the ovarian follicle pool and a decrease in the ovarian reserve are the primary causes of the female reproductive ability decline in humans [13]. Despite uterine and neuroendocrine factors, it is well characterized that ovaries and ovarian follicles are outstanding regulators of reproductive aging. This statement is substantiated by oocyte donation from younger women in the treatment of age-related infertility [10, 14].

It is widely accepted that female mammals are born with a finite supply of primordial follicles (PMFs), which are gradually depleted over the course of their lives [15]. A follicle reserve is formed in the fetal or early postnatal ovaries. Composed of pregranulosa cells and primary oocytes arrested in the diplotene stage of meiotic prophase I. These latter are formed from primordial germ cells (PGCs), which originate outside the gonadal anlages and migrate into the forming ovaries [16]. After establishment, each PMF has three developmental options: I remain quiescent, (ii) die directly from the quiescent state, or (iii) be recruited into a growing follicle pool via a process known as follicle activation, which contributes to cyclic endocrine secretion.

The size of the ovarian PMF pool is estimated to be 7 million oogonia by the fifth month of prenatal development (Sadler, 2011). Except for a small number near the ovarian surface, many oogonia and primary oocytes become atretic at this time. During the female fertile age, a cohort of primordial follicles is recruited month by month in order to develop a single dominant follicle and ovulate its fertile oocyte. The dormant oocyte is arrested in prophase I in primordial follicles and is surrounded by a single layer of flattened granulose cells (GCs) [17]. Primordial follicle recruitment causes the oocyte to activate and mature, as well as the proliferation and differentiation of surrounding GCs, resulting in the formation of primary follicles, which are distinguished by a single layer of cuboidal GCs surrounding the oocyte. In secondary follicles, GC layers continue to proliferate. They differentiate into cumulus cells (CCs), which are cells contiguous with the maturing oocyte [18, 19]. CCs are also important in the recruitment of androgen-producing theca cells (later segregated into theca interna and externa layers) from the ovarian mesenchyme and mesonephros progenitor pools [20]. Folliculogenesis is a paracrine signaling gonadotropin-independent unit comprised of multiple locally active growth factors and small molecules secreted by early follicle GCs until the formation of the preantral follicle [21].

Maturing follicles eventually express gonadotropin receptors and become responsive to gonadotropins, first to follicle-stimulating hormone (FSH) and then to luteinizing hormone (LH).

Follicles become hormone-secreting units during this gonadotropin-dependent phase of folliculogenesis.

FSH promotes GC growth, estradiol production, and dormant follicle selection [22], whereas LH is in charge of androgen secretion from cholesterol, meiosis I completion in the oocyte, germinal vesicle breakdown [23, 24], and subsequent progression to metaphase II [25]. With the production of a mature oocyte capable of fertilization, ovulation marks the end of folliculogenesis [26].

Multiple follicles are arrested at different stages of the highly regulated and well-orchestrated folliculogenesis process and undergo irreversible atretic degeneration with increasing speed after the mid-30s [27, 28].

The development of an antral follicle from a dormant primordial follicle into a mature, healthy oocyte that is prepared for fertilization is a carefully orchestrated, complicated process that requires the precise synchronized timing of intraovarian molecules and cells. Aging causes progressive deterioration in follicle function and capacity to form an oocyte capable of fertilization. Age-related disruption in folliculogenesis is attributed to several changes that occur concurrently. Bioenergetics dysfunction, shortened telomere length, decreased DNA repair capacity with loss of chromosome cohesion and spindle aberration increase the risk of mutations and meiotic errors have been identified in aged oocytes [29, 30]. Additionally, the number of GCs surrounding the oocyte declines with aging as a result of decreased proliferation [31] and elevated GC apoptosis [32], which is accompanied by altered production of locally active growth factors [33], and disrupted steroidogenesis [34].

The decline in steroid hormone biosynthesis with age is primarily due to a decrease in the number of ovarian follicles, and thus a decrease in functional steroid-producing cells. Markers associated with reproductive aging and senescence in women are based on a decline in granulosa cell activity, such as a decrease in circulating levels of the anti-Müllerian hormone (AMH; produced by immature granulosa cells), decreased levels of estrogen (produced by mature granulosa cells), and elevated levels of FSH (due to a lack of inhibin production by granulosa cells).

AMH, also known as Mullerian Inhibitory Substance, is a peptide belonging to the TGF superfamily that functions by binding to the AMHR2 receptor. Beginning at roughly 36 weeks of gestation in female fetuses, AMH expression in the ovary reaches a peak in the middle of the 20s and then gradually declines until menopause [35–37]. The majority of AMH produced by antral follicles is released by CCs [38]. AMH and its receptor AMHR2 are largely expressed in the GCs of mature follicles in the ovary, with the levels of expression varying depending on the stage [38, 39]. Beginning in primary follicle GCs, AMH expression rises steadily until it reaches its peak in small antral follicles less than 6 mm in size [35].

Regarding AMH's function in preventing the formation of primordial follicles, human studies on primordial reserve using ovarian cortex biopsies are still controversial [38]. AMH expression during fetal gonadal development has a detrimental effect on healthy ovarian and follicular pool development, AMH inhibits the developing follicle during the early gonadotropin-dependent and gonadotropin-independent phases of follicular development [36]. AMH is essential for choosing cyclic antral follicles as well [40]. AMH knockout mouse models recruit noticeably more developing follicles with ovarian stimulation than the control group [36]. AMH regulation and the production of its receptors are intricate processes that still need more research.

4. Vascular aging

In humans, vascular endothelial dysfunction appears to occur with aging even in the absence of clinical cardiovascular disease (CVD) and significant CVD risk factors, according to a number of lines of research. Older humans, rodents, and non-human primates have all shown signs of impaired endothelium-dependent dilation, reduced fibrinolytic activity, increased leukocyte adhesion, altered permeability, and/or other markers of endothelial dysfunction [41]. The function of the macro- and microvascular endothelium declines gradually with age [42] rarefaction, which affects the systemic microvasculature in all organs, being a crucial indicator of aging [43–47]. It is believed that decreased endothelium turnover and enhanced apoptosis cell death are two factors in age-related microvascular rarefaction. Age-related microvascular rarefaction causes blood flow to decrease, which worsens ischemia injury, especially in tissues with high metabolic activity like the brain and heart. This loss in blood flow also diminishes metabolic support and decreases microvascular flexibility and the circulatory system's capacity to adapt to variations in metabolic demand [48].

Although more data are needed to link ovarian aging and vascular rarefaction, indirect evidence suggests a relationship between oocyte maturation, aging, and vasculature. As previously stated, follicular vasculature begins to develop inside the theca cell layer at the secondary follicle stage, with the GC layer remaining avascular and separated by the basement membrane.

The normal function of the ovaries and ovarian follicles is maintained by continuous angiogenesis, which is the development of new blood vessels from existing ones. Endothelial and mural cells become destabilized in response to an angiogenic stimulation such as hypoxia or injury. Following that, they migrate toward angiogenic stimuli and grow, resulting in the formation of a new vessel [49]. Follicular vasculature seems to be crucial in achieving dominance by the follicle. It is well known that dominant follicles ingest more serum gonadotrophins than other follicles, in addition to having a more vascular theca [50].

Microvasculature is critical for the follicle nutrients and oxygen, as well as ensuring an adequate supply of gonadotropins, steroid precursors, and other regulators. VEGF is thought to be crucial for follicular growth and for the formation of the antrum thecal angiogenesis and guarantee vascular permeability.

Microvasculature determines follicular dominance because the dominant follicle has more plentiful vasculature in its theca layer than other follicles in the same cohort. Oocytes derived from follicles with adequate vascularization and oxygen content (3%) had increased fertilization and developmental potential in prospective research based on pulsed Doppler ultrasonographic examination [51]. Studies of perifollicular vascularity also revealed a positive correlation between high-grade vascularity and better results during IVF cycles [52].

A diminished oxygen supply to the leading follicle, which is a state dependent on a defective perifollicular vascularization, was proposed as a possible representation of a key environmental component responsible for oocyte senescence [53, 54]. In fact, it has been noted that alterations in older MII oocytes, such as aberrant chromosome and spindle structure, are similar to those in young oocytes derived from Graafian follicles with lower perifollicular vascularization and oxygen concentration [54, 55].

Growing follicles definitely require a sufficient ingrowth of capillaries into the theca, as opposed to primordial and preantral follicles, which obtain their blood supply from the stromal arteries.

There is no question that VEGF and its receptors, VEGFR1 and VEGFR2 are regulatory factors in mammalian ovarian folliculogenesis controlling both follicular and luteal angiogenesis as well as new capillary creation within the ovulatory follicle. Its blockage causes a significant reduction in endothelial and granulosa cell proliferation in growing antral follicles, as well as inhibition of follicular growth and ovulation [56].

Small preantral follicles in the ovarian cortex lack their own blood supply and must rely on passive diffusion from stromal tissue for nourishment and oxygenation. Beginning with secondary follicles, outer stromal cells surrounding the oocyte develop into theca cells during follicular maturation [57]. For the follicle to expand, the inner theca layer, which is separated from the granulosa cell layer by a basement membrane, creates a capillary network [58, 59]. Direct injection of VEGF into the ovarian blood supply can improve angiogenesis, increase the number of primary and secondary follicles, and decrease follicular atresia [60, 61].

VEGF levels in follicular fluid rise with age in both natural and in vitro fertilization (IVF) cycles [33, 62–65]. This aging-related rise in VEGF levels could be a result of selective gonadotropin elevation in older reproductive-age women, a compensatory response to follicular hypoxia, and a decrease in energy synthesis in the presence of impaired mitochondrial function [21].

Nitric oxide is an important angiogenesis mediator. NO is pro-angiogenic because it increases endothelial cell survival, proliferation, and migration. VEGF, FGF, and other growth factors increase endothelial NO synthesis, which is a significant mediator of their actions. Angiogenesis is hampered by NOS pathway abnormalities caused by pharmacological, metabolic, or genetic factors. Similarly, ADMA, an endogenous NOS inhibitor, functions as a natural anti-angiogenic agent [66].

The NOS pathway's activity is thus critical in the response to endogenous or therapeutic angiogenic drugs. Manipulation of the NOS pathway could provide another strategy for therapeutically modify angiogenesis in folliculogenesis. Multiple isoenzymes of NO synthase (NOS) catalyze the oxidation of L-arginine to L-citrulline in a nicotinamide adenine dinucleotide phosphate reduced form (NADPH) and oxygen-dependent reaction in mammals. NOS1, NOS2, and NOS3 are the three NOS isoforms. The product of the NOS1 gene is known as neuronal NOS (nNOS), whereas the product of the NOS3 gene is known as endothelial NOS (eNOS). These isoforms are calcium-dependent and constitutive. The third isoform produced by the NOS2 gene is an inducible NOS (iNOS) that is calcium-independent. Only cytokines such as lipopolysaccharide, interleukin 1, and tumor necrosis factor-alpha (TNF) activate iNOS [67].

NO exerts remarkable functions within the ovary, including the control of steroidogenesis, folliculogenesis, and oocyte competence. NO can be produced in the ovary not only by ovarian cells but also by the ovarian vasculature and resident or invading macrophages [68].

In rats, eNOS is found in mural granulosa cells, theca layer, ovarian stroma, and ovarian blood vessels [69], but iNOS is found only in somatic cells of primary, secondary, and small antral follicles, as well as luteal cells.

In contrast, both eNOS and iNOS are expressed in theca and granulosa cells of the mouse ovary [69]. eNOS is expressed in theca and granulosa cells, as well as the surface epithelium and luteal cells, in the bovine ovary [70]. Additionally, eNOS is discovered more frequently than iNOS in granulosa cells in the porcine ovary [71]. Human granulosa and luteal cells have been shown to contain inducible NOS and eNOS [72].

NO represents a key regulator in ovarian steroidogenesis, NO exerts its inhibitory effect on aromatase activity, a key enzyme in the steroidogenic pathway. The direct inhibitory effect on the enzyme is mediated by the formation of a nitrosothiol group in the cysteine residue of the aromatase enzyme [73].

Age-related endothelium dysfunction is primarily caused by at least three NO-related events, including changed NOS enzyme expression and activity, decreased vascular antioxidant capacity, and NO consumption by excessive O_2.

NO has been linked favorably to delaying oocyte aging. As previously presented NO is a common molecule that plays a crucial role in the microenvironment of the oocyte from folliculogenesis to early embryo development.

When fresh oocytes are exposed to superoxide, the zona pellucida dissolution time of these oocytes increases significantly. Further, superoxide exposure of fresh oocytes exhibited increased ooplasm microtubule dynamics (OMD) and major CG loss. Both old and fresh oocytes exposed to NO have a considerable decrease in OMD and the zona pellucida dissolution time, as well as a reduction in spontaneous CG loss. Additionally, NO exposure lowers the frequency of aberrant spindles. Because of its capacity to neutralize peroxyl lipid radicals and cytotoxic ROS, NO may act as an unusual antioxidant. Through the activation of guanylate cyclase, which increases the generation of cyclic guanosine monophosphate and might greatly reduce zona pellucida dissolution time and OMD, NO may also contribute to the delay of oocyte aging. Overall, NO slows down oocyte aging and strengthens the microtubular spindle apparatus in older oocytes [74].

5. Mitochondria

A defining contributing factor in aging has been for a long time mitochondrial dysfunction [75, 76]. Deterioration of pleiotropic activities is the result of mitochondrial malfunction, which is linked to a number of characteristics of aging including dysregulation of cell signaling and inefficient energy production [77, 78]. The accumulation of somatic mtDNA mutations, decreased OXPHOS activity, increased oxidative damage, altered mitochondrial quality control, ineffective mitochondrial biogenesis or clearance, and dysregulation of mitochondrial dynamics are all aspects of mitochondrial dysfunction that have been linked to aging [79–81].

ROS formation occurs naturally as a byproduct of energy production in the mitochondria [40, 82]. The majority of endogenous ROS are produced by mitochondrial OXPHOS, which serves as the final step in the metabolism of substrates and the creation of ATP [83, 84].

The hypothesis for why mtDNA is more susceptible to oxidative damage than nuclear DNA is that it is close to the respiratory chain, lacks histones, and has ineffective repair mechanisms [47]. It was shown that the production of ROS, oxidative damage, and chronological age are all strongly correlated [48]. mtDNA mutations are expected to build up over time, causing cells to have less oxidative energy and, eventually, an aging phenotype. In reproductive cells, it has been hypothesized that age-related ROS buildup and oxidative damage in mtDNA cause a reduction in the rate of oocyte fertilization and developmental potential [49].

This hypothesis can not be confirmed because several studies have obtained contradictory results or even no differences in the frequency of mtDNA changes in the oocytes of older women [85–90]. Furthermore, no increase in mtDNA mutations was observed in embryo samples from women above the age of 40 [91].

Because of inconsistencies in human data, accepting the free radical hypothesis of aging as a final mechanical explanation for ovarian aging is difficult (reviewed in [92]).

Mitochondrial dynamics are defined by fission and fusion. Fission produces smaller mitochondria, which could be better at driving cell proliferation and causing ROS, whereas fusion improves communication with the endoplasmic reticulum and dilutes accumulated mtDNA mutations and oxidized proteins [93]. Fission and fusion abnormalities have serious implications for ovarian aging. In C57BL/6 mice, oocyte-specific deletion of the mitochondrial fusion protein Mitofusin (Mfn1) results in rapid depletion of the ovarian follicular reserve. Based on immunofluorescence, it was shown that ceramide, a membrane sphingolipid involved in apoptosis and cell cycle arrest, was elevated in Mfn1−/− mice oocytes, suggesting that it is probably a factor in the mechanism of decreased ovarian reserve in this mouse model. Myriocin, a ceramide synthesis inhibitor, was administered to mice every day for 21 days in a row, which increased follicular growth and allowed the production of antral follicles, partially reversing the reproductive phenotype [94].

A vital and intricate homeostatic coordination mechanism of the nuclear and mitochondrial genomes is necessarily necessary to drive correct mitochondrial biogenesis.

It is reliant on nuclear genes encoding nuclear respiratory factor-1 and -2, estrogen-related receptor (ERR), peroxisome proliferator-activated receptor (PPAR) coactivator 1 (PGC-1), and PGC-1 (NRF-1, 2). Additionally, the mitochondrial-localized sirtuin (SIRT) family genes SIRT3, SIRT4, and SIRT5 are involved. The most thoroughly studied sirtuin, SIRT3, has been discovered to interact with PGC-1, a crucial regulator of mitochondrial biogenesis, suppress intracellular ROS, and perhaps even control longevity and aging phenotypes [95]. The primary regulator of mitochondrial homeostasis and a promoter of mitochondrial biogenesis is AMP-activated protein kinase (AMPK). In particular, AMPK interacts with PGC-1 in a variety of ways [96]. Mitophagy, the selective autophagic eradication of defective mitochondria, controls mitochondrial biogenesis. PTEN-induced kinase 1 (PINK1)-Parkin pathway as well as AMPK both have a role in controling mitophagy [97, 98].

Critical to ovarian function is mitochondrial biogenesis. From the immature germinal vesicle stage to the mature oocyte, there is a dramatic increase in mitochondrial biogenesis. A single egg contains hundreds of thousands of mitochondria at the time of fertilization, providing enough ATP to enable fertilization and support development until implantation when mitochondrial replication picks back up in the blastocyst.

During ovarian aging, decreasing mtDNA content, which indicates decreased mitochondrial biogenesis, is frequently seen. Premature ovarian aging patients had the lowest amounts of mtDNA, followed by IVF recipients who respond normally and recipients who do not respond well to IVF [99].

In humans undergoing in vitro fertilization (IVF), sirtuin 3 (SIRT3) active protein co-localized to mitochondria in follicular granulosa and cumulus cells. SIRT3 mRNA levels were also lower in advanced maternal-age women compared to control women [100]. Advanced maternal-age women showed lower PGC-1 expression in cumulus cells along with lower mtDNA concentration in cumulus and oocyte cells when compared to women with normal ovarian reserve women [101]. These correlations provide evidence in favor of the hypothesis that poor oocyte competence in IVF may be caused by insufficient mitochondrial biogenesis during oocyte maturation [102].

mtDNA copy number has lately been the subject of several research because it is one of the mitochondrial factors that may represent the reproductive capability of gametes and embryos.

Mammalian models have shown that mtDNA levels dramatically rise during oogenesis [103] remain constant during fertilization, and then resume replication at the blastocyst stage [104, 105].

As a result, each time a cell divides in the early preimplantation embryo, mtDNA is distributed among the different blastomeres [106] and the total amount of mtDNA in cleavage-stage embryos corresponds to the mtDNA content of the oocyte [107, 108].

In an effort to identify a reliable biomarker for the implantation potential of euploid embryos, several researchers looked at the mtDNA content of biopsy samples from the cleavage and blastocyst stages of euploid embryos. In the initial study, Fragouli et al. used a combination of array-comparative genomic hybridization, real-time quantitative polymerase chain reaction, and next-generation sequencing to examine day-3 and day-5 embryos. They found that older women's embryos contained much more copies of mtDNA. Higher amounts of mtDNA, which were age-independent, were also seen in aneuploid embryos [91]. Importantly, they identified a threshold for mtDNA beyond which euploid embryos did not implant. Diez Juan et al. discovered poor implantation potential for day-3 and day-5 euploid embryos with higher quantities of mtDNA in a later investigation that also examined day-3 blastomere and day-5 trophectoderm biopsies. However, unlike Fragouli et al., Diez Juan et al. did not discover a rise in mtDNA copy number in embryos from older vs. younger reproductive-age women [109]. These results supported the quiet embryo hypothesis, which holds that under ideal circumstances, embryos would have little metabolic activity whereas under stress, embryos would boost mitochondrial replication as a coping mechanism [110] but no clear differences in embryos from women with advanced reproductive age.

6. Methods to prolong reproductive life and slow down ovarian aging

There are currently few therapy options available to help women with their ovarian reserve and oocyte quality. Infertility patients can get Coenzyme Q10 (CoQ10), Dehydroepiandrosterone (DHEA), vitamins including vitamins C and D, or dietary or supplement isoflavones as therapies for diminished ovarian reserve.

No study has categorically validated the routine administration of these bioactive substances, despite the possibility that they have some therapeutic effects on DOR. Therefore, more study is required to develop novel therapeutic approaches that will improve patients' reproductive results.

6.1 Mitochondrial support therapy

It has been demonstrated that the mitochondrial electron transport chain component CoQ10 reduces mitochondrial dysfunction in infertile mice [111]. A 2014 human study evaluated the post-meiotic aneuploidy rates in embryos of IVF patients treated with 600 mg per day of CoQ10 versus placebo and found that the two groups had respective aneuploidy rates of 46.5% and 62.8%, respectively. CoQ10 is a soluble lipid transporter that is essential for complex III stability. Furthermore, it is a strong cellular antioxidant. Normal tissues produce their own supply, however, it has been found that tissue concentration decreases with aging [112]. In mice, research on the potential effects of CoQ10 supplementation on fertility found that it may boost mitochondrial activity, reduce ROS levels, and postpone the loss of ovarian reserve while also restoring the expression of the mitochondrial gene in oocytes [111, 113, 114]. Importantly, early results of a stopped (and solely existing) human research due to worries about the effects of polar body biopsy on embryos. The trial was halted, and statistical significance was not reached although suggested that CoQ10 supplementation might reduce aneuploidy rates [115, 116].

Several members of the sirtuin deacetylase family function as anti-aging agents in mammalian cells [117]. Sirtuin 3 (SIRT3) activation enhances mitochondrial activity [100]. Similar to this, ovarian reserve is improved both quantitatively and qualitatively when SIRT1 expression is activated by resveratrol [118, 119]. In oocytes, mtDNA concentrations, membrane potential, and ATP production were discovered to be elevated by the anti-aging chemical resveratrol [120, 121]. Additionally, resveratrol was discovered to increase the quantity and quality of oocytes in mice, protecting against the decline in fertility brought on by aging of the reproductive system [122]. Melatonin is thought to activate sirtuin [123, 124]. Melatonin and SIRT3 posttranslationally collaborate for the regulation of free radical equilibrium in mitochondria, increasing the size of the primordial follicle pool and delaying ovarian aging [125, 126]. Melatonin is a chemical that functions as both a direct antioxidant and a modulator of the mechanisms defending cells against oxidative stress. It was initially utilized in reproductive medicine to treat endometriosis and adenomyosis-related infertility [33, 34, 127, 128]. Since then, fresh research has shown how melatonin may delay the aging of the ovary [36]. Melatonin administration is clearly advised for women with age-related ovarian decay or POI even though the mechanism underlying the hormone's anti-aging effect in the human ovary still needs to be fully understood [36]. It has no serious side effects and offers additional benefits to patients who receive it.

Multiple observations have revealed that aging-related pathologies are also significantly influenced by the mTOR signaling system [129]. Rapamycin, an inhibitor of mTOR, controls the sirtuin and mTOR pathways and prevents the first activation of follicles [130]. Rapamycin is being researched as a potential preventative agent against early ovarian failure and reproductive aging after it was discovered to partially reverse the infertile phenotype in Clpp knockout mice [92].

A potent antioxidant and mitochondrial metabolic facilitator, alpha-lipoic acid [131], has been shown to enhance in vitro follicular growth and oocyte maturation while reducing follicular ROS generation by improving mitochondrial metabolism [132, 133].

Overall, significant progress has been made in understanding the nutrients that could enhance mitochondrial activity, slow the aging of the ovaries, and benefit women with DOR or early ovarian insufficiency. A protective effect has not yet been demonstrated, though.

6.2 HGH administration

The first treatment proven to be effective in older women was GH injection during ovarian stimulation.

In a randomized controlled trial, 100 women over the age of 40 who were receiving treatment for assisted reproduction were randomly assigned to receive growth hormone treatment or a placebo, and the results showed that the GH arm had significantly higher delivery and live birth rates than the placebo arm [134]. These results were supported by subsequent research, which also expanded the use of GH therapy to include younger women with POI [135, 136].

The cell signaling pathways involved in cellular defense against oxidative stress are affected by GH [137], and adult GH deficiency results in insufficient cellular response to radical generation. This explains why ovarian degradation can be influenced by age-related or early GH insufficiency, even when it is largely brought on by other factors. GH might help a subset of patients who do not respond well to treatment—women with poor oocyte and/or embryonic development. Therefore, in women who have both age-related ovarian decline and POI, GH may be used as an adjuvant therapy during ovarian stimulation [136].

6.3 Dehydroepiandrosterone supplementation

The zona reticularis layer of the adrenal cortex and the theca cells of the ovary create DHEA, an important prohormone, when they synthesize testosterone and estradiol from cholesterol [138]. Its levels are seen to be high, particularly in the early stages of reproduction, and to decrease with age [116, 139]. Several phases of folliculogenesis have seen the identification of androgen receptors (AR) [140]. By stimulating primordial follicles in monkeys [141, 142] and mouse models, androgens were found to increase the number of primary follicles [143]. Additionally, they influence the development of preovulatory follicles, follicle maturation, and FSH-R mRNA synthesis in primate and mouse models [144, 145] as well as GC proliferation in vitro [146].

DHEA was shown to be crucial for folliculogenesis, just as androgens, and its administration may enhance the success of IVF, particularly in populations with DOR or weak ovarian response. One of the first to discuss the advantages of DHEA with DOR was Casson et al. They observed an increase in peak estradiol levels [147, 148] as well as an increase in ovarian responsiveness to gonadotropin stimulation. Following Casson's original study, numerous studies in mice and humans with poor responders were carried out using different doses (10–80 mg per day) of DHEA administration for various lengths of time (pre-IVF treatment or concurrently with ovarian stimulation), and it was found that improved ovarian function was associated with an increase in ovarian response and a decrease in the number of atretic follicles [123, 139]. When DHEA was pretreated for at least 8 weeks prior to IVF treatment, Li et al. found that the CCs of women older than 38 years produced more energy and had higher-quality oocytes [124]. A premature ovarian insufficiency rat model with subfertility, decreased follicular number, and increased atresia was used in a different investigation by Sozen et al. Primal follicular recruitment and follicular development were both stimulated by DHEA [149].

One of the mechanisms by which DHEA can have positive effects, has been identified to be secondary to its involvement in raising IGF1, which may then improve responsiveness to gonadotropins and may have favorable effects on oocyte quality, particularly in those who respond poorly to these hormones [150]. Additionally, Zhang et al. [151] confirmed that 2-month DHEA supplementation enhanced BMP15 levels in cases of inadequate ovarian response. DHEA is also known to control AR expression and boost follicular development and recruitment [152]. Another mechanism for DHEA's effects on aged follicles is that it enhances mitochondrial hemostasis, transports oxidative phosphorylation, increases cumulus cells' mitochondrial oxygen consumption, and switches energy generation from anaerobic metabolism to aerobic metabolism [124] preventing mitochondrial malfunction with the alternating expression of mitochondrial dynamics genes. With DHEA administration in human CCs, it was observed that the expression of MFN1, a mitochondrial fusion gene, was elevated while PINK1 and PRKN, important proteins for mitophagy, were downregulated [153]. DHEA can also reduce the rate of CC apoptosis in aged follicles [154]. It is believed that DHEA will improve the ovarian microenvironment and reduce age-related embryonic aneuploidy [139].

Testosterone is another androgen that can be used as a potential modifier of folliculogenesis. Lower serum testosterone levels have been linked to reproductive aging [155]. The effects of testosterone supplementation in ovarian aging mammalian models or among older women undergoing IVF, however, are not currently known. As an aromatase inhibitor, letrozole prevents the conversion of testosterone to estrogen, which raises the levels of testosterone. It has been shown to increase the number of retrieved oocytes and the rate of implantation in poor responders [156] and lower IVF expenditures by reducing gonadotropin dosage [157, 158]. Data on its impact on clinical pregnancy rates or live birth rates, however, are limited [159].

6.4 Vitamin D

Vitamin D (VD) is a fat-soluble secosteroid. VD regulates the transcription of genes involved in a variety of cellular processes, including pro-differentiation, anti-proliferation, pro-apoptosis, immunosuppressive, and anti-inflammation activities, in target cells via binding to specific VD receptors (VDR). There is a growing understanding that VD is crucial for optimal folliculogenesis and maximizing women's reproductive potential, in addition to its critical function in bone physiology and health [160, 161].

Ovarian follicles display VD production and signaling mechanisms [161]. VD administration enhanced follicle survival, size, and function as well as oocyte maturation and AMH production, according to in vitro experiments carried out on rhesus monkeys [162]. They also verified that VD production and signaling control follicular growth, raising the possibility that VD has endocrine, paracrine, and autocrine effects in the ovary. Reduced ovarian aromatase activity in VDR null mutant mice leads to compromised folliculogenesis [163]. Less oocytes were recovered from oviducts after gonadotropin stimulation in VD-deficient diets, which also delayed follicular development and lengthened estrous cycles [164]. Serum AMH levels have demonstrated a relationship between VD levels and ovarian reserve. The connection between circulating VD and AMH in premenopausal women with regular menstrual cycles suggests that VD deficit may be linked to a reduced ovarian reserve in late-reproductive-aged women [165]. Patients with uterine fibroids also showed an inverse correlation between blood VD levels and ovarian reserve [166]. Additionally, a VDR polymorphism was linked to lower antral follicle numbers in women receiving ovarian stimulation [167].

The capacity for and results of reproduction seem to be influenced by VD levels.

Higher FF levels of 25-hydroxyvitamin D were shown to be substantially related to greater clinical pregnancy and implantation rates in a study examining infertile women undergoing IVF [168]. The number of mature oocytes retrieved and the success rates of oocyte fertilization in patients undergoing IVF were favorably connected with blood VD levels in various prospective studies [65]. The same study's multivariable logistic regression analysis found FF levels of VD as an independent predictor of an IVF cycle's success after correcting for age, BMI, ethnicity, and the number of embryos transferred (Esencan et al., 2022).

The adjusted odds ratio for clinical pregnancy in women with vitamin D levels of 20 ng/mL was considerably higher as compared to women with serum levels of 20 ng/mL in another study [169] examining a cohort of women undergoing IVF. According to a subgroup study, women with the highest serum levels (> 30 ng/mL) had the best probability of getting pregnant [163]. However, there has been a lack of consistency in research evaluating the predictive usefulness of FF VD on IVF results. Despite the fact that a prospective cohort study by Kinuta et al., found that women with higher serum and FF vitamin D levels were significantly more likely to experience clinical pregnancy after IVF-embryo transfer, a different study found lower-quality embryos and significantly lower clinical pregnancy rates with higher levels of follicular VD [164].

7. Cell therapy

Stem cells' therapeutic effects are carried out by differentiation, homing, and paracrine activation. The injured ovary attracts stem cells on their own, where they adhere and grow under a variety of conditions. Recent studies suggest that paracrine mechanisms may be in charge of the therapeutic effect of stem cell transplantation. Surrounding cells release a variety of physiologically active substances, such as cytokines, growth factors, regulatory factors, and signal peptides, in order to influence nearby cells. Injured ovaries' health is improved by this technique through immunological modulation, angiogenesis, antiapoptosis, antifibrosis, and anti-inflammation, as presented in **Figure 1**.

Studies have thus far focused on providing women with weakened ovarian reserves with a suitable environment in an effort to restore the damaged ovarian niche. Autologous stem cells produced from various organs have drawn the attention of many researchers. As a result of the paracrine secretion of soluble factors [171] playing a role in the activation of primordial follicles in impaired ovaries, other researchers have concentrated their attention on various approaches, such as platelet-rich plasma (PRP) [172].

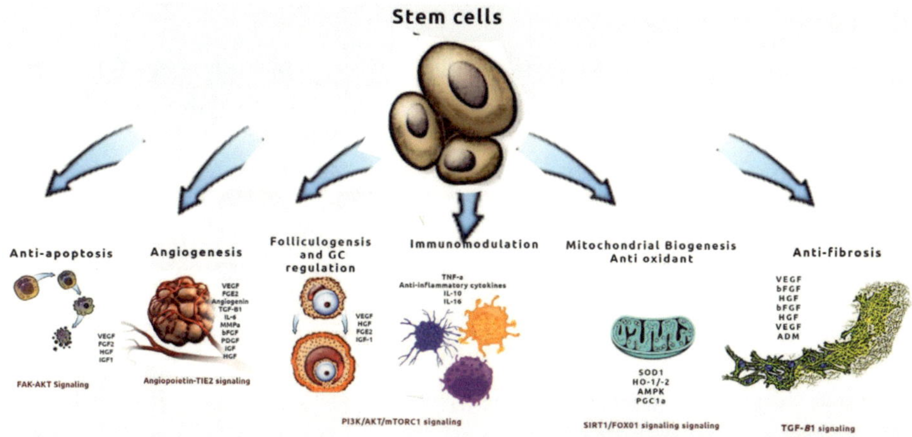

Figure 1.
Mechanisms involved in stem cell-based therapies in POF. Adapted from [170].

8. Platelet-rich plasma (PRP)

Platelet-rich plasma (PRP) is produced by centrifugation and separation of its various components from whole blood, which contains plasma (55%), red blood cells (41%), platelets, and white blood cells (4%). Red blood cells are removed during the centrifugation and separation process, and plasma is created with a 5–10 times higher concentration of growth factors [173]. Alpha granules, which are found in platelets in PRP, produce a variety of substances that promote angiogenesis, cell proliferation, and growth when triggered [174]. It has been demonstrated that the growth factors in PRP are crucial for promoting collagen synthesis, bone cell proliferation, fibroblast chemotaxis, macrophage activation, angiogenesis, immune cell chemotaxis, endothelial cell migration and mitosis, epithelial cell differentiation, and cytokine secretion by mesenchymal and epithelial cells. **Table 1** summarizes the composition of PRP [175].

After a venous blood sample, autologous PRP therapy administers injections of the patient's own concentrated platelets and plasma. The natural healing process is the body's initial response to tissue injury by sending activated platelets and releasing growth factors, according to the theory underlying the use of this method for treatment. Over the past ten years, the clinical application of PRP has grown significantly, and it is currently used to treat conditions like alopecia, musculoskeletal injuries, arthritis, periorbital rejuvenation, regenerative dentistry, and wound healing [176]. For women who have a poor ovarian reserve (POR), premature ovarian insufficiency (POI), or even menopause, PRP treatment has recently been employed as an adjuvant in assisted reproductive technology, in particular, as an intraovarian injection in conjunction with in vitro fertilization (IVF). Reviewed in [172].

The impact of PRP on the development and viability of isolated early human follicles was examined in one experimental research [177]. After brain death was determined in three postmortem women under the age of 35, ovarian tissue samples were taken. After removing the ovarian cortex tissue, half of the sample was vitrified for future research while the other half was used right away. Following that, ovarian follicle isolation was carried out under a stereomicroscope. Fresh samples' follicles were grown in fetal bovine serum (FBS), platelet-rich plasma (PRP), or PRP + FBS. Additionally, FBS, PRP, PRP + FBS, or human serum albumin were cultured with the follicles from

Function	Factors
Adhesive proteins	Von Willebrand factor, fibrinogen, trombospondin-1, trombospondin-2, laminin-8
Angiogenic factors	Vascular endothelium growth factor (VEGF), platelet-derived growth factor (PDGF), fibroblast growth factor (FGF)
Chemokines	CCL5 (RANTES), CCL-3 (MIP-1a), CCL-2 (MCP-1), CCL-7 (MCP-3), CXCL8 (IL-8), CXCL2 (MIP-2), CXCL6 (LIX), CXCL-1 (GRO-a), CXCL5 (ENA-78), CXCL-12 (SDF-1a), CXCL4 (PF4)
Clotting factors and their inhibitors	Factor V, factor IX, antithrombin, factor S, protease nexin-1, protease nexin-2, tissue factor pathway inhibitor,
Growth factors	Epidermal growth factor (EGF), insulin-like growth factor 1 (IGF-1), hepatocyte growth factor (HGF), transforming growth factor ß (TGF-ß)
Immune mediators	Complement C3 precursor, complement C4 precursor, factor D, factor H, C1 inhibitor, IgG
Integral membrane proteins	Integrin aIIb3, GPIba-IX-V, GPVI, TLT-1, p-selectin

Table 1.
Platelet granule content [175].

vitrified-thawed samples. A 5 ml of blood was taken into tubes containing 0.5 ml of acid citrate solution to prepare PRP (anticoagulant). The top and middle layers of the blood were transferred to fresh tubes and centrifuged at 3000 g for 15 minutes after the blood had been centrifuged at 200 g for 20 min at 20°C. The remaining 0.5 mL of plasma with precipitated platelets was mixed uniformly and utilized for PRP after the supernatant plasma was discarded. To release the growth factor from the platelets, 20 IU/mL thrombin was added to the PRP, causing it to clot. The platelet fragments were finally removed from the clot by centrifuging it at 4000 g for 5 minutes. The samples were compared after 10 days of cultivation. Sixty primordial follicles in all were extracted and cultivated from the fresh samples. The PRP alone group demonstrated the greatest changes in size ($p < 0.001$) and viability ($p < 0.05$) after 10 days, with 91.4% 1.86 vs. 61% 0.89 in the fresh group with FBS and 82% 1.70 vs. 59% 1.00 in the vitrified group with FBS. The follicles' sizes also significantly increased ($p < 0.001$) after 10 days in all groups. A total of 240 primordial follicles were extracted and cultivated from the vitrified-thaw group. Once more, the follicles that received PRP supplementation changed the most in size and viability. Fresh samples displayed a greater growth rate and more viable follicles when compared to vitrified-thawed ones. These findings suggest that PRP more effectively supports the vitality and proliferation of human primordial and primary follicles that have been separated and/or enclosed.

The results of this well-conducted study may not be extended to infertile patients beyond the age of 35 because the study was only able to include three participants and relatively younger patients without an infertility diagnosis. There is a need for additional research to ascertain whether the use of thrombin had an impact on the outcomes compared to the use of pure PRP without thrombin in that study's modification of PRP to release growth factors.

Non-autologous PRP was investigated by Ahmadian et al. in rats given gonadotoxic IP chemical agents [178]. Female rats were used in the non-autologous production of PRP. The relative expression of the angiogenic-related genes ANGPT2 and KDR was used to study how dramatically PRP reduced follicular atresia and inflammatory response. After PRP, the birth rate in POI rats also increased. Due to the use of intraovarian PRP (rather than IP) and the reporting of birth rate, this study has greater clinical value (which is the end goal of this therapy). In order to treat mice models of gonadotoxin-induced POI, Vural et al. combined non-autologous PRP with rat mesenchymal stem cells (MSCs) from adipose tissue [179]. AMH and estradiol (E2) levels considerably increased when MSC was introduced to PRP. The expressions of CXCL12, BMP-4, TGF-, and IGF-1 (insulin-like growth factor-1) were likewise elevated in that group. CXCL12 stands for C-X-C motif chemokine ligand 12. The study came to the conclusion that PRP alone did not increase follicular regeneration, whereas MSC with or without PRP did.

The first controlled trial incorporating ovarian PRP injection was released by Stojkovska et al. [180]. This prospective, controlled, non-randomized pilot trial included 40 patients who met the POR requirements (at least two of the Bologna criteria) and had normal partner semen tests. The population under study was 35–42 years old.

PRP was administered intravenously in the intervention group, and IVF was carried out in the control and PRP groups two months later. There was no statistically significant difference between the groups in terms of clinical pregnancies and live birth rate. Clinical pregnancy and live birth rates were, respectively, 33.33 ± 44.99, 40.00 ± 50.71, and 10.71 ± 28.95, 14.29 ± 36.31, in the PRP group and 10.71 ± 28.95, 14.29 ± 36.31, and in the control group. Hormone levels also did not considerably improve. Only individuals whose IVF procedures finally led to an embryo transfer were included in the study, which is a significant limitation.

Another prospective, controlled, non-randomized pilot trial using intraovarian PRP injection and 120 patients who were monitored for three months was published by Sfakianoudis et al. [181]. POR (matching Bologna criteria), POI (age 40, amenorrhea at least 4 months, and increased FSH > 25 IU/L), perimenopause (age 40, irregular menstrual cycles), or menopause (age 45–55, with amenorrhea at least 1 year without HRT, and FSH > 30 IU/L) were the criteria for inclusion. In each of these four distinct study groups, bilateral ovaries received an injection of 4 mL of activated PRP with $1X10^9$ platelets/mL. In 60% of POI patients, menstruation returned, and levels of AMH, FSH, and AFC showed statistically significant improvement. In the menopausal group, 43% of the women had lowered FSH or started menstruating again. For 80% of the perimenopausal women, normal menstruation, increased hormone levels, and AFC were noted. Within the study groups, conceptions through IVF and natural means were both successful. The results showed a considerable improvement in the POR group's hormonal profile, ovarian reserve indicators, and ICSI cycle performance.

The actual understanding of PRP administration therapy seems to have a non-negligible encouraging effect on women who had previously displayed decreased ovarian function, and it should not be disregarded as a potential therapeutic option that may increase the chance for both natural conception and IVF conception, as well as even improvement of perimenopausal symptoms. PRP injection is thought to activate some of the ovaries' latent oocytes, hence enhancing hormonal profiles and any symptoms of estrogen deficiency. Finally, to ascertain whether autologous intraovarian PRP injection is advantageous in female reproduction, particularly for women with POR, POI, and early menopause, it needs to be researched on a larger scale in a clinical trial setting with standardized preparation, injection, and follow-up techniques [176].

9. Adult stem cells

Mesenchymal stem cells (MSCs) can be detected in a variety of adult tissues and exhibit strong replication capability as well as in vitro differentiation potential into chondrocytes, osteocytes, and adipocytes [182].

Liu et al. [183] used human amniotic fluid MSCs in a POF mice model based on cyclophosphamide to conduct the first study on the ability of human MSCs to survive, engraft, and proliferate into the ovaries. By lowering atresia, preserving the growth of surviving follicles, and reestablishing estrous cyclicity, direct ovarian infusion of mouse amniotic fluid MSCs enhances ovarian function and permits the production of offspring and short-term fertility recovery [184]. After delivery, amniotic membranes can also be easily separated from amniotic epithelial cells (AEC) and amniotic mesenchymal cells (AMSCs), allowing the recovery of clinically important cell values. In mice with various degrees of chemotherapy-induced ovarian damage, ranging from DOR to established POF, human AECs and AMSCs have both been successfully evaluated [185]. After the infusion of hAECs, it has been reported that hormone synthesis, differentiation into granulosa cells, and restoration of folliculogenesis have all returned [185], though hAMSCs have even more positive effects. MSCs have been successfully extracted from umbilical cord blood, which has shown promise in treating a number of non-reproductive degenerative illnesses. Umbilical cord blood MSCs injected into ovaries shield follicular cells from death [186], boosting follicle development and estradiol release. These findings, which have been confirmed in perimenopausal rat ovaries treated with chemotherapy and aged naturally, appear to be mediated by an indirect effect on the ovarian epithelium and niche via expression of key regulators for apoptosis and folliculogenesis, such as cytokeratin 8/18, transforming growth factor (TGF-b), and proliferating cell nuclear antigen [171].

The lack of an autologous source for these MSCs, however, should be viewed as a con to their use for cell treatment in already old and POI patients without previously cryopreserved umbilical cord blood or amniotic membranes, as well as in the absence of menses, such as women with POI. Other autologous cell sources, including adipose tissue and bone marrow, have been investigated as a result of these problems. Adipose MSCs actually induce the expression of POF-related genes and the production of paracrine cytokines, which reduce ovarian apoptosis and restore ovulation in a chemoablated mouse model [187, 188]. However, ovarian effects appear to be smaller than those seen for MSCs generated from amniotic tissue [189].

Recent clinical findings show that stem cell therapy improves ovarian function as seen by resumed menstruation, controlled hormone levels, and, in very rare circumstances, the capacity to become pregnant. It is crucial to choose the right individuals while conducting an analysis of stem cells' therapeutic effects. The inclusion and exclusion criteria were mostly comparable among the clinical studies included in **Table 2**. The majority of studies comprised patients with FSH levels above 20 or 25, who were younger than 40, had a normal karyotype, and were diagnosed with POI.

Studies using animal models and clinical trials have previously demonstrated the therapeutic benefits of stem cells. It is clear that stem cells can support and restore ovarian function, which in turn has a favorable impact on folliculogenesis, guard against GC apoptosis, and manages ovarian hormones (**Figure 1**). The use of stem cells does present significant ethical and technical challenges, and stem cell therapies are still illegal in several nations. Although employing MSCs instead of ESCs can address ethical issues about their use, there are still some unanswered safety questions with the extraction and transplantation of stem cells for therapeutic purposes. Minimally

Stem cell type	Sponsor	Clinical Trial Number
OCT4 marker measured	Al-Azhar University	NCT02151890
hUCMSC and hCBMNC transplantation	Shenzhen Beike Bio-Technology Co., Ltd	NCT01742533
autologous MSCs injection	El-Rayadh Fertility Centre	NCT02043743
autologous MSCs treatment + OCT4 marker measured	Sayed Bakry	NCT02062931
BMSC treatment directly to ovary	University of Illinois at Chicago	NCT02696889
embryonic stem cell-derived MSC-like cell transplantation directly into bilateral ovaries	Chinese Academy of Sciences	NCT03877471
VSELs from the patient's peripheral blood injected in bilateral oviducts + hormone and menstrual conditions measured	Fuda Cancer Hospital, Guangzhou	NCT03985462
Derivation of hESC lines	Hadassah Medical Organization	NCT00353197

hUCMSC human umbilical cord mesenchymal stem cell, hCBMNC human cord blood-mononuclear cells, BMSC bone marrow derived mesenchymal stem cells, VSEL very small embryonic-like stem cell, hESC human embryonic stem cell.

Table 2.
Clinical study of stem cell therapy on POF (192).

invasive techniques that do not injure the donor can be used to extract MSCs from adipose cells, the placenta, or the umbilical cord. Direct transplantation can be invasive and may result in adverse reactions such as immunological responses. Additional in vivo research and clinical trials should be conducted to assess these problems.

Author details

Antonio Díez-Juan[1]* and Iavor K. Vladimirov[2,3]

1 Igenomix R & D, Valencia, Spain

2 IVF Unit, SBALAGRM, Sofia, Bulgaria

3 Faculty of Biology, Sofia University "St. Kliment Ohridski", Bulgaria

*Address all correspondence to: antonio.diez@igenomix.com

References

[1] Leidal AM, Levine B, Debnath J. Autophagy and the cell biology of age-related disease. Nature Cell Biology. 2018;**20**:1338-1348

[2] Comizzoli P, Ottinger MA. Understanding reproductive aging in wildlife to improve animal conservation and human reproductive health. Frontiers in Cell and Development Biology. 2021;**9**:680471

[3] Quesada-Candela C, Loose J, Ghazi A, Yanowitz JL. Molecular basis of reproductive senescence: Insights from model organisms. Journal of Assisted Reproduction and Genetics. 2021;**38**(1):17-32

[4] Vom Saal FS. Natural history and mechanisms of reproductive aging in humans, laboratory rodents, and other selected vertebrates. Physiology of Reproduction. 1994;**2**:1213-1314

[5] Hernandez-Segura A, Nehme J, Demaria M. Hallmarks of cellular senescence. Trends in Cell Biology. 2018;**28**:436-453

[6] Ahmed TA, Ahmed SM, El-Gammal Z, Shouman S, Ahmed A, Mansour R, et al. Oocyte aging: The role of cellular and environmental factors and impact on female fertility. Advances in Experimental Medicine and Biology. 2020;**1247**:109-123

[7] Secomandi L, Borghesan M, Velarde M, Demaria M. The role of cellular senescence in female reproductive aging and the potential for senotherapeutic interventions. Human Reproduction Update. 2022;**28**:172-189

[8] Kaufman JM, Lapauw B, Mahmoud A, T'Sjoen G, Huhtaniemi IT. Aging and the male reproductive system Endocrine Rev. 2019;**40**:906-972

[9] Hamet P, Tremblay J. Genes of aging. Metabolism. 2003;**52**:5-9

[10] Velde P. The variability of female reproductive ageing. Human Reproduction Update. 2002;**8**:141-154

[11] Tan TY, Lau SK, Loh SF, Tan HH. Female ageing and reproductive outcome in assisted reproduction cycles. Singapore Medical Journal. 2014;**55**:305-309

[12] Crawford NM, Steiner AZ. Age-related infertility. Obstetrics and Gynecology Clinics of North America. 2015;**42**:15-25

[13] Faddy MJ. Follicle dynamics during ovarian ageing. Molecular and Cellular Endocrinology. 2000;**163**:43-48

[14] Sauer MV, Paulson RJ, Lobo RA. A preliminary report on oocyte donation extending reproductive potential to women over 40. The New England Journal of Medicine. 1990;**323**:1157-1160

[15] Mandl AM, Zuckerman S. The relation of age to numbers of oocytes. The Journal of Endocrinology. 1951;**7**(2):190-193

[16] Felici M. The formation and migration of primordial germ cells in mouse and man. Results Probl Cell Differ. 2016;**58**:23-46. DOI: 10.1007/978-3-319-31973-5_2

[17] Gougeon A. Regulation of ovarian follicular development in primates: Facts and hypotheses. Endocrine Reviews. 1996;**17**(2):121-155

[18] Matzuk MM, Burns KH, Viveiros MM, Eppig JJ. Intercellular

communication in the mammalian ovary: Oocytes carry the conversation. Science. 2002;**296**(5576):2178-2180

[19] Anderson E, Wilkinson RF, Lee G, Meller S. A correlative microscopical analysis of differentiating ovarian follicles of mammals. Journal of Morphology. 1978;**156**(3):339-366

[20] Liu C, Peng J, Matzuk MM, Yao HH. Lineage specification of ovarian theca cells requires multicellular interactions via oocyte and granulosa cells. Nature Communications. 2015;**6**:6934

[21] Babayev E, Duncan FE. Age-associated changes in cumulus cells and follicular fluid: The local oocyte microenvironment as a determinant of gamete quality. Biology of Reproduction. 2022;**106**(2):351-365

[22] Zeleznik AJ. Follicle selection in primates: "Many are called but few are chosen". Biology of Reproduction. 2001;**65**(3):655-659

[23] Canipari R, Palombi F, Riminucci M, Mangia F. Early programming of maturation competence in mouse oogenesis. Developmental Biology. 1984;**102**(2):519-524

[24] Eppig JJ, Chesnel F, Hirao Y, O'Brien MJ, Pendola FL, Watanabe S. Oocyte control of granulosa cell development: How and why. Human Reproduction. 1997;**12**(11):127-132

[25] Sorensen RA, Wassarman PM. Relationship between growth and meiotic maturation of the mouse oocyte. Developmental Biology. 1976;**50**(2):531-536

[26] Edson MA, Nagaraja AK, Matzuk MM. The mammalian ovary from genesis to revelation. Endocrine Reviews. 2009;**30**(6):624-712

[27] Tal R, Seifer DB. Ovarian reserve testing: A user's guide. American Journal of Obstetrics and Gynecology. 2017;**217**:129-140

[28] Hsueh AJ, Billig H, Tsafriri A. Ovarian follicle atresia: A hormonally controlled apoptotic process. Endocrine Reviews. 1994;**15**(6):707-724

[29] Eichenlaub-Ritter U. Oocyte ageing and its cellular basis. The International Journal of Developmental Biology. 2012;**56**(10-12):841-852

[30] Kordowitzki P. Oxidative stress induces telomere dysfunction and shortening in human oocytes of advanced age donors. Cell. 2021;**10**(8):1866. DOI: 10.3390.10081.866

[31] Seifer DB, Charland C, Berlinsky D, Penzias AS, Jr RVH, Naftolin F. Proliferative index of human luteinized granulosa cells varies as a function of ovarian reserve. American Journal of Obstetrics and Gynecology. 1993;**169**(6):1531-1535

[32] Seifer DB, Gardiner AC, Ferreira KA, Peluso JJ. Apoptosis as a function of ovarian reserve in women undergoing in vitro fertilization. Fertility and Sterility. 1996;**66**(4):593-598

[33] Klein NA, Battaglia DE, Woodruff TK, Padmanabhan V, Giudice LC, Bremner WJ, et al. Ovarian follicular concentrations of activin, follistatin, inhibin, insulin-like growth factor I (IGF-I. age). The Journal of Clinical Endocrinology and Metabolism. 2000;**85**:2

[34] Pellicer A, Mari M, Santos MJ, Simon C, Remohi J, Tarin JJ. Effects of aging on the human ovary: The secretion of immunoreactive alphainhibin and progesterone. Fertility and Sterility. 1994;**61**(4):663-668

[35] Weenen C, Laven JS, Bergh AR, Cranfield M, Groome NP, Visser JA. Anti-Mullerian hormone expression pattern in the human ovary: Potential implications for initial and cyclic follicle recruitment. Mol Hum Reprod. 2004;**10**:77-83

[36] Durlinger AL, Gruijters MJ, Kramer P, Karels B, Ingraham HA, Nachtigal MW. Anti-Mullerian hormone inhibits initiation of primordial follicle growth in the mouse ovary. Endocrinol. 2002;**143**(3):1076-1084

[37] Rajpert-De Meyts E, Jørgensen N, Graem N, Müller J, Cate RL, Skakkebaek NE. Expression of anti-Mullerian hormone during normal and pathological gonadal development: Association with differentiation of Sertoli and granulosa cells. The Journal of Clinical Endocrinology and Metabolism. 1999;**84**(10):3836-3844

[38] Clemente N, Racine C, Pierre A, Taieb J. Anti-Mullerian hormone in female reproduction. Endocrine Reviews. 2021;**42**(6):753-782

[39] La Marca A, Sighinolfi G, Radi D, Argento C, Baraldi E, Artenisio AC, et al. Anti-Mullerian hormone (AMH) as a predictive marker in assisted reproductive technology (ART). Human Reproduction Update. 2010;**16**(2):113-130

[40] Hayes E, Kushnir V, Ma X, Biswas A, Prizant H, Gleicher N. Intracellular mechanism of anti-Mullerian hormone (AMH) in regulation of follicular development. Molecular and Cellular Endocrinology. 2016;**433**:56-65

[41] de Mora JF, Juan AD. The decay of stem cell nourishment at the niche. Rejuvenation Research. 2013;**16**(6):487-494

[42] Ungvari Z, Tarantini S, Donato AJ, Galvan V, Csiszar A. Mechanisms of vascular aging. Circulation Research. 2018;**123**(7):849-867

[43] Damber JE, Bergh A, Widmark A. Age-related differences in testicular microcirculation. International Journal of Andrology. 1990;**13**:197-206

[44] Mieno S, Boodhwani M, Clements RT, Ramlawi B, Sodha NR, Li J, et al. Aging is associated with an impaired coronary microvascular response to vascular endothelial growth factor in patients. The Journal of Thoracic and Cardiovascular Surgery. 2006;**132**:1348-1355

[45] Payne GW, Bearden SE. The microcirculation of skeletal muscle in aging. Microcirculation. 2006;**13**:275-277

[46] Hunter JM, Kwan J, Malek-Ahmadi M, Maarouf CL, Kokjohn TA, Belden C, et al. Morphological and pathological evolution of the brain microcirculation in aging and Alzheimer's disease. PLoS One. 2012;7:e36893

[47] Urbieta-Caceres VH, Syed FA, Lin J, Zhu XY, Jordan KL, Bell CC, et al. Age-dependent renal cortical microvascular loss in female mice. American Journal of Physiology. Endocrinology and Metabolism. 2012;**302**:979-986

[48] Faber JE, Zhang H, Lassance-Soares RM, Prabhakar P, Najafi AH, Burnett MS, et al. Aging causes collateral rarefaction and increased severity of ischemic injury in multiple tissues. Arteriosclerosis, Thrombosis, and Vascular Biology. 2011;**31**:1748-1756

[49] Robinson RS, Woad KJ, Hammond AJ, Laird M, Hunter MG, Mann GE. Angiogenesis and vascular

function in the ovary. Reprod. 2009;**138**(6):869-881

[50] Redmer AD, Reynolds LP. Angiogenesis in the ovary. Reviews of Reproduction. 1996;**1**:182-192

[51] Huey S, Abuhamad A, Barroso G, Hsu MI, Kolm P, Mayer J, et al. Perifollicular blood flow Doppler indices, but not follicular pO2, pCO2, or pH, predict oocyte developmental competence in in vitro fertilization. Fertil Steril. 1999;**72**:707-712

[52] Bhal PS, Pugh ND, Chui DK, Gregory L, Walker SM, Shaw RW. The use of transvaginal power Doppler ultrasonography to evaluate the relationship between perifollicular vascularity and outcome in in-vitro fertilization treatment cycles. Human Reproduction. 1999;**14**:939-945

[53] Fujino Y, Ozaki K, Yamamasu S, Ito F, Matsuoka I, Hayashi E, et al. DNA fragmentation of oocytes in aged mice. Human Reproduction. 1996;**11**:1480

[54] Blerkom J, Antczak M, Schrader R. The developmental potential of the human oocyte is related to the dissolved oxygen content of follicular fluid: Association with vascular endothelial growth factor levels and perifollicular blood flow characteristics. Human Reproduction. 1997;**12**(5):1047-1055

[55] Blerkom J. The influence of intrinsic and extrinsic factors on the developmental potential and chromosomal normality of the human oocyte. Journal of the Society for Gynecologic Investigation. 1996;**3**:3-11

[56] Fraser HM, Duncan WC. Vascular morphogenesis in the primate ovary. Angiogenesis. 2005;**8**(2):101-116

[57] Bruno JB, Celestino JJ, Lima-Verde IB, Lima LF, Matos MH, Araujo VR. Expression of vascular endothelial growth factor (VEGF) receptor in goat ovaries and improvement of in vitro caprine preantral follicle survival and growth with VEGF. Reprod Fertil Dev. 2009;**21**:679-687

[58] Suzuki T, Sasano H, Takaya R, Fukaya T, Yajima A, Nagura H. Cyclic changes of vasculature and vascular phenotypes in normal human ovaries. Human Reproduction. 1998;**13**(4):953-959

[59] Kaczmarek MM, Schams D, Ziecik AJ. Role of vascular endothelial growth factor in ovarian physiology - an overview. Reproductive Biology. 2005;**5**(2):111-136

[60] Danforth DR, Arbogast LK, Ghosh S, Dickerman A, Rofagha R, Friedman CI. Vascular endothelial growth factor stimulates preantral follicle growth in the rat ovary. Biology of Reproduction. 2003;**68**(5):1736-1741

[61] Quintana R, Kopcow L, Sueldo C, Marconi G, Rueda NG, Baranao RI. Direct injection of vascular endothelial growth factor into the ovary of mice promotes follicular development. Fertility and Sterility. 2004;**82**(3): 1101-1105

[62] Friedman CI, Danforth DR, Herbosa-Encarnacion C, Arbogast L, Alak BM, Seifer DB. Follicular fluid vascular endothelial growth factor concentrations are elevated in women of advanced reproductive age undergoing ovulation induction. Fertility and Sterility. 1997;**68**(4):607-612

[63] Manau D, Balasch J, Jimenez W, Fabregues F, Civico S, Casamitjana R. Follicular fluid concentrations of adrenomedullin, vascular endothelial growth factor and nitric oxide in IVF cycles: Relationship to ovarian

response. Human Reproduction. 2000;**15**(6):1295-1299

[64] Fujii EY, Nakayama M. The measurements of RAGE, VEGF, and AGEs in the plasma and follicular fluid of reproductive women: The influence of aging. Fertility and Sterility. 2010;**94**(2):694-700

[65] Esencan E, Beroukhim G, Seifer DB. Age-related changes in Folliculogenesis and potential modifiers to improve fertility outcomes-a narrative review. Reproductive Biology and Endocrinology. 2022;**20**(1):1-18

[66] Cooke JP. NO and angiogenesis. Atherosclerosis. Supplements. 2003;**4**(4):53-60

[67] Budani MC, Tiboni GM. Novel insights on the role of nitric oxide in the ovary: A review of the literature. International Journal of Environmental Research and Public Health. 2021;**18**(3):980

[68] Dave S, Farrance DP, Whitehead SA. Evidence that nitric oxide inhibits steroidogenesis in cultured rat granulosa cells. Clinical Science. 1997;**92**:277-284

[69] Nath P, Maitra S. Physiological relevance of nitric oxide in ovarian functions: An overview. General and Comparative Endocrinology. 2019;**279**:35-44

[70] Basini G, Grasselli F. Nitric oxide in follicle development and oocyte competence. Reproduction. 2015;**150**:1-9

[71] Grasselli F, Ponderato N, Basini G, Tamanini C. Nitric oxide synthase expression and nitric oxide/cyclic GMP pathway in swine granulosa cells. Domestic Animal Endocrinology. 2001;**20**:241-252

[72] Voorhis BJ, Dunn MS, Snyder GD, Weiner CP. Nitric oxide: An autocrine regulator of human granulosa-luteal cell steroidogenesis. Endocrinology. 1994;**135**:1799-1806

[73] Kagabu S, Kodama H, Fukuda J, Karube A, Murata M, Tanaka T. Inhibitory effects of nitric oxide on the expression and activity of aromatase in human granulosa cells. Molecular Human Reproduction. 1999;**5**:396-401

[74] Goud AP, Goud PT, Diamond MP, Abu-Soud HM. Nitric oxide delays oocyte aging. Biochemistry. 2005;**44**(34):11361-11368

[75] Srivastava S. The mitochondrial basis of aging and age-related disorders. Genes (Basel). 2017;**8**(12):398

[76] López-Otín C, Kroemer G. Hallmarks of health. Cell. 2021;**184**:33-63

[77] Bratic A, Larsson NG. The role of mitochondria in aging. The Journal of Clinical Investigation. 2013;**123**(3):951-957

[78] Tilly JL, Sinclair DA. Germline energetics, aging, and female infertility. Cell Metabolism. 2013;**17**:838-850

[79] Velarde MC, Flynn JM, Day NU, Melov S, Campisi J. Mitochondrial oxidative stress caused by Sod2 deficiency promotes cellular senescence and aging phenotypes in the skin. Aging (Albany NY). 2012;**4**(1):3-12

[80] Sun N, Youle RJ, Finkel T. The mitochondrial basis of aging. Molecular Cell. 2016;**61**:654-666

[81] Kauppila TES, Kauppila JHK, Larsson NG. Mammalian mitochondria and aging: An update. Cell Metabolism. 2017;**25**(1):57-71

[82] Balaban RS, Nemoto S. Mitochondria, oxidants, aging. Cell. 2005;**120**(4):483-495

[83] Rigoulet M, Yoboue ED, Devin A. Mitochondrial ROS generation and its regulation: Mechanisms involved in H2O2 signaling. Antioxidants & Redox Signaling. 2011;**14**(3):459-468

[84] Quinlan CL, Perevoshchikova HM IV, Hey-Mogensen M, Orr AL, Brand MD. Sites of reactive oxygen species generation by mitochondria oxidizing different substrates. Redox Biology. 2013;**1**:304-312

[85] Keefe DL, Niven-Fairchild T, Powell S, Buradagunta S. Mitochondrial deoxyribonucleic acid deletions in oocytes and reproductive aging in women. Fertility and Sterility. 1995;**64**(3):577-583

[86] Brenner CA, Wolny YM, Barritt JA, Matt DW, Munné S, Cohen J. Mitochondrial DNA deletion in human oocytes and embryos. Molecular Human Reproduction. 1998;**4**(9):887-892

[87] Barritt JA, Brenner CA, Cohen J, Matt DW. Mitochondrial DNA rearrangements in human oocytes and embryos. Molecular Human Reproduction. 1999;**5**(10):927-933

[88] Barritt JA, Cohen J, Brenner CA. Mitochondrial DNA point mutation in human oocytes is associated with maternal age. Reproductive Biomedicine Online. 2000;**1**(3):96-100

[89] Chan CC, Liu VW, Lau EY, Yeung WS, Ng EH, Ho PC. Mitochondrial DNA content and 4977 bp deletion in unfertilized oocytes. Molecular Human Reproduction. 2005;**11**:843-846

[90] Chan CC, Liu VW, Lau EY, Yeung WS, Ng EH, Ho PC. Mitochondrial DNA deletion in granulosa and cumulus oophorus cells. Fertility and Sterility. 2006;**85**(3):780-782

[91] Fragouli E, Spath K, Alfarawati S, Kaper F, Craig A, Michel CE, et al. Altered levels of mitochondrial DNA are associated with female age, aneuploidy, and provide an independent measure of embryonic implantation potential. PLoS Genetics. 2015;**11**(6):e1005241

[92] Kasapoğlu I, Seli E. Mitochondrial dysfunction and ovarian aging. Endocrinology. 2020;**161**(2):bqaa001

[93] Archer SL. Mitochondrial dynamics — Mitochondrial fission and fusion in human diseases. The New England Journal of Medicine. 2013;**369**:2236-2251

[94] Zhang M, Bener MB, Jiang Z, Wang T, Esencan E, Scott R. Mitofusin 2 plays a role in oocyte and follicle development, and is required to maintain ovarian follicular reserve during reproductive aging. Aging (Albany NY). 2019;**11**(12):3919-3938

[95] Lombard DB, Tishkoff DX, Bao J. Mitochondrial Sirtuins in the regulation of mitochondrial activity and metabolic adaptation. Handb Exp Pharmacol. 2011;**206**:163-188. DOI: 10.1007/978-3-642-21631-2_8

[96] Mottis A, Herzig S, Auwerx J. Mitocellular communication: Shaping health and disease. Science. 2019;**366**:827-832

[97] Wang T, Zhang M, Jiang Z, Seli E. Mitochondrial dysfunction and ovarian aging. American Journal of Reproductive Immunology. 2017;**77**:12651

[98] Herzig S, Shaw RJ. AMPK: Guardian of metabolism and mitochondrial homeostasis. Nature Reviews. Molecular Cell Biology. 2018;**19**:121-135

[99] Bonomi M, Somigliana E, Cacciatore C, Busnelli M, Rossetti R, Bonetti S, et al. Blood cell mitochondrial DNA content and premature ovarian aging. PLoS One. 2012;7:42423

[100] Pacella-Ince L, Zander-Fox DL, Lan M. Mitochondrial SIRT3 and its target glutamate dehydrogenase are altered in follicular cells of women with reduced ovarian reserve or advanced maternal age. Human Reproduction. 2014;**29**(7):1490-1499

[101] Boucret L, Barca JM, Moriniere C, Desquiret V, Ferre-L'Hotellier V, Descamps P, et al. Relationship between diminished ovarian reserve and mitochondrial biogenesis in cumulus cells. Human Reproduction. 2015;**30**:1653-1664

[102] May-Panloup P, Boucret L, Barca JM, Desquiret-Dumas V, Ferré-L'Hotellier V, Morinière C, et al. Ovarian ageing: The role of mitochondria in oocytes and follicles. Human Reproduction Update. 2016;**22**:725-743

[103] Michaels GS, Hauswirth WW, Laipis PJ. Mitochondrial DNA copy number in bovine oocytes and somatic cells. Developmental Biology. 1982;**94**:246-251

[104] St John JC, Facucho-Oliveira J, Jiang Y, Kelly R, Salah R. Mitochondrial DNA transmission, replication and inheritance: A journey from the gamete through the embryo and into offspring and embryonic stem cells. Human Reproduction Update. 2010;**16**(5):488-509

[105] Wai T, Ao A, Zhang X, Cyr D, Dufort D, Shoubridge EA. The role of mitochondrial DNA copy number in mammalian fertility. Biology of Reproduction. 2010;**83**(1):52-62

[106] Cree LM, Samuels DC, Sousa Lopes SC. A reduction of mitochondrial DNA molecules during embryogenesis explains the rapid segregation of genotypes. Nature Genetics. 2008;**40**(2):249-254

[107] Piko L, Taylor KD. Amounts of mitochondrial DNA and abundance of some mitochondrial gene transcripts in early mouse embryos. Developmental Biology. 1987;**123**(2):364-374

[108] Reynier P, May-Panloup P, Chrétien MF. Mitochondrial DNA content affects the fertilizability of human oocytes. Molecular Human Reproduction. 2001;7(5):425-429

[109] Diez-Juan A, Rubio C, Marin C, Martinez S, Al-Asmar N, Riboldi M, et al. Mitochondrial DNA content as a viability score in human euploid embryos: Less is better. Fertility and Sterility. 2015;**104**(3):534-41.e1

[110] Leese HJ. Quiet please, do not disturb: A hypothesis of embryo metabolism and viability. BioEssays. 2002;**24**(9):845-849

[111] Ben-Meir A. Coenzyme Q10 restores oocyte mitochondrial function and fertility during reproductive aging. Aging Cell. 2015;**14**:887-895. DOI: 10.1111/acel.12368

[112] Pignatti C, Cocchi M, Weiss H. Coenzyme Q10 levels in rat heart of different age. Biochemistry and Experimental Biology. 1980;**16**(1):39-42

[113] Abdulhasan MK, Li Q, Dai J, Abu-Soud HM, Puscheck EE, Rappolee DA. CoQ10 increases mitochondrial mass and polarization, ATP and Oct4 potency levels, and bovine oocyte MII during IVM while decreasing AMPK activity and oocyte death. Journal of Assisted Reproduction and Genetics. 2017;**34**(12):1595-1607

[114] Boots CE, Boudoures A, Zhang W, Drury A, Moley KH. Obesity-induced oocyte mitochondrial defects are partially prevented and rescued by supplementation with co-enzyme Q10 in

a mouse model. Human Reproduction. 2016;**31**(9):2090-2097

[115] Bentov Y, Casper RF. The aging oocyte—Can mitochondrial function be improved? Fertility and Sterility. 2013;**99**(1):18-22

[116] Mamas L, Mamas E. Premature ovarian failure and dehydroepiand rosterone. Fertility and Sterility. 2009;**91**(2):644-646

[117] Zhang J, Chen Q, Du D. Can ovarian aging be delayed by pharmacological strategies? Aging (Albany NY). 2019;**11**(2):817-832

[118] Chen ZG, Luo LL, Xu JJ, Zhuang XL, Kong FXX, Y.C. Effects of plant polyphenols on ovarian follicular reserve in aging rats. Biochemistry and Cell Biology. 2010;**88**(4):737-745

[119] Liu Y. Resveratrol protects mouse oocytes from methylglyoxal-induced oxidative damage. PLoS One. 2013;**8**:e77960. DOI: 10.1371/journal.pone.0077960

[120] Sugiyama M, Kawahara-Miki R, Kawana H, Shirasuna K, Kuwayama T, Iwata H. Resveratrol-induced mitochondrial synthesis and autophagy in oocytes derived from early antral follicles of aged cows. The Journal of Reproduction and Development. 2015;**61**(4):251-259

[121] Takeo S, Sato D, Kimura K. Resveratrol improves the mitochondrial function and fertilization outcome of bovine oocytes. The Journal of Reproduction and Development. 2014;**60**(2):92-99

[122] Liu M, Yin Y, Ye X. Resveratrol protects against ageassociated infertility in mice. Human Reproduction. 2013;**28**(3):707-717

[123] Neves AR, Montoya-Botero P, Polyzos NP. The role of androgen supplementation in women with diminished ovarian reserve: Time to randomize, not meta-analyze. Front Endocrinol (Lausanne). 2021;**12**:653857

[124] Li CJ, Lin LT, Tsui KH. Dehydroepiandrosterone shifts energy metabolism to increase mitochondrial biogenesis in female fertility with advancing age. Nutrients. 2021;**13**(7):2449. DOI: 10.3390.13072449

[125] Reiter RJ, Tan DX, Rosales-Corral S, Galano A, Zhou XJ, Xu B. Mitochondria: Central organelles for melatonins antioxidant and anti-aging actions. Molecules. 2018;**23**(2):509

[126] Tamura H, Kawamoto M, Sato S. Long-term melatonin treatment delays ovarian aging. Journal of Pineal Research. 2017;**62**(2):e12380

[127] Li Y, Hung SW, Zhang R, Man GCW, Zhang T, Chung JPW, et al. Melatonin in endometriosis: Mechanistic understanding and clinical insight. Nutrients. 2022;**14**(19):4087

[128] Mosher AA, Tsoulis MW, Lim J, Tan C, Agarwal SK, Leyland NA, et al. Melatonin activity and receptor expression in endometrial tissue and endometriosis. Human Reproduction. 2019;**34**(7):1215-1224

[129] Albert V, Hall MN. mTOR signaling in cellular and organismal energetics. Current Opinion in Cell Biology. 2015;**33**:55-66

[130] Adhikari D, Risal S, Liu K, Shen Y. Pharmacological inhibition of mTORC1 prevents over-activation of the primordial follicle pool in response to elevated PI3K signaling. PLoS One. 2013;**8**(1):e53810

[131] Packer L, Witt EH, Tritschler HJ. Alpha-lipoic acid as a biological antioxidant. Free Radical Biology & Medicine. 1995;**19**(2):227-250

[132] Talebi A, Zavareh S, Kashani MH, Lashgarbluki T, Karimi I. The effect of alpha lipoic acid on the developmental competence of mouse isolated preantral follicles. Journal of Assisted Reproduction and Genetics. 2012;**29**(2):175-183

[133] Zhang H, Wu B, Liu H. Improving development of cloned goat embryos by supplementing α-lipoic acid to oocyte in vitro maturation medium. Theriogenology. 2013;**80**(3):228-233

[134] Tesarik J, Hazout A, Mendoza C. Improvement of delivery and live birth rates after ICSI in women aged >40 years by ovarian co-stimulation with growth hormone. Human Reproduction. 2005;**20**(9):2536-2541

[135] Tesarik J, Galán-Lázaro M, Conde-López C, Chiara-Rapisarda AM, Mendoza-Tesarik R. The effect of GH administration on oocyte and zygote quality in young women with repeated implantation failure after IVF. Front Endocrinol (Lausanne). 2020;**11**:519572

[136] Tesarik J, Mendoza-Tesarik R. New criteria for the use of growth hormone in the treatment of female infertility: Minireview and a case series. EC Gynaecology. 2020;**9**(3):1-4

[137] Hart RJ. Use of growth hormone in the IVF treatment of women with poor ovarian reserve. Front Endocrinol (Lausanne). 2019;**10**:500

[138] Burger HG. Androgen production in women. Fertility and Sterility. 2002;**77**(4):3-5

[139] Gleicher N, Barad DH. Dehydroepiandrosterone (DHEA) supplementation in diminished ovarian reserve (DOR). Reproductive Biology and Endocrinology. 2011;**9**:67

[140] Walters KA. Role of androgens in normal and pathological ovarian function. Reprod. 2015;**149**(4):193-218

[141] Vendola K, Zhou J, Wang J, Famuyiwa OA, Bievre M, Bondy CA. Androgens promote oocyte insulin-like growth factor I expression and initiation of follicle development in the primate ovary. Biology of Reproduction. 1999;**61**(2):353-357

[142] Vendola KA, Zhou J, Adesanya OO, Weil SJ, Bondy CA. Androgens stimulate early stages of follicular growth in the primate ovary. The Journal of Clinical Investigation. 1998;**101**(12):2622-2629

[143] Yang JL, Zhang CP, Li L, Huang L, Ji SY, Lu CL. Testosterone induces redistribution of forkhead box-3a and down-regulation of growth and differentiation factor 9 messenger ribonucleic acid expression at early stage of mouse folliculogenesis. Endocrinol. 2010;**151**(2):774-782

[144] Fujibe Y, Baba T, Nagao S, Adachi S, Ikeda K, Morishita M. Androgen potentiates the expression of FSH receptor and supports preantral follicle development in mice. J Ovarian Res. 2019;**12**(1):31

[145] Weil S, Vendola K, Zhou J, Bondy CA. Androgen and follicle-stimulating hormone interactions in primate ovarian follicle development. The Journal of Clinical Endocrinology and Metabolism. 1999;**84**(8):2951-2956

[146] Laird M, Thomson K, Fenwick M, Mora J, Franks S, Hardy K. Androgen stimulates growth of mouse Preantral follicles in vitro: Interaction with follicle-stimulating hormone and with growth

factors of the TGFbeta superfamily. Endocrinol. 2017;**158**(4):920-935

[147] Casson PR, Lindsay MS, Pisarska MD, Carson SA, Buster JE. Dehydroepiandrosterone supplementation augments ovarian stimulation in poor responders: A case series. Human Reproduction. 2000;**15**(10):2129-2132

[148] Casson PR, Santoro N, Elkind-Hirsch K, Carson SA, Hornsby PJ, Abraham G. Postmenopausal dehydroepiandrosterone administration increases free insulin-like growth factor-I and decreases high-density lipoprotein: A six-month trial. Fertility and Sterility. 1998;**70**(1):107-110

[149] Sozen B, Ozekinci M, Erman M, Gunduz T, Demir N, Akouri R. Dehydroepiandrosteronesupplementation attenuates ovarian ageing in a galactose-induced primary ovarian insufficiency rat model. Journal of Assisted Reproduction and Genetics. 2019;**36**(10):2181-2189

[150] Xie M, Zhong Y, Xue Q, Wu M, Deng X, Santos HO. Impact of dehydroepianrosterone (DHEA) supplementation on serum levels of insulin-like growth factor 1 (IGF-1): A dose-response meta-analysis of randomized controlled trials. Experimental Gerontology. 2020;**136**:110949

[151] Zhang HH, Xu PY, Wu J, Zou WW, Xu XM, Cao XY. Dehydroepiand rosterone improves follicular fluid bone morphogenetic protein-15 and accumulated embryo score of infertility patients with diminished ovarian reserve undergoing in vitro fertilization: A randomized controlled trial. J Ovarian Res. 2014;**7**:93

[152] Sen A, Hammes S. Granulosa cell-specific androgen receptors are critical regulators of ovarian development and function. Molecular Endocrinology. 2010;**24**(7):1393-1403

[153] Li CJ, Chen SN, Lin LT, Chern CU, Wang PH, Wen ZH, et al. Dehydroepiandrosterone ameliorates abnormal mitochondrial dynamics and Mitophagy of cumulus cells in poor ovarian responders. Journal of Clinical Medicine. 2018;**7**(10):293. DOI: 10.3390.71.00293

[154] Sonmezer M, Ozmen B, Cil AP, Ozkavukcu S, Tasci T, Olmus H. Dehydroepiandrosterone supplementation improves ovarian response and cycle outcome in poor responders. Reproductive Biomedicine Online. 2009;**19**(4):508-513

[155] Meldrum DR, Chang RJ, Giudice LC, Balasch J, Barbieri RL. Role of decreased androgens in the ovarian response to stimulation in older women. Fertility and Sterility. 2013;**99**(1):5-11

[156] Frattarelli JL, Gerber MD. Basal and cycle androgen levels correlate with in vitro fertilization stimulation parameters but do not predict pregnancy outcome. Fertility and Sterility. 2006;**86**(1):51-57

[157] Goswami SK, Das T, Chattopadhyay R, Sawhney V, Kumar J, Chaudhury K. A randomized single-blind controlled trial of letrozole as a lowcost IVF protocol in women with poor ovarian response: A preliminary report. Human Reproduction. 2004;**19**(9):2031-2035

[158] Ozmen B, Sonmezer M, Atabekoglu CS, Olmus H. Use of aromatase inhibitors in poor-responder patients receiving GnRH antagonist protocols. Reproductive Biomedicine Online. 2009;**19**(4):478-485

[159] Sunkara SK, Pundir J, Khalaf Y. Effect of androgen supplementation

or modulation on ovarian stimulation outcome in poor responders: A meta-analysis. Reproductive Biomedicine Online. 2011;**22**(6):545-555

[160] Holick MF. Vitamin D deficiency. The New England Journal of Medicine. 2007;**357**(3):266-281

[161] Xu J, Lawson MS, Xu F, Du Y, Tkachenko OY, Bishop CV. Vitamin D3 regulates follicular development and Intrafollicular vitamin D biosynthesis and signaling in the primate ovary. Frontiers in Physiology. 2018;**9**:1600

[162] Xu J, Hennebold JD, Seifer DB. Direct vitamin D3 actions on rhesus macaque follicles in three-dimensional culture: Assessment of follicle survival, growth, steroid, and antimullerian hormone production. Fertility and Sterility. 2016;**106**(7):1815-20.e1

[163] Kinuta K, Tanaka H, Moriwake T, Aya K, Kato S, Seino Y. Vitamin D is an important factor in estrogen biosynthesis of both female and male gonads. Endocrinol. 2000;**141**(4):1317-1324

[164] Dicken CL, Israel DD, Davis JB, Sun Y, Shu J, Hardin J. Peripubertal vitamin D (3) deficiency delays puberty and disrupts the estrous cycle in adult female mice. Biology of Reproduction. 2012;**87**(2):51

[165] Merhi ZO, Seifer DB, Weedon J, Adeyemi O, Holman S, Anastos K. Circulating vitamin D correlates with serum antimullerian hormone levels in late-reproductive-aged women: Women's interagency HIV study. Fertility and Sterility. 2012;**98**(1):228-234

[166] Jukic AM, Steiner AZ, Baird DD. Association between serum 25-hydroxyvitamin D and ovarian reserve in premenopausal women. Menopause. 2015;**22**(3):312-316

[167] Reginatto MW, Pizarro BM, Antunes RA, Mancebo ACA, Hoffmann L, Fernandes P. Vitamin D receptor TaqI polymorphism is associated with reduced follicle number in women utilizing assisted reproductive technologies. Front Endocrinol (Lausanne). 2018;**9**:252

[168] Ozkan S, Jindal S, Greenseid K, Shu J, Zeitlian G, Hickmon C. Replete vitamin D stores predict reproductive success following in vitro fertilization. Fertility and Sterility. 2010;**94**(4):1314-1319

[169] Anifandis GM, Dafopoulos K, Messini CI, Chalvatzas N, Liakos N, Pournaras S. Prognostic value of follicular fluid 25-OH vitamin D and glucose levels in the IVF outcome. Reproductive Biology and Endocrinology. 2010;**8**:91

[170] Ali I, Padhiar AA, Wang T, He L, Chen M, Wu S, et al. Stem cell-based therapeutic strategies for premature ovarian insufficiency and infertility: A focus on aging. Cell. 2022;**11**(23):3713

[171] Herraiz S, Pellicer N, Romeu M, Pellicer A. Treatment potential of bone marrow-derived stem cells in women with diminished ovarian reserves and premature ovarian failure. Current Opinion in Obstetrics & Gynecology. 2019 Jun;**31**(3):156-162

[172] Sills ES. Ovarian recovery via autologous platelet-rich plasma: New benchmarks for condensed cytokine applications to reverse reproductive aging. Aging Med (Milton). 2022;**5**(1):63-67

[173] Holcomb JB, Tilley BC, Baraniuk S, Fox EE, Wade CE, Podbielski JM, et al. Transfusion of plasma, platelets, and red blood cells in a 1:1:1 vs a 1:1:2 ratio and mortality in patients with severe trauma:

The PROPPR randomized clinical trial. Journal of the American Medical Association. 2015;**313**(5):471-482

[174] Sills ES, Wood SH. Autologous activated platelet-rich plasma injection into adult human ovary tissue: Molecular mechanism, analysis, and discussion of reproductive response. Bioscience Reports. 2019;**39**(6):20190805

[175] Pavlovic V, Ciric M, Jovanovic V, Stojanovic P. Platelet rich plasma: A short overview of certain bioactive components. Open Med (Wars). 2016;**11**(1):242-247

[176] Seckin S, Ramadan H, Mouanness M, Kohansieh M, Merhi Z. Ovarian response to intraovarian platelet-rich plasma (PRP) administration: Hypotheses and potential mechanisms of action. Journal of Assisted Reproduction and Genetics. 2022;**39**(1):37-61

[177] Hosseini L, Shirazi A, Naderi MM, Shams-Esfandabadi N, Borjian Boroujeni S, Sarvari A, et al. Platelet-rich plasma promotes the development of isolated human primordial and primary follicles to the preantral stage. Reproductive Biomedicine Online. 2017;**35**(4):343-350

[178] Ahmadian S, Sheshpari S, Pazhang M, Bedate AM, Beheshti R, Abbasi MM, et al. Intra-ovarian injection of platelet-rich plasma into ovarian tissue promoted rejuvenation in the rat model of premature ovarian insufficiency and restored ovulation rate via angiogenesis modulation. Reproductive Biology and Endocrinology. 2020;**18**(1):78

[179] Vural B, Duruksu G, Vural F, Gorguc M, Karaoz E. Effects of VEGF (+) mesenchymal stem cells and platelet-rich plasma on inbred rat ovarian functions in cyclophosphamide-induced premature ovarian insufficiency model. Stem Cell Reviews and Reports. 2019;**15**(4):558-573

[180] Stojkovska S, Dimitrov G, Stamenkovska N, Hadzi-Lega M, Petanovski Z. Live birth rates in poor responders' group after previous treatment with autologous platelet-rich plasma and low dose ovarian stimulation compared with poor responders used only low dose ovarian stimulation before in vitro fertilization. Open Access Maced J Med Sci. 2019;**7**(19):3184-3188

[181] Sfakianoudis K, Simopoulou M, Grigoriadis S, Pantou A, Tsioulou P, Maziotis E, et al. Reactivating ovarian function through autologous platelet-rich plasma intraovarian infusion: Pilot data on premature ovarian insufficiency, perimenopausal, menopausal, and poor responder women. Journal of Clinical Medicine. 2020;**9**(6):1809

[182] Friedenstein AJ, Petrakova KV, Kurolesova AI, Frolova GP. Heterotopic of bone marrow. Analysis of precursor cells for osteogenic and hematopoietic tissues. Transplantation. 1968;**6**:230-247

[183] Liu T, Huang Y, Guo L, Cheng W, Zou G. CD44+/CD105+ human amniotic fluid mesenchymal stem cells survive and proliferate in the ovary long-term in a mouse model of chemotherapy-induced premature ovarian failure. International Journal of Medical Sciences. 2012;**9**(7):592-602

[184] Xiao GY, Liu IH, Cheng CC. Amniotic fluid stem cells prevent follicle atresia and rescue fertility of mice with premature ovarian failure induced by chemotherapy. PLoS One. 2014;**9**:e106538

[185] Ding C, Li H, Wang Y. Different therapeutic effects of cells derived from human amniotic membrane on premature ovarian aging depend on distinct cellular biological characteristics. Stem Cell Research & Therapy. 2017;**8**:173

[186] Wang S, Yu L, Sun M, Mu S, Wang C, Wang D, et al. The therapeutic potential of umbilical cord mesenchymal stem cells in mice premature ovarian failure. BioMed Research International. 2013;**2013**:690491

[187] Zuk PA, Zhu M, Ashjian P. Human adipose tissue is a source of multipotent stem cells. Molecular Biology of the Cell. 2002;**13**:4279-4295

[188] Sun M, Wang S, Li Y. Adipose-derived stem cells improved mouse ovary function after chemotherapy-induced ovary failure. Stem Cell Research & Therapy. 2013;**4**:80

[189] Satija NK, Singh VK, Verma YK. Mesenchymal stem cell-based therapy: A new paradigm in regenerative medicine. Journal of Cellular and Molecular Medicine. 2009;**13**:4385-4402